The

Encyclopedia

of

BACH

FLOWER

THERAPY

Encyclopedia

of

BACH
FLOWER
THERAPY

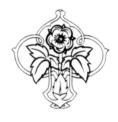

MECHTHILD SCHEFFER

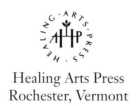

Healing Arts Press
Rochester, Vermont

Healing Arts Press
One Park Street
Rochester, Vermont 05767
www.InnerTraditions.com

Healing Arts Press is a division of Inner Traditions International

Originally published in Germany as *Die Original Bach-Blütentherapie: Das gesamte theoretische und praktische Bach-Blütenwissen*
Copyright © 1999 Heinrich Hugendubel Verlag

English translation copyright © 2001 by Inner Traditions International

Note to the reader: This book is intended as an informational guide. The remedies, approaches, and techniques described herein are meant to supplement, and not to be a substitute for, professional medical care or treatment. They should not be used to treat a serious ailment without prior consultation with a qualified health care professional.

Library of Congress Cataloging-in-Publication Data

Scheffer, Mechthild.
   [Bach Blütentherapie. English]
   The encyclopedia of Bach flower therapy / Mechthild Scheffer.
      p.   cm.
Includes bibliographical references.
   ISBN 0-89281-941-3
   1. Flowers—Therapeutic use. I. Title.
   RX615 .F55 S3413 2001
   615' .321—dc21

                          2001001925

Printed and bound in Hong Kong

10 9 8 7 6 5 4

Text design and layout by Priscilla Baker
This book was typeset in Janson

Contents

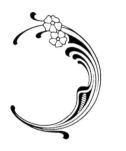

Author's Note

The Original Bach Flower Therapy was developed over sixty years ago by the English physician Edward Bach to serve as a simple form of preventive health care. Today it enjoys a worldwide reputation.

Bach Flower Therapy helps us to deal more constructively with the negative behavior patterns of human nature such as jealousy, impatience, inability to say no, timidity, and inappropriate guilt—patterns that are seen, by Bach as well as many others, as a deeper cause of physical illness.

By better understanding and correcting the "mental errors" underlying our negative behavior patterns, we can reconnect with our own true nature. With the help of Bach Flowers we regain access to our spiritual healing forces, which strengthen our immune system and support our overall health.

Bach Flowers may also be used to support professional psychological or medical treatment—but cannot take their place.

Note: The phrases in this book that coincide with medical terms such as *diagnosis*, *patient*, *therapy*, and *healing* are not to be interpreted in a legal sense.

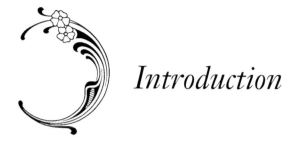

Introduction

"You Have a Mission"

The development of Bach Flower Therapy in German-speaking countries during the last twenty years is well highlighted by two events.

In 1979 I asked John Ramsell, the curator of the English Bach Centre, for contacts on Bach Flowers in German-speaking countries. I received only two addresses.

In 1996 a popular Swiss magazine featured a crossword puzzle with one clue reading Bach *Blüte mit drei Buchstaben* (Bach Flower, three letters). Obviously, Bach Flowers had found their way into general public knowledge in the interim.

In 1973, at a naturopathic school where I was taking classes outside of my career as an artist, one of my fellow students asked whether I had heard of Bach Flowers.

I replied, "No, what are they?"

She said, "No idea, but they're supposed to be great."

At that time I would not have been able to explain to anybody why I stopped at the Watkins Book Shop on Charing Cross Road on my next visit to London, asking for books on Bach Flower Remedies. The person at the counter thought for quite a while and then pointed to the bottom shelves on the right. Lo and behold, I found two slightly dusty books there: *The Medical Discoveries of Dr. Edward Bach* by Nora Weeks and *The Handbook of the Bach Flower Remedies* by Philip Chancellor.

At that time my interest in natural medicine was focused on classical homeopathy, more specifically on "mentals" (mental symptoms) in that field. I was shocked when I opened the book by Philip Chancellor. It consisted entirely of easily understood descriptions of mental symptoms. Could Bach Flower Remedies really be as simple as that? If they were, this I wanted to see.

On a nice summer day in the same year, I went by rail to Oxford and visited Mount Vernon, the

English Bach Centre. I can recall my first meeting with John Ramsell, a small, very friendly man who looked at me, smiled, and said, "You have a mission." Then he considered which Flower might be best for me and gave me Vervain. At that time, neither of us could have anticipated the enormous unfolding and expansion that Bach Flower Therapy would experience in the coming years. Our meeting was most likely the real beginning of the active use of Bach Flower Therapy in German-speaking countries.

With great enthusiasm, I immediately started to experiment with Bach Flowers. I tried them on myself, my friends, and acquaintances and the results were surprisingly positive. In a newsletter from the English Bach Centre I learned about a private seminar on Bach Flowers to be held in London by Melanie Reinhard. After that I took advantage of every opportunity to meet with experts on Bach Flowers, including Bonnie Spalato in Holland and Johanna Salajan in Spain.

In 1979 John Ramsell published a note in his newsletter: "People interested in Bach Flowers in German-speaking countries can contact Mechthild Scheffer." While I did not receive a single letter that year, by 1980 patients and other interested people from all over Germany had begun seeking me out in my naturopathic (Heilpraktiker) practice in Hamburg-Eppendorf. Among insiders word had spread about the amazing effect of Bach Flowers. The demand increased for material written in German, and I decided to translate a booklet by Julian Barnard,

whom I had visited in London. He was just about to leave for Australia but gave my plans his okay. While I was translating his text I became aware that there was more to be said on Bach Flower Therapy. Thus I started to evaluate my own notes, tapes, and patient records, which I had accumulated over six years, as well as all other existing literature on the subject. In the fall of 1980 the Hugendubel Company published the original writings of Edward Bach under the title *Blumen, die durch die Seele heilen* with *Heal Thyself* translated by Wulfing von Rohr.

I asked the publisher if he would consider taking on another book on Bach Flower Remedies. "You'll have it in three months," I promised. "We'll need it in six months," smiled the publisher when he found out that I'd never written a book before. Two months went by, then three and almost four, and I had written less than twenty pages. There were professional and private reasons of all kinds that kept me from writing. Finally, only two months from my deadline, I canceled all my activities and wrote day and night to finish the book. For each of the thirty-eight Flowers I had only one day—twenty-four hours, minus four hours of sleep—to cull through my writer's box full of fragmented text, mostly in English, to complete detailed descriptions of the Flower's positive potential and "supportive measures." During this process I drifted more and more into altered states: I felt as if I were living in a different world. For example, one night I discovered a grumpy elf sitting on the oleander bush that was spending the winter in my hallway—but it didn't surprise me at all! While I was describing Impatiens I was barely able to sit on my chair. It was then that I first noticed that this work made me experience every negative inner state and its transformations. Today I have no idea what gave me the strength—even as an Oak type—to survive my task.

One thing became increasingly obvious: I was not writing alone. Specifically, when I chose my material and final expressions, I had the inspiration and growing mental support of Bach's spiritual consciousness. Later I recognized this to be the reason that people would write to me again and again to tell me that they experienced a harmonizing effect simply by reading one or another of the Flowers' descriptions. Likewise, the psychology student who was typing my text—and who clearly had at that time no openness to spiritual thinking—began crying one morning in front of the typewriter. While preparing the text on Wild Oat she was so profoundly moved that it took her hours to complete the pages.

These are just some of the reasons why I have incorporated Bach's philosophical foundations and the Bach-inspired formulations of my original book in the new book presented here. Despite some dramatic circumstances (the final correction of the book was even lost in the mail and had to be completely redone), the book was finally published in German in the fall of 1981.

Over twenty years have passed since then. They have been filled with surprising experiences, major challenges, extensive research and learning, and many uplifting moments that would easily fill another book. In retrospect, the Bach Flowers would not have become established so quickly in German-speaking countries without the active and energetic participation of the Bach Flowers themselves through their effect on those who used them.

For me it was fascinating to discover that we reach our Higher Selves only through an emotionally harmonious state.

As the daughter of parents whose families had for generations produced professionals in the fields of law and theology, I experienced few real emotions during my entire childhood. Sharp analysis (Beech) or a kind of helpless otherworldliness (Clematis and Wild Rose) dominated the atmosphere at home. These contributed to me being somewhat uptight and insecure. My saving grace was that after spending boringly dry mornings at a humanist high school I found compensation in the afternoons in the world of dance. After graduating from high school, I wanted to become a choreographer. To my great disappointment and my parents' relief, however, there was yet no school at that time where I could study within the field. Following ten years of unsatisfactory attempts in different fields of study and work (Wild Oat), I found my much-longed-for satisfaction, success, and appreciation as a creative consultant. Already during these years I moved constantly between different worlds. I can see now that without trying or even caring about it, I was learning to receive inspiration and pass on ideas and information in ways that others could readily use.

It was during my various activities in connection with the work of Dr. Bach that I first began taking a closer personal look at the negative behavior patterns of human nature. It was a good thing for me. Constant change among my various activities in therapy, writing, and developing a business—together with the influence on me of the "happy fellows of the plant world"—finally had a stabilizing effect on my personality. I became more realistic and learned to keep both feet firmly planted on the ground.

During the past two decades there has been a great shift in the understanding of health and illness for a broad spectrum of the population, particularly among women and younger people. It has been my intention during these years to make Bach Flower Therapy accessible to people of all walks of life, which was Bach's original vision, and to legalize the importation and sales of Bach Flower Remedies. Due to different pharmacological regulations in Germany, Austria, and Switzerland, I was finally forced, at great personal and material cost, to open and run three independent offices. At that time, some of my actions were misunderstood by some who were not aware of the requirements of business and pharmacological law. These problems weighed heavily on me, but upholding Bach's original vision was my overriding objective, and it kept me working. That this goal was achieved and has

been sustained for over twenty years now is something I am very proud of.

Altogether, I'm glad I didn't miss a single hour of the past two amazing decades. In this period I was privileged to directly experience more and more people opening up to the work of Dr. Bach—not only colleagues and seminar participants but also journalists, lawyers, and public officials.

Today, it is much more widely accepted that it is the individual and not the illness that must be the center of attention in medical treatment. Bach Flower Therapy continues to contribute strongly to this development because it's so readily available and easily understood, and allows each person to have his or her own personal, positive experience.

The seeds that Bach planted have grown profusely—but not always with the best result. Their rapid and unexpected development sparked the interest of the media. Every magazine had to have an article on Bach Flowers, no talk show could be without discussions of the subject. In addition, most bigger publishing houses produced self-help books on Bach Flowers that borrowed liberally from previously published materials, and many self-appointed Bach Flower Therapists took advantage of the trend, distorting Dr. Bach's work to match their own ideas. This development has unfortunately led to some of Bach's medical peers—whom he meant to introduce to a more humane kind of medicine—to become skeptical of his ideas without having tested them carefully enough to recognize their enormous potential.

Some have also discarded or belittled Bach Flower Therapy as "housewives' medicine." The term has resulted in a misinterpretation of Bach's ideas that is painful for me and many others to observe. However, even Bach predicted this kind of development in his now famous essay, "Distortion." He wrote the following to a close associate, not long before his death:

> It is proof of the value of our work when material agencies arise to distort it, because distortion is a far greater weapon than attempted destruction.
>
> Mankind asked for free will, which God granted him, hence mankind must always have a choice. As soon as a teacher has given his work to the world, a contorted version of the same must arise. Such has happened even from the humblest like ourselves, who have dedicated our work to the good of our fellow men. . . . The contortion must be raised for people to be able to choose between the gold and the dross.
>
> Our work is steadfastly to adhere to the simplicity and purity of this method of healing.

At the other end of the spectrum, a group of open-minded doctors who were mainly students of mine* established the world's first medical association for Bach Flower Therapy: the Österreichisch-Deutsche Ärztegesellschaft Dr. med. E. Bach. (Austrian-German doctor's association—Dr. med. Edward Bach)

Today the most important task for all serious practitioners of Bach Flower Therapy is to maintain the simplicity and purity of Bach's original work. This is so vital because the market has been flooded with so-called Bach Flower Therapists and independently produced "Flower Remedies According to Bach," of widely varying quality.

There are also those who question whether or not Bach Flower Therapy has moved past its apex. On the contrary, I believe it stands at the threshold of a totally new phase of development. While it may be that the number of fans and devotees caught up in the initial excitement will shrink to a healthy level, it appears that a deeper, more solid base is growing of those who make good, responsible use of Bach's gift.

This book aims to place the essence of Bach's teachings into the context of today's world, enriched through the objective study and experience of the past twenty-five years. The inspiring original quotes from Bach that appear in this volume have been collected from several of his books and shortened so that his spirit may come to life in this book.

---

* In 1982 I created the first complete training program for Bach Flower Therapy and in the following years opened the Research and Education Institutes for Bach Flower Therapy in Hamburg, Vienna, and Zurich.

Re-Harmony: The Message and Contributions of Bach Flower Therapy

Not long ago I was asked by a young child:

What are Bach Flowers?

They're soul helpers—they bring messengers from another world.

From which world?

They bring helpful messages and information from the world of plants.

How do they help me?

You have another world within you too, and if the entrance to your other world has fallen shut, they'll help you reopen it.

What kind of a world is it?

It's the beautiful world that we all travel to sometimes at night. A land you wish you could stay in, where you find peace and quiet but also find new things.

I've been there already!

Of course you have. We all live in that world as well as in the normal everyday one. This other world provides you with your important personal information when you have problems in your everyday world or when you don't know what to do.

What is "my important personal information"?

It's the answer to questions like these: What do I really want? What's the best thing to do now so I don't make a mistake?

That I know anyway.

True, but do you always? How do you feel at times when you don't?

I feel bad. I don't want to do anything! Sometimes I get so angry that I want to break everything.

And then what do you do to make things better?

I ask somebody . . . or just ask my inner voice.

Your inner voice is where you get your important personal information.

Really?

Definitely! How do you feel after you find an answer?

I feel great again, I feel light and have a lot of energy.

Do you always hear your inner voice?

No. . . . Sometimes it's very far away.

Right. That's when Bach Flowers will help you. It's like making a telephone call to communicate with your inner voice if you can't hear it anymore.

Why is it so far away sometimes?

Because you get cut off from your other world.

The world where my important personal information is located?

. . . and that the Bach Flowers can help you to contact again.

The eternal truths that underlie the effectiveness of Bach Flower Therapy can be expressed in many ways. When interviewing someone, my goal is to communicate these principles, in whatever words, pictures, or examples I can come up with, until they are clearly understand, so that through this understanding, my interview partner can restore a resonance with his or her inner voice. This, I believe—along with a mature personality and a solid knowledge of the material—may be the most important ability of the Bach Flower practitioner.

At first glance Bach's message might appear unrealistic, a distant, ideal world—but it's a world that really does exist. The material world (at the level of the personality, including its struggles and crises) and the spiritual world (the Soul and the Higher Self) are constantly interpenetrating each other, mutually dependent like inhalation and exhalation, day and night. What we must learn is to keep these worlds in balance since every excess in one world will be followed by a shortage in the other. Too little attention to the material world (Clematis) results in a distorted connection to the Higher Self just as paying too much attention to the material level does (Crab Apple).

Whenever this kind of imbalance takes hold, illness or a crisis is sure to result. This causes the necessary chaos out of which energy and new life can arise, making possible the next step in our life's journey. The ordering and harmonizing impulses of the "happy fellows of the plant world" bring us the good news: You can do it differently! Taking the proper Remedy creates the relevant experience. Depending on the nature of the imbalance, Bach Flower Remedies can either broaden our field of vision to allow us a larger perspective, or help us focus on a specific need.

This process of harmonization follows naturally without further human influence, providing that the right Flower has been chosen. This aspect is for me the most exciting and special part of Bach Flower Therapy. The macrocosm itself acts to re-tune the human microcosm in the same way that walking in the woods or witnessing a sunrise does. This happens very subtly, nearly imperceptibly, and draws on specifically what is possible and necessary at any given moment.

Even in a diagnostic interview (done in the way Bach recommended), both partners tune into the macrocosm and our higher nature. Thus they subordinate themselves to spiritual law, call upon positive forces, and mobilize them. Therefore the diagnostic interview provides a vital initial spark that is then consolidated through the effect of the Bach Flower Remedies. Indeed, every Bach Flower interview is also an act of practical brotherly love, inspiring and elevating both partners.

Without fail, over time, the involvement with Bach Flower Therapy brings us more in tune with nature as a whole as well as our own true inner nature. This awakens a love and understanding for all creation, as well as tolerance for the individuality of the people around us. Taking Bach Flower Remedies strengthens our positive motivation and spiritual defense forces.

Our sense of personal responsibility grows, helping us to be more grown-up in the best sense of the word. This cannot help but have a positive influence on our environment, within our family, and among friends and acquaintances. On an even larger scale, every Bach Flower interview contributes to the greater whole as it improves the spiritual climate of the planet and helps to cleanse it of today's massive amount of mental and emotional pollution.

To my understanding, this is one of the most important reasons that more and more people continue to be drawn to Bach Flower Therapy. For the same reason, I am confident that it will survive any distortions or fashionable trends—if enough people come to apply the remedies according to the principles of Dr. Bach.

How to Make the Best Use of This Book

The information in this book is organized on three levels in order to accommodate the multilevel approach of Edward Bach's work:

1. The philosophical and spiritual levels— chapters 1 through 5.

2. The psychological and spiritual levels— chapters 5, 6, 7, and 9.

3. The pragmatic, practical level—chapters 6 through 11.

Start at the level of most interest to you. Many people will simply open the book and begin reading the description of whatever Flower they find on that page.

At the end of most chapters you will find the questions that most frequently have been asked on the subject. For the answers to these questions, refer to appendix A. Please match the *italicized terms* in the questions with the terms in the list of alphabetized issues in the appendix.

For more in-depth information on any of the various topics in this book, I recommend the following books, as well as those listed in appendix B:

❀ For information on the philosophical/ spiritual background of Bach Flower Remedies, see Edward Bach's *Heal Thyself, The Twelve Healers, Original Writings of Edward Bach* (Saffron Walden, Essex, England: C. W. Daniel Company, 1990)

❀ For a deeper understanding of specific Bach Flower patterns, see my *Keys to the Soul: A Workbook for Self-Diagnosis Using the Bach Flowers* (Saffron Walden, Essex, England: C. W. Daniel Company, 1998).

❀ For case studies and experiences from over one hundred practitioners, see my *Original Bach-Blütentherapi: Lehrbuch für die Arzt und Naturheilpraxis* (Neckarsulm, 1996) and *Erfahrungen mit der Bach-Blütentherapie* (München, 1995).

Materials for practical use such as questionnaires are located in chapter 10. Addresses and other contact information for institutes offering seminars and continuing education can be found in appendix B.

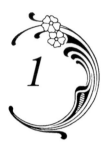

Soul Therapy through Flower Energy

The Vision of Dr. Edward Bach

When we come to the problem of healing, we can understand that this will have to keep pace with the times and change its methods from those of gross materialism to those of a science founded upon the realities of truth and governed by the same divine laws that rule our very natures. Healing will pass from the domain of physical methods of treating the physical body to that of spiritual and mental healing, which by bringing about harmony between the Soul and mind will eradicate the very basic cause of disease and then allow such physical means to be used as may be necessary to complete the cure of the body.

So that the physician of the future will have two great aims:

The first will be to assist the patient to a knowledge of himself and to point out to him the fundamental mistakes he may be making.

Such a physician will have to be a great student of the laws governing humanity and of human nature itself, so that he may recognize in all who come to him those elements that are causing a conflict between the Soul and the personality.

He must be able to advise the sufferer how best to bring about the harmony required, what actions against unity he must cease to perform, and the necessary virtues he must develop to wipe out his defects.

Each case will need a careful study, and it will be only those who have devoted much of their life to the knowledge of mankind and in whose heart burns the desire to help who will be able to undertake successfully this glorious and divine work for humanity, to open the eyes of a sufferer and enlighten him on the reason of his being, and to inspire hope, comfort, and faith that will enable him to conquer his malady.

In correct healing nothing must be used that

relieves the patient of his own responsibility: but such means only must be adopted that help him overcome his faults.

The second duty of the physician will be to administer such remedies as will help the physical body to gain strength and assist the mind to become calm, widen its outlook, and strive toward perfection, thus bringing peace and harmony to the whole personality.

Such remedies are in nature, placed there by the mercy of the Divine Creator for the healing and comfort of mankind. A few of these are known and more of them are sought at the present time by physicians in different parts of the world, especially in our Mother India, and there is no doubt that when such researches have become more developed we shall regain much of the knowledge that was known more than two thousand years ago.

Let not the simplicity of this method deter you from its use, for you will find that the farther your researches advance, the greater you will realize the simplicity of all creation.

Edward Bach

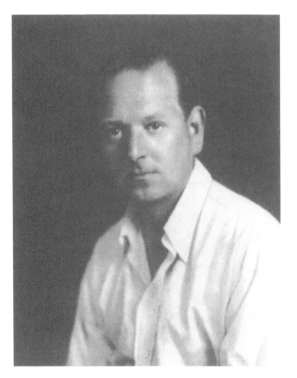

Edward Bach, 1886–1936

Listening to Your Intuition

Has it ever occurred to you that God gave you an individuality? Yet he certainly did.

He gave you a personality of your very own, a treasure to be kept to your very own self. He gave you a life to lead that you and only you should lead. He gave you work to do that you and only you can do. He placed you in this world, a divine being, a child of himself—to learn how to become perfect, to gain all knowledge possible, to grow gentle and kind, and to help others.

And it's not so difficult as it may at first appear; we are simply expected to do our best, and we know that this is possible for all of us if we will but listen to the dictates of our own Souls. Life does not demand of us unthinkable sacrifice; it asks us to travel its journey with joy in our hearts.

Many of us in our childhood and early life are much nearer to our own Soul than we are in later years. We have then clearer ideas of our work in life, the endeavors we're expected to make, and the characters we are required to develop.

And has it ever occurred to you how God speaks to you and tells you of your own individuality, and of your very own work, of how to steer your ship true to its own course? He speaks to you through your own desires, which are the instincts of your Soul. How else could he speak?

If we but listen to and obey our own desires, uninfluenced by any other personality, we shall always be led rightly.

Our Souls (the still small voice, God's own voice) speak to us through our intuition, our instincts, our desires, our ideals, our ordinary likes and dislikes, in whichever way it's easiest for us individually to hear.

All true knowledge comes only from within ourselves *in silent communication with our Souls.*

Neither is it a difficult, faraway attainment to hear the voice of our own Souls; it has all been made simple for us if we will but acknowledge it. Simplicity is the keynote of all creation.

Truth has no need to be analyzed, argued about, or wrapped up in many words. It's realized in a flash. It's part of us.

Only about the unessential, complicated things of life do we need much convincing. This has led to the development of intellect.

The things that count are simple; they're the ones that make us say, "Why, that's true, I seem to have known that always." So is the realization of the happiness that comes to us when we're in harmony with our spiritual selves, and the closer the union, the more intense the joy.

We can judge our health by our happiness,

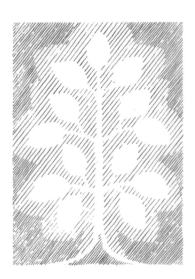

Life Plan of the Higher Self for the development of the personality

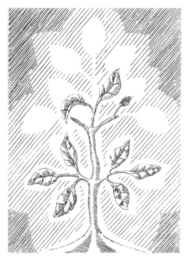

Imperfectly developed personality: potential not fully utilized

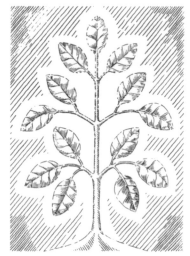

Ideal state of the personality: perfectly realized Life Plan

Genius and Compassion

No written account of Edward Bach's life exists other than a biography by his assistant, Nora Weeks. The highlights of his life listed below are based on her account.

The daughter of one of Bach's colleagues, J. F. Wheeler (Bach was responsible for saving her life with his Flowers when she was a child), once told me, "First and foremost, he was always working hard." Wheeler himself related the following:

> In Edward Bach genius was combined with a joyousness and simplicity of nature, a great humility and lack of self-pride in his achievements which endeared him to all those with whom he worked or came in contact.
>
> His striking personality, his intuitive knowledge and understanding of human nature, his certainty of his own purpose in life and disregard of all that might interfere with that mission, made him one of those outstanding characters who are remembered and loved for themselves and their work throughout the world's history.

The Road to Bach Flowers: An Abbreviated Résumé

September 24, 1886: Edward Bach is born in Moseley near Birmingham, the first of three children. His family came from Wales and owned a brass foundry.

1903–1906: Edward Bach works as an apprentice in his father's company. His observations of physical illnesses and their connections with psychological conflicts among the workers, along with his desire to help, make this the key, formative experience for his future work. For a long time he vacillates between studying theology and medicine.

1906–1913: He studies medicine in Birmingham and London. Soon he is licensed as a physician and works as the head of the emergency department at University College Hospital. Later he takes the position of assistant in the department of bacteriology and immunology. He recognizes the connection between certain types of bacteria in the colon and chronic disease. He successfully isolates and prepares different types of these bacteria as vaccines.

1917: Edward Bach suffers a major breakdown. A malignant tumor is removed from his spleen, and the prognosis suggests he has three months to live. However, he completely overcomes this crisis within only three months due to his absolute desire to finish his research.

1918–1922: After recovery, Bach accepts a position at the Homeopathic Hospital in London. He's introduced to the book *Organon* by Samuel Hahnemann and realizes that Hahnemann's term *Psora* is identical to what he himself called *colon-toxemia.* Thereafter he prepares his vaccines in the form of homeopathic nosodes, which he separates into seven major groups. (Later they are named after him: Bach Nosodes.) Bach works out the symptoms of the homeopathic "mentals" and finally matches each group of bacteria (nosodes) with a specific disharmonious state.

1920–1928: Bach opens a laboratory, a private practice, and a separate office offering free treatment to the poor in London. He recognizes that the seven nosodes can only heal the symptoms summarized under the term *Psora*, but not the symptoms of other chronic diseases. This encourages him to seek out new preparations as well as a purer way to make them all—using none of the diseased bacteria that he was still using in his nosodes. He searches for and discovers plants that have vibrations similar to those of the nosodes but initially fails to match their polarity. Plants prepared by homeopathic methods show positive polarity, while effective nosodes taken from the colon have a negative polarity.

Beginning in 1928: Bach increasingly observes the psychic components in physical illnesses, which leads to his understanding that they are tied to certain personality types and to specific negative reaction patterns of our human nature. He sees that, depending on their personality type, people would show the same or similar reactions to physical illnesses of any kind.

Beginning in 1930: At the peak of his medical career, Bach decides to sell his practice and labo-ratory in London in order to concentrate fully on studying the different personality types and finding the corresponding healing plants. Together with his assistant, Nora Weeks, he discovers and prepares the first nine of the plants that will eventually be called the Twelve Healers: Impatiens, Mimulus, Clematis, Agrimony, Chicory, Vervain, Centaury, Cerato, and Scler-anthus. A new production process (the sun method) used in making the preparations also solves the problem of polarity. In his major work, *Heal Thyself,* Bach formulates his findings and philosophy in plain language so that they can be understood by the general public. Former colleagues try out his Flower Remedies and encourage him to proceed with his work.

Beginning in 1931: Edward Bach discovers the last three remedies of the Twelve Healers: Water Violet, Gentian, and Rock Rose.

1932: The medical association reacts to his work by threatening to expel him from its register should he continue working with laymen or promote his findings publicly. Bach successfully holds to his beliefs and practices.

1933: Bach experiences an increased level of sensitivity, helping him to discover and prepare additional flowers, which he calls the Four Helpers: Gorse, Oak, Heather, and Rock Water. Bach offers his mother tinctures (see chapter 4, page 30) free of charge to two large homeopathic pharmacies in London, instructing them to pass on the remedies as inexpensively as possible.

1934–1935: Bach discovers the last three flowers of his first series of remedies: Wild Oat, Olive, and Vine. He creates his well-known first-aid remedy, Rescue, and finally settles down in the little village of Sotwell in the Thames valley, where grow most of the plants that he has already found. Bach's sensitivity increases to an extreme level; he experiences further negative human states, which lead him to discover corresponding plants. After preparing and taking their essences, the negative states disappear within hours. Aided by Nora Weeks, he is able to discover another nineteen remedies, which he prepares largely according to the newly discovered boiling method.

1936: Bach is convinced that his system is now complete and his work finished. He plans to travel and give lectures about his therapy and findings. He holds his first on his birthday, September 24.

November 27, 1936: Edward Bach dies in his sleep.

Bach had already appointed Nora Weeks and Victor Bullen as his successors and they preserved and continued his work until 1978. They in turn appointed the next custodians of Bach's work, the children of whom are still administering the Bach Centre in Sotwell.

Simplicity: Eight Points That Highlight the Uniqueness of Bach Flower Therapy

Even today it is very difficult to categorize the Bach Flower System. One could say that the Bach Flower Remedies rank among the subtle methods of healing, similar to the classical homeopathy of Samuel Hahnemann, anthroposophical medicine, and spagyric medicine because they do not act via the physical body but at more subtle levels that directly influence the human energy system.

Before he developed his Flower Remedies, Bach was a highly successful bacteriologist and homeopathic physician.* He felt a spiritual link with Hippocrates, Paracelsus, and Samuel Hahnemann, sharing their view that "there are no diseases, but only sick people." Yet it would be taking too narrow a view of him and his work to call him the "present-day Hahnemann," as contemporary colleagues had done.

Eight points differentiate the Bach Flower System from other subtle healing systems in the West:

1. **The conceptual basis.** Bach's approach is rooted in a frame of reference that rises above the boundaries of a single human

---

* For those interested in homeopathy, it may be curious to know that Bach had already laid out his fundamental philosophy by the time he was introduced to the work by Samuel Hahnemann.

personality to extend into spiritual dimensions.

2. **The therapeutic goal: "Heal thyself."** Edward Bach calls upon each person to take responsibility for his or her own life. He states that all human beings hold within whatever they need for their own healing. Thus there is no longer a reason to fear illness.

3. **The new form of diagnosis.** Instead of concentrating on physical symptoms, the Bach Flower System relies solely on "disharmonies" or negative human behavior patterns—similar to but more comprehensive than homeopathic "mentals."

4. **The criteria for the choice of plants.** Bach used only "plants with high vibrations" (see page 29).

5. **The method of production.** Bach's simple, natural means of production differ from all other methods known to Western medicine. The methods he developed—the sun method and the boiling method—release the healing energy of the Flowers from their material form, which allows this energy to bind to the substance of the carrier (water). This produces a much more stable energetic pattern than those found in homeopathic remedies.

6. **The gentle, self-regulating effects.** Bach Flower Essences work as subtle, nonmaterial impulses. They communicate information through specific, high vibrations that stimulate our emotional and mental self-healing forces. They produce no side effects and are compatible with all other forms of therapy.

7. **The larger number of possible users.** Their harmless effects make Bach Flower Remedies a risk-free system to use in self-healing, and therefore available to far more people than other subtle healing systems. The states described by Bach are archetypal behavior patterns of human nature; they aren't symptoms of illness. Therefore it is not necessary to undergo medical training to be a successful practitioner of Bach Flower Therapy. Characteristics and abilities that are much more important are maturity combined with a clear grasp of the human condition, perceptiveness, sensitivity, and an honest compassion for others. Bach's vision was that the Flower Essences would someday find their way into the medicine chest of every household.

8. **Simplicity as a basic principle.** As the world grows more and more complex, the word *simplicity* can easily be mistaken for *primitive*. Simplicity relates to fundamental principles such as unity, perfection,

and harmony. Everybody is attracted—though not necessarily consciously—to the simple things in life. To grasp the unity and simplicity that lie behind our complex world, it is necessary to have not only objectivity and perceptiveness but also a fundamental readiness to see oneself as part of a whole, a part that in the final instance is governed by a simple, holistic creative principle. It cannot be without reason that most of the great scientists have embraced this kind of view at the end of their lives.

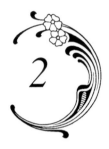

Heal Thyself: The Theoretical Foundations of Bach Flower Therapy

Disease is solely and purely corrective: it is neither vindictive nor cruel; but it is the means adopted by our Souls to point out to us our faults; to prevent our making greater errors; to hinder us from doing more harm; and to bring us back to that path of truth and light from which we should never have strayed.

Edward Bach

To many people this understanding of disease may at first sound improbable, but it becomes perfectly clear if the premise on which Bach based his line of thought*—similar to that of Hippocrates, Hahnemann, and Paracelsus, great men of like spirit—is understood and accepted.

Creation and Destiny

❀ Human life on this planet is part of a greater concept of creation. We live within a wider frame of reference, a more com-prehensive unity, more or less like a cell within a human body.

❀ Every person is two things: a unique individual and a vital and essential part of the greater unity, the greater whole.

❀ Because there is unity in all things, each of us is connected to everything else by a common, higher, more powerful energy vibration that has been given many names, such as the creative force, universal Life principle, cosmic principle, love, and simply, God.

❀ Just as everything else in our universe, from frost patterns on our windows to the generation and death of whole planetary systems, the development of every individual human being follows an inner programmed course of unfolding. Every human being has a

---

* Thoroughly explained in *Heal Thyself*, Bach's major work of only fifty-nine pages (Saffron Walden, Essex, England, 1931).

specific Life Plan, a mission, task, destiny, *karma*, or whatever we may call it.

❀ Being part of the great plan of creation, every human being has an immortal Soul—a real Self—and a mortal personality that we live in here on earth.

❀ Closely related to the Soul is our Higher Self—the Inner Guidance that mediates between the Soul and the personality.

❀ The Soul is aware of a person's particular mission. With the aid of the Higher Self and through the flesh and blood personality, it seeks to express the mission and make it a concrete reality.

❀ Initially, the personality is not aware of its Life Plan.

Virtues and Vices

❀ The potential goals our Soul wishes to realize through the personality are not material. They are in fact higher, ideal qualities that Edward Bach referred to as "the virtues of our Higher Nature." They include gentleness, firmness, courage, constancy, wisdom, joyfulness, and purposefulness. Poets of all ages have praised these as noble qualities of character. They could also be called the ideal archetypal Soul qualities of mankind whose realization as part of the big picture embodies our true happiness.

❀ If these potential qualities are unrealized, sooner or later the opposite feeling— unhappiness—will develop. The virtues that we have failed to realize now show themselves from their shadow side as vices such as pride, cruelty, hatred, self-love, ignorance, and greed. Bach referred to these vices as the primary diseases of mankind, and states that they are the ground from which physical illness grows.

Health and Disease

Everyone has the unconscious desire to live in harmony because nature, as a great cosmic field of energy, is constantly driven to achieve an efficient and therefore harmonious state of energy.

Health

If the personality could and would act in complete harmony with its Soul, then humans would live in perfect harmony. The universal energy of creation would flow freely and express itself in the life of the personality. Humanity would be strong, healthy, and happy, a harmoniously vibrating part of the great cosmic field of energy.

Disease

In every situation in which the personality is not in complete harmony with its Soul and the cosmic field of energy, we find disharmony, disturbance, friction, distortion, and energy loss. These problems first show up as negative moods and thoughts; later they manifest in physical weakness, and finally in established disease. Physical illness serves as a last corrective factor. It's a warning light, indicating with force that something has to be changed immediately in order to prevent complete dysfunction from setting in.

Causes of Disease

What are the reasons for the disharmony between Soul and personality that leads to disease? It's not only Bach who points to mental errors and disregard of spiritual laws. These same factors are noted in the teachings of many philosophies from many ages.

- ✹ **The first error.** The personality fails to pay attention to its Higher Self or Inner Guidance and does not act in accordance with its Life Plan. It lives under the illusion that it can be entirely independent.

  In the most extreme case, the personality is unable to even recognize the existence of its Soul or Higher Self, materialistically accepting only what can be seen and touched. In doing so, the personality cuts its own cosmic umbilical cord, desiccates, and destroys itself.

  More often, though, the personality merely misunderstands parts of the Soul's intentions and then acts according to its limited understanding of the situation.

  In all the areas where the personality has turned away from its cosmic connection—or, as Bach said, "away from love"*—it loses touch with its Inner Guidance. It loses sight of its Life Plan and access to its positive potential. It then drops to a lower vibration and falls prey to the primary diseases of mankind, the symptoms of which are expressed in Bach's thirty-eight negative archetypal behavior patterns.

- ✹ **The second error.** The personality acts against the principle of Unity.

  By acting against the intentions of its Higher Self and Soul, the personality is automatically acting against the interest of the greater Unity because its Soul is energetically connected to this Unity.

  Above all, however, the personality is acting against the principle of Unity if it attempts to force its own will on another being. This not only impedes the development of another, but also upsets the entire cosmic energy field and the development of mankind as a whole.

The Healing Strategy of Edward Bach

Bach's healing strategy could be summarized with the formula: "Don't fight it, transform it."

---

* "Righteousness without love makes us hard. Faith without love makes us fanatical. Power without love makes us brutal. Duty without love makes us grumpy. Orderliness without love makes us petty." These words by Laotzu say this perfectly.

1. Recognize character weaknesses and mental errors, and the resulting negative behavior patterns.

2. Don't fight the condition. Acknowledge its existence without judgment.

3. Find the appropriate supportive Flowers and take them.

4. Now reorient yourself toward the greater Unity, spiritual laws, your Inner Guidance and your own Life Plan.

5. Lovingly apply the corresponding positive behavior patterns to reconnect with your Higher Self and unlock your positive potential.

But when we realize . . . that, as we have already seen, the real cause of disease lies in our own personality and is within our control, then have we reason to go about without dread and fearless, knowing that the remedy lies within ourselves.

Healing must come from within ourselves, by acknowledging and correcting our faults, and harmonizing our being with the divine plan.

Be it remembered that when the fault is found, the remedy lies not in a battle against this and not in a use of willpower and energy to suppress a wrong, but in a steady development of the opposite virtue, thus automatically washing from our natures all trace of the offender.

To struggle against a fault increases its power; keeps our attention riveted on its presence, and brings us a battle indeed.

To forget the failing and consciously to strive to develop the virtue that would make the former impossible—this is true victory.

At first this may be a little difficult, but only just at first, for it is remarkable how rapidly a true encouraged virtue will increase.

Edward Bach

An Example

A young woman's Higher Self would like to express its potential creativity and self-assurance in her personality, and sends appropriate impulses. The young woman repeatedly has the idea that she would like to open a flower shop. In the ideal case she will use the energy that comes to her from her Higher Self to ponder this. Finally she decides in favor of the idea and after having all the positive and negative experiences that are part of opening a business, she becomes a contented florist.

What has happened? The potential of the Higher Self has been expressed successfully in the personality of this woman, and her personality has been enriched.

However, the impulses of the Higher Self won't always be accepted and fulfilled so unreservedly by an individual. The following might also occur: The young woman receives the impulse from her Higher Self and feels good about it. At the same time, though, she experiences a contrary feeling. A picture of her father flashes up in her memory; many years ago he had gone into bankruptcy with a flower business. She thinks, "I won't be able to do this. Nothing will

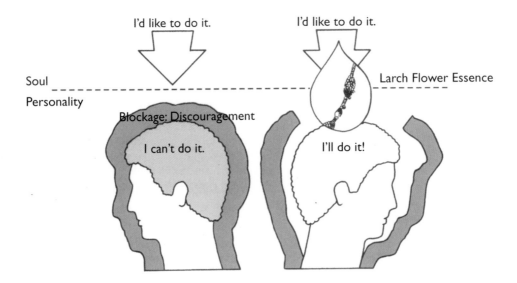

I'd like to do it. I'd like to do it.

Soul
Personality

Larch Flower Essence

Blockage: Discouragement

I can't do it. I'll do it!

come of this!" Then she gets a serious case of the flu and finally rejects the idea. Later she tells a girlfriend that she doesn't feel competent enough to open a flower shop: "Others may be able to do such a thing, but not me. Anyway, flower shops aren't what they used to be."

The result is that the energy impulse of her Higher Self is now blocked. The potential cannot be actualized.

What Error Has the Personality Made in This Case?

The young woman does not pay attention to her Inner Guidance, believing instead that the experience of her father is more relevant. She doesn't understand that she would not receive the steady impulse from her Higher Self to open a flower shop if it wasn't part of her Life Plan. The block that she unknowingly is setting up against her Inner Guidance causes the opposite

to happen. What started out as creative energy turns into discouragement and the feeling of inability: I can't do it. Not only does this not enrich the personality; it makes it twice the poorer.

First, a part of the woman's potential and Life Plan remain unfulfilled and valuable creative energy is blocked. Second, the ensuing inner conflict regularly uses up additional psychic energy—energy that does not come from the inexhaustible source of the Soul, but rather draws on the resources of the personality, which then deprives other areas of the energy they need for further development.

If this prospective florist takes Bach Larch Flower Essence, however—"for those who feel inferior to others"—what would be the effect? Having the same vibration as the energy potential of the Higher Self that wishes to express itself, it is able to make direct contact with this energy potential. It washes out the blockage, which is at a lower, disharmonious frequency, flooding it with its own higher, harmonious frequency.

The potential of the Higher Self is thus supported, and in turn the correct message gets through to the young woman and completely dissolves the rest of the blockage.

In this example the young woman becomes aware of her lack of self-esteem and starts to see things differently. She might tell herself, "What happened to my father doesn't need to happen to me. Why shouldn't I be capable of opening a store? I'll try it and see what happens. If it doesn't work, at least I will have learned a great deal from it."

Of course, the whole process will never be as straightforward as has been depicted here, and obviously there will be setbacks and obstacles to overcome, but ultimately once the blockage has been resolved, the energy from the Higher Self can be used fully by the personality. At the same time the individual again has creative energy at her disposal that was previously spent on the daily maintenance of the negative avoidance reaction. The personality has become doubly enriched.

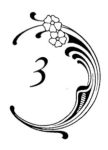

3

How Bach Flowers Work

The actions of certain flowers, shrubs, and trees that grow in the wild raise our vibrations and open our channels for the reception of the Spiritual Self to flood our natures with the particular virtue we need, and wash out from us the fault that is causing the harm. They are able, like beautiful music or any glorious uplifting thing that gives us inspiration, to raise our very natures to bring us nearer to our Souls, and by that very act bring us peace and relieve our sufferings. They cure not by attacking the disease, but by flooding our bodies with the beautiful vibrations of our higher nature, in the presence of which disease melts away as snow in the sunshine. There is no true healing unless there is a change in outlook, peace of mind, and inner happiness.*

Edward Bach

---

* See also my *Keys to the Soul: A Workbook on Self-Diagnosis Using the Bach Flowers* (Saffron Walden, Essex, England: C. W. Daniel Company, 1998).

Traditional scientists will find Dr. Bach's words difficult to accept, although in light of recent research in the fields of biophysics and psycho-neuro-immunology, we can assume that in a few years we will be able to measure the effect of Bach Flowers objectively. Therefore, it may be useful to look from several different perspectives at how Bach Flowers work.

Philosophical/Spiritual Interpretation

The Flowers that Bach used are "plants of higher order." Each of them embodies a certain potential of the Soul that is expressed through its particular vibration. Each of these "floral" vibrational patterns corresponds to a matching Soul frequency within the human energy field. The human Soul carries in principle all of Bach's thirty-eight potentials in the form of virtues—the archetypal repertoire of harmonic behavior patterns—although they are balanced differently in each of us.

If for a potential such as self-confidence there is a misunderstanding between the Soul's intentions and the understanding of the personality, the frequency of the potential will be distorted and will become evident as a negative behavior pattern in the personality—presenting, for example, as a lack of trust in our own abilities.

The frequency of the Flower Essence Larch corresponds to the potential that has to do with self-esteem. Taking Larch sends a harmonizing impulse into the specific area of the human energy field that is distorting this potential and, when taken over time, re-harmonizes and reestablishes the positive behavior pattern: lack of confidence transforms into self-esteem.

In other words, the Bach Flower acts as a catalyst, reconnecting the specific, blocked contact between the Soul and the personality. The Soul can be "heard" again by the personality. Where there were disharmony and rigidity, life flows once again. Or, as Bach put it, "A person that 'wasn't quite himself anymore' is now restored to be 'fully himself.'"

Through the support of the Bach Flower frequencies, the personality finds its way out of its oh-so-human confusion and limitation and back to the Soul's potentials, or virtues, that give meaning and harmony to our existence on this planet.

Bach Flowers in the Human Energy Field

The human bioenergetic field incorporates the layers of the human field of energy that are located beyond the physical body and are invisible to most of us. Traditionally they are called the *aura*. These layers influence and complement each other and each vibrates at a specific frequency.

At the first, or etheric, level of the aura, energies are collected and distributed from centers known as *chakras*. These are related to the other levels of the energy field and rotate at different frequencies, which those who are sensitive are

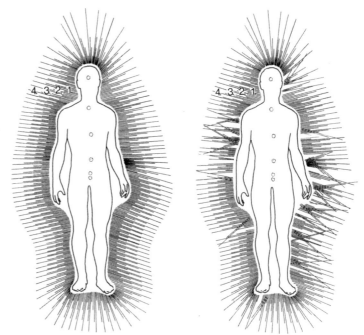

1. Etheric; 2. Emotional; 3. Mental; 4. Transpersonal

able to perceive as different colors and patterns. Modern photography techniques, such as the color-plate method, are making these layers of energy more and more visible to normal sight.

The aura encompasses all of a personality's levels of consciousness and experience. On the aura's transpersonal level, the Higher Self forms the bridge between the personality and the Soul.

- ❁ **Health** in an ideal sense is the harmonious vibrational balance within and between all layers of the aura and the Higher Self.

- ❁ **Disease** is, according to this interpretation, disharmony or the distortion of frequencies within or between different levels of the aura and the Higher Self. The information pattern of the distortion shows itself at the etheric level—which obeys different laws of time than the physical body—for weeks, months, or even years before it is manifested in the body.

Some sensitive people are able to perceive evidence of these disharmonies in the form of shadows, others experience them as disharmonious energy radiations. If these disharmonies are corrected at the etheric level by using subtle methods of healing, they will not manifest in the physical body. This explains why Bach referred constantly to the prophylactic value of the Remedies.

The deeper reasons for most disease can be detected within the emotional and mental levels of the aura as well, where subconscious and perceived reactions to feelings and thoughts are either blocked or overstimulated.

This leads to distortions in the energy frequencies and hence to negative states such as fear, hate, jealousy, anger, impatience, and sadness. These act through the etheric level, first on the nervous system of the physical body and later on the organs.

Bach says that the Flower Essences open our channels to the messages of our Higher Self and that they act in all layers of the aura. While Bach Flowers are active as "divine impulses" reaching all levels of vibration, other drugs and therapies affect only certain levels, mainly in the physical body.

Some sensitive healers see or feel enhanced activity within the whole aura immediately after a patient has taken a Flower Remedy. Many sensitive patients experience an immediate reaction in one particular chakra, which is sometimes accompanied by the sensation of color. Still others spontaneously think of the specific potential that's addressed by the Flower energy, even if they didn't know which Flower they were taking.

A Hypothesis from the Naturopathic Point of View

From the viewpoint of natural healing, Bach Flower Therapy can be seen as a cleansing and re-tuning therapy. Just as the metabolic waste products and leftovers from bad nutrition weigh on the physical body and can cause disease, so can psychological "waste"—psycho-toxins—hinder our psychological metabolism and the adequate assimilation of mental and emotional impressions and responses. These psycho-toxins are washed away or transformed through the consumption of Bach Flowers. Through this psychological re-harmonization we are able to reconnect with our psychological and physical self-healing forces.

Bach Flowers and the Immune System

Researchers in immunology have shown that negative feelings and stress weaken our immune response. The number of killer cells in the blood that destroy viruses and bacteria, for example, is significantly reduced in people who are depressed or resigned. Thus it's more difficult for these people to cope with illness-causing agents. If the negative feelings are harmonized, however, the immune system will be strengthened and can deal more effectively with incoming pathogens.

From this point of view, Bach Flower Therapy can be seen as a new and effective form of psychological preventive health care.

A Female Patient's Testimony on the Effect of Bach Flowers

"This therapy seems to have the most effect in parts of our consciousness that we are not aware of and that have not been transformed. Miraculously, it helps us be true to the phrase 'Become what you are!' I sensed the effect mostly on an emotional level and through inner experience.

"After I took my first Flower combination, everything became much clearer to me. Now I experience daily an increased awareness of the different layers of my entire being. All of myself is getting to be more individualized. When I take the Flower Essences and when I think about them, I often experience deep gratitude for this gift and feel an increasing love for all living beings and plants.

"Bach Flowers help me to better understand the wide variety of human character traits. The result is an increased tolerance toward others and the opportunity to accept all individuals for who they are. The healing of the physical body appears to be simply a by-product of this inner process; this work unfolds from the inside to the outside.

"On the physical level I sometimes feel the activity of the Bach Flowers in certain localized areas that in the past were areas of illness—for instance, pains around scars from past operations, or headaches. For a while my hair would stand straight out, and I wondered if it was a sign of the extreme activity inside my head.

"What impresses me the most is the fact that Bach Flowers work in such a clear and simple way without any unnatural or manipulative interference. However, the flowers can only stimulate our developmental process, they cannot force it."

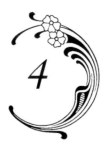

4

Edward Bach's Soul Flowers

Flowering Plants and Human Unfolding

"Are you searching for the Highest, the Greatest, look to the plant, it will be able to teach you. What it is without a will of its own, you must intend to be, that is all." In these words German poet Friedrich Schiller captured the essence of Edward Bach's Flower Therapy—one hundred years before Bach himself defined it!

The mature flower in bloom has been a symbol of beauty and superior abilities through the ages. Examples are the rose of the Rosicrucians and the lotus of a thousand petals in Indian philosophy. C. G. Jung called plants "beings of light" (*Lichtwesen*), and the blooming part of the plant was his symbol for the Self. The highest, most energy-laden potential of a plant is embodied in the flower at its peak of maturity.

Tibetan masters relate that there is a direct link between our unconscious and the plant kingdom. We are therefore able to contact our own Higher Self at an unconscious level through the plant world and thereby restore harmony within ourselves. According to Rudolf Steiner, the flowering process in plants corresponds to metabolism in humans. It is interesting to note that Edward Bach started his career as a researcher studying the degeneration of metabolic processes in the colon. Certainly we can assume that Bach was able to intuitively draw from the collective knowledge of his Celtic ancestors from Wales, who had for generations processed wild plants together with water and the sun for healing purposes.

Wolf-Dieter Storl, one of my coauthors of another book, stresses that Edward Bach took his Flower Essences from a dimension in the macrocosm where vital life processes touch our mental and spiritual processes.* In humans, the analogous effect can be observed in the limbic

---

* More detail on this subject can be found in my and Wolf-Dieter Storl's *Die Seelenpflanzen des Edward Bach* (Heinrich Hugendubel Verlag: Munich, 1995).

system and in the midbrain; here there is a seam where our emotions very delicately cross over into physiological reactions. The Flowers initiate their action at a point where nothing has yet been fixed, where everything is in between, anything is still possible, and what might become difficult later is still easy to rectify.

Bach's Criteria for Choosing His Plants

Plants are of three types. The first group is relatively below that of man in their evolution; of such are the primitive varieties, the seaweeds, the cactus, the dodder, etc.

A second class is on the same relative scale as man, which are harmless and may be used as food.

But there is a third group relatively high or higher than average mankind. Of these we must choose our remedies, for they have been given the power to heal and to bless.

These plants are there to extend a helping hand to man in those dark hours of forgetfulness, when he loses sight of his divinity, and allows the cloud of fear or pain to obscure his vision.

Edward Bach

When Bach decided to replace his nosodes (see chapter 1) with purer remedies, he looked for specific plants with high vibrations. He did this because he differentiated between plants of me-

dicinal value for physical ailments—most of the official medicinal plants we use today—and those that heal beyond the physical level. He called the latter "plants of higher order."

Bach found the Flowers intuitively and called them "the happy fellows of the plant world." At this point his sensitivity was developed to such an extreme that he needed only to place a single petal of a particular flower on his tongue to experience specific reactions on his body, mind, and emotions.

Bach intentionally chose plants whose Flowers contained no poisonous substances and those that were not food-producing plants. His chosen plants were less noticeable species that were often referred to as weeds. Many of the plants, in particular the trees, had comparable symbolic properties in folk medicine. For example, the beech tree is in many places associated with tolerance and the oak has a worldwide reputation as standing for strength and stability.

It is important to gather these plants from the wild, where nature's forces are very strong. If they were cultivated, they would lose some of their "divine" healing power. After six years of searching for Flowers in different parts of England, Bach located most of the plants in the Thames valley, in places with particularly strong energy. These locations are where the Flowers are still collected today. Some of them are on the grounds of the English Bach Centre, and others are in a natural preserve not far from it. Bach asked some friends in Switzerland and Italy to prepare Olive and Vine Essences for him; today both are harvested and prepared in Spain.

New and Simple Ways of Potentizing: Sun Method and Boiling Method

As simple as most of Bach's plants are, so are the methods of potentizing them* that Bach discovered, or rather rediscovered—Native American healers are reported to have used similar methods. In order to coax the "essence," [†] or the Soul information of the plant, from the physical body of the plant, Edward Bach used the sun method and the boiling method.

He employed the sun method with the plants that bloom in late spring or in summer, when the sun reaches its greatest strength: As many plants as possible are collected—all of the same variety—during the morning of a sunny day with cloudless skies, when the plants are in full bloom. There are, however, only a few perfect days a year when these two conditions coincide. To pick the flowers, a leaf is folded between thumb and index finger to protect the blooming parts from contact with human skin. Then, enough flowers to crowd the surface are placed in a bowl of springwater. The bowl is left in the sun for three or four hours until the wilting of the flowers and bubbles forming in the water indicate that the essence of the flowers has crossed into the springwater. The water that has been "impregnated" in this fashion is now poured into a bottle and is topped off with an equal amount of grape alcohol. This "essence bottle" or "mother tincture" keeps its potency indefinitely. Its contents are the basis for Bach's stock bottles, each of which contained 1 part of mother tincture to 240 parts of brandy.

The boiling method is mostly used to harvest the essence of flowers from trees, bushes, and shrubs that bloom early in the year before the sun has reached its full strength. The flowers are collected in the same manner as for the sun method. They are boiled in water for approximately thirty minutes, filtered repeatedly, and poured into bottles as described above.

Bach saw the following advantages to his simple method of potentizing as compared with the process of dynamization in homeopathy or with the methods of production used for spagyric or anthroposophic remedies:

❀ No destruction or harm to the plant is necessary. The flower, which holds the Soul's information, is harvested at its point of fullest development—just before it falls from the plant.

---

* The term *potentizing* is not to be confused with the procedure of the same name in classic homeopathy. More detailed explanations of Dr. Bach's methods are to be found in *The Bach Flower Remedies: Illustrations and Preparations* by Nora Weeks and Victor Bullen (Saffron Walden, Essex, England, Essex, England: C. W. Daniel Company, 1964).

† This term does not correspond with the term *essence* in chemistry.

❀ The time interval between the picking of the flowers and their preparation is kept to a minimum so that hardly any energy is lost. The whole is a harmonious process of natural alchemy, involving the tremendous powers of all four elements. Earth and air have brought the plant to the point of ripeness. The sun, or the element of fire, is used to liberate the Soul of the plant from its body. Water serves as the vehicle for the flower's information.

The Happy Fellows of the Plant World: Characteristics and Locations

The following information has been adapted and condensed from the book *Bach Flower Remedies: Illustrations and Preparations* by Nora Weeks and Victor Bullen,* two of Bach's closest associates.

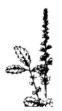

1. Agrimony
(*Agrimonia eupatoria*)

Description: Grows to a height of 1 to 2 feet (30–60 cm), mainly in fields, hedgerows, and on uncultivated lands. It flowers between June and August, producing a tall conical spike of small yellow flowers. Each stand

---

* See the first footnote on page 30.

blooms for only three days.
Preparation: Sun method

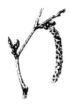

2. Aspen
(*Populus tremula*)

Description: A slender tree with flattened leafstalks. The pendant male flowers and the smaller round female catkins appear in March or April, before the leaves.
Preparation: Boiling method

3. Beech
(*Fagus sylvatica*)

Description: A handsome tree reaching a height of up to 100 feet (30 m). Formerly known as "the mother of the wood." Male and female flowers develop on the same tree. It flowers in April or May, as the leaves come out.
Preparation: Boiling method

4. Centaury
(*Centaurium umbellatum*)

Description: A very upright annual, 2 to 12 inches (5–30 cm) in height, growing in dry fields, along roadsides, and on uncultivated ground. The small pink flowers form tight stalked clusters at the top of the plant. They

appear between June and August, opening only on bright days.
Preparation: Sun method

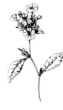

5. Cerato
(*Ceratostigma willmottiana*)

Description: This flowering plant from the Himalayas reaches about 2 feet (60 cm) in height. It does not grow wild in Western countries, but is cultivated in private gardens. The pale blue tubular flowers are less than $1/2$ inch (1 cm) in length. They are gathered in August and September.
Preparation: Sun method

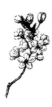

6. Cherry Plum
(*Prunus cerasifera*)

Description: The thornless young shoots of a tree or shrub growing to a height of 9 to 12 feet (3–4 m) that is often planted in rows to provide a windbreak. The flowers are pure white, slightly larger than those of blackthorn or hawthorn, and open in February to April, before the leaves appear.
Preparation: Boiling method

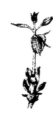

7. Chestnut Bud
(*Aesculus hippocastanum*)

Description: The same tree also provides White Chestnut Essence from the flowers. In the present case the glossy buds are used, their resinous outer layer of fourteen overlapping scales enveloping both flower and leaves.
Preparation: Boiling method

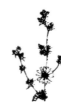

8. Chicory
(*Chicorium intybus*)

Description: A much branched perennial, up to 3 feet (90 cm) in height, found on gravel, chalk, and fallow land, as well as on the open borders of roadsides and fields. Only a few of the starlike bright blue flowers open at a time. They're very delicate, wilting as soon as they're picked.
Preparation: Sun method

9. Clematis
(*Clematis vitalba*)

Description: A woody climber found on chalky soils and limestone, on embankments, and in hedges, thickets, and woodlands. The stem of an older plant may

be up to 40 feet (12 m) in length and is ropelike. It flowers from July to September. Four greenish white downy sepals surround the fragrant flowers. In autumn the stamens develop into long, silvery, threadlike filaments like gray hair, hence its common name old man's beard.
Preparation: Sun method

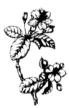

10. Crab Apple
(Malus pumila, M. sylvestris)

Description: Probably a cultivated apple tree that has gone wild. Spreading crown; short, thornlike shoots; maximum height 30 to 35 feet (10 m). The tree grows in hedgerows, thickets, and woodland clearings. The heart-shaped petals are a rich pink on the outside and white with just a tinge of pink inside. It flowers in May.
Preparation: Boiling method

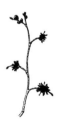

11. Elm
(Ulmus procera)

Description: Flowers between February and April, depending on the weather, in woodlands and hedgerows. The small, very numerous purplish brown flowers growing in clusters open before the leaves. Elms have become rare due to disease.
Preparation: Boiling method

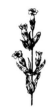

12. Gentian
(Gentianella amarella)

Description: A biennial, 6 to 8 inches (15–20 cm) in height, growing on dry hilly pasturelands, cliffs, and dunes. The numerous flowers range from blue to purple in color. They are gathered from August to October.
Preparation: Sun method

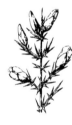

13. Gorse
(Ulex europaeus)

Description: Native to Europe, Gorse grows on stony ground, dry pastureland, and heath. Fragrant yellow flowers bloom from February to June.
Preparation: Sun method

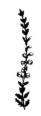

14. Heather
(Calluna vulgaris)

Description: Not to be confused with the red-flowering *Erica* genus, Heather flowers July to

September, with mauve, pink, and occasionally white flowers on heaths, dry moors, and in open barren places.

Preparation: Sun method

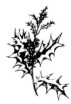

15. Holly
(*Ilex aquifolium*)

Description: This tree or shrub with glossy evergreen leaves and brilliant red berries grows in woodlands and hedgerows. The white, slightly fragrant male and female flowers usually grow on different trees. Both types of blossoms open in May and June.

Preparation: Boiling method

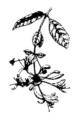

16. Honeysuckle
(*Lonicera caprifolium*)

Description: A vigorous, fragrant climber found in woodlands, on the edges of forests, and on heaths. The petals, reddish outside and white inside, turn yellow upon pollination. Less common than the yellow-flowering Honeysuckle, it blooms from June to August.

Preparation: Sun method

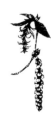

17. Hornbeam
(*Carpinus betulus*)

Description: A tree that is at first sight similar to the Beech but smaller and greener, growing singly or in groups in woods and coppices. The pendant male flowers and upright female flowers are green-brown and open in April or May.

Preparation: Boiling method

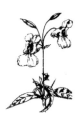

18. Impatiens (*Impatiens glandulifera, I. roylei*)

Description: A fleshy annual, up to 6 feet (2 m) in height, growing on river- and canalbanks and on damp, lower ground. Flowers are pale or reddish mauve and appear between July and September.

Preparation: Sun method

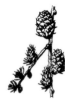

19. Larch
(*Larix decidua*)

Description: A graceful tree reaching a height of up to 100 feet (30 m). It prefers hills and the edges of woods. Male and female flowers grow on the same tree. They open when the needles just become visible as tiny bright green tufts.

Preparation: Boiling method

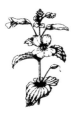

20. Mimulus
(*Mimulus guttatus*)

Description: Native to North America, this perennial, about 1 foot (30 cm) in height, grows along brooks, streams, and in damp places. The large solitary yellow flowers open between June and August.

Preparation: Sun method

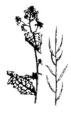

21. Mustard (*Sinapis arvensis*)

Description: An annual 1 to 2 feet (30–60 cm) in height growing in fields and by the wayside. The brilliant yellow flowers first form short spikes, which soon develop into long, beaded pods. It flowers from May to July.

Preparation: Sun method

22. Oak (*Quercus robur*)

Description: Our forefathers considered the Oak a holy tree. It grows in woodlands and on grasslands. Male and female flowers develop on the same tree, blooming between the end of April and early May.

Preparation: Sun method

23. Olive (*Olea europoea*)

Description: The Olive tree, an evergreen native to the Mediterranean, flowers in different spring months according to the climate of the country where the tree grows. The inflorescence consists of twenty or thirty inconspicuous white flowers.

Preparation: Sun method

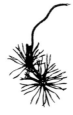

24. Pine (*Pinus sylvestris*)

Description: This slender tree reaches a height of up to 100 feet (30 m). Its bark is brown-red lower down and orange-brown in the upper crown. It grows in forests and on heaths, preferring sandy soil. The male and female flowers grow on the same tree; the male is thickly covered with yellow pollen.

Preparation: Boiling method

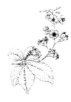

25. Red Chestnut (*Aesculus carnea*)

Description: The plant is more delicate and less robust than the White Horse Chestnut. The flowers are a good strong rose-pink, appearing in large pyramidal inflorescences in late May or early June.

Preparation: Boiling method

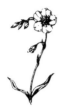

26. Rock Rose
(*Helianthemum nummularium*)

Description: A freely branching undershrub growing on chalky uplands, preferring limestone and gravelly soils. The radiant yellow flowers open from June to September, usually only one or two at a time.
Preparation: Sun method

27. Rock Water
(springwater with
healing properties)

Description: This is not a plant but rather water from natural springs located in areas un-touched by civilization and known for their power to heal the sick. Such half-forgotten wells, exposed only to the free interplay of sun and wind as they bubble up among trees and grasses, may still be found in many parts of the world.

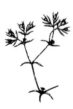

28. Scleranthus
(*Scleranthus annuus*)

Description: A low annual, bushy or creeping, reaching a height up to 2 1/2 feet (70 cm)

with numerous tangled stems. It grows in wheat fields and on sandy and gravelly soils. The flowers appear in clusters, pale to dark green, between July and September.
Preparation: Sun method

29. Star of Bethlehem
(*Ornithogalum umbellatum*)

Description: This plant is related to the onion and to garlic and is found in woodlands and meadows, growing to a height of 6 to 12 inches (15–30 cm). Each of its slender leaves shows a white line running down the center, and its flowers—which open only when the sun is out, between April and May—are striped green on the outside and are pure white inside.
Preparation: Boiling method

30. Sweet Chestnut
(*Castanea sativa*)

Description: This tree grows to a height of about 65 feet (20 m) in open woodlands, on loose soils with a moderate degree of moisture. The catkinlike, sickly scented flowers appear after the

leaves, in June to August, later than on other trees.
Preparation: Boiling method

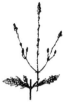

31. Vervain *(Verbena officinalis)*

Description: Up to 2 feet (60 cm) in height, this robust upright perennial may be found by the roadside, on dry waste ground, and in sunny pastures. The small lilac or mauve flowers open between July and September.
Preparation: Sun method

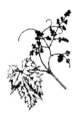

32. Vine *(Vitis vinifera)*

Description: A climbing plant, growing to a length of 45 feet (15 m) or more, Vine grows in countries with a warmer climate. The small, fragrant green flowers grow in dense clusters. The flowering time varies with the climate.
Preparation: Sun method

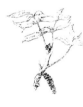

33. Walnut *(Juglans regia)*

Description: This tree grows to a height of up to 100 feet (30 m) and does well in protected areas, by hedges, and in orchards. Male and female flowers grow on the same tree, the males in much greater number than the greenish females. The tree blooms in April or May, before or just as the leaf buds burst.
Preparation: Boiling method

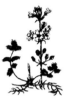

34. Water Violet *(Hottonia palustris)*

Description: This is a member of the primrose family, flowering in May and June and growing in slow-moving or stagnant water, pools, and ditches. The pale lilac flowers with yellow centers grow in whorls around the leafless stalk. The finely divided leaves remain below the surface of the water.
Preparation: Sun method

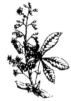

35. White Chestnut *(Aesculus hippocastanum)*

Description: This is the Horse Chestnut, flowering at the end of May or in early June. The male flowers tend to be at the top of the "candelabra," the female lower down. The color of the flowers is creamy white splashed and dotted with crimson and yellow.
Preparation: Sun method

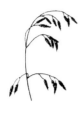

36. Wild Oat *(Bromus ramosus)*

Description: A grass commonly found in damp woods, thickets, and by roadsides. Scales in their spikelets enclose the hermaphrodite flowers.
Preparation: Sun method

37. Wild Rose *(Rosa canina)*

Description: The ancestor of many cultivated roses, the Wild Rose likes to grow in the sun, on the fringes of woods, in hedgerows, and on stony slopes. The flowers are white, pale pink, or deep pink, with five large heart-shaped petals. They open singly or in clusters of three between June and August.
Preparation: Boiling method

38. Willow *(Salix vitellina)*

Description: There are many different Willow species, but this one is easily recognized in winter, when its branches turn a bright orange-yellow. It likes to grow on moist and low-lying ground. Male and female flowers open early in May on separate trees.
Preparation: Boiling method

Bach's Seven Groups

Bach discovered his Soul plants in three stages. First he discovered the Twelve Healers,* then the Four Helpers, and finally twenty-two additional Flowers, trees, and shrubs. After each step he was convinced that he had found and defined all negative archetypal behavior patterns of our human nature. However, each time he became aware of even subtler behavior patterns and, thus, more appropriate Flowers to be found. He discovered his last remedy just half a year before his death and declared at that time that his work was finished.

Based on his research on the seven nosodes, he classified the thirty-eight Flowers in seven groups.

1. For those who have fear: Rock Rose, Mimulus, Cherry Plum, Aspen, Red Chestnut.

2. For those who suffer from uncertainty: Cerato, Scleranthus, Gentian, Wild Oat, Gorse, Hornbeam.

3. For those who lack sufficient interest in present circumstances: Clematis, Honeysuckle, Wild Rose, Olive, White Chestnut, Chestnut Bud, Mustard.

4. For those who feel lonely: Water Violet, Impatiens, Heather.

* See also Edward Bach's *Heal Thyself, The Twelve Healers, Original Writings of Edward Bach* (Saffron Walden, Essex, England: C. W. Daniel Company, 1990).

5. For those who are oversensitive to others' influences and ideas: Agrimony, Centaury, Walnut, Holly.

6. For those who are suffering from despondency and despair: Larch, Pine, Elm, Sweet Chestnut, Star of Bethlehem, Willow, Oak, Crab Apple.

7. For those who over-care for the welfare of others: Chicory, Vervain, Vine, Beech, Rock Water.

However, the author Philip Chancellor, in his 1971 book on Bach's work, had already discontinued the use of this classification of the different Flowers. During the decades following Bach's death, so many additional facets of the Flowers and the behavior patterns connected to them have been revealed that in some cases the classification becomes difficult to follow and, in these cases, seems to limit the understanding of each Flower.

Frequently Asked Questions

For further information, please match the *italicized terms* in the following questions with those from the alphabetized list of issues found in appendix A.

How are the Bach Flowers *produced today*?

Does the quality of Bach Flowers suffer because of *pollution*?

How long will the supplies from *original locations* last in the light of increasing worldwide use of Bach Flower Remedies?

In what ways do the *original locations* of the plants that supply Bach Flowers differ from other locations where the same plants grow?

In what ways do *new Flower Essences* differ from the original Bach Essences?

Is the effectiveness of Bach Flowers influenced by *changes in the earth's energy field*?

Is it more effective to make *tea* from the Flowers of Bach plants or to eat them raw?

How compatible are the subtle frequencies of Bach Flowers and the oils used in *aromatherapy*?

Is it advisable to treat *plants* with Bach Flower Essences?

Do we know why *Bach didn't include certain flowers* in his system that may have fit his criteria, such as linden flowers?

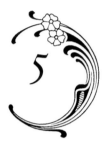

The Bach Flower System

How to Use These Flower Descriptions

Every Bach Flower represents a virtue, or a human Soul quality. For instance, Agrimony represents honesty. This quality can be observed either as a positive potential (positive behavior pattern) or, in its distorted form, as a negative behavior pattern. The Essence corresponding to the quality or virtue acts to re-harmonize it. In a step-by-step process the distorted behavior pattern is brought back to the positive potential. In this chapter the title phrases for each Flower summarize this process. Thus the first Flower reads, "Agrimony: The Honesty Flower—From Pretended Harmony to Inner Peace."

The introductory text for each Flower gives various examples of how the negative behavior pattern presents itself in different types of people and in different life situations. It then goes on to explain why the distortion may have arisen and in what way the positive potential expresses itself. For each Flower the section on Key Symptoms summarizes the negative pattern as it has been

observed most frequently. You will not always identify with a key symptom as given. If you already have been consciously working with it, you will have seen it at an earlier stage and it will express itself more subtly in you.

The section on the Behavior Pattern in the Blocked State is a collection of various shades of reaction in a given pattern that people might experience depending upon their circumstances and level of consciousness. Its important to note that the list is not all-inconclusive—it would be endless if it were to include every individual expression based on factors such as generational differences, local attitudes, and a particular cultural or moral milieu. Therefore it's important not to cling to a strict interpretation of the descriptions here and instead to seek over time to develop a personal "feeling sense" for both the blocked states and the positive quality behind them.*

* See also my *Keys to the Soul: A Workbook on Self-Diagnosis for Using the Bach Flowers* (Saffron Walden, Essex, England: C. W. Daniel Company, 1998).

Upon reading the long list of reactions, people tend to believe that their need of a particular Flower is directly proportional to the number of reactions they can identify with. This is not the case; under any given Flower, even if only one or two of the reactions described precisely match your present situation, that Flower is one you need.

The section called Positive Potential may be the most important of each Flower's description. This gives examples of how the positive potential is experienced and expressed in human life as positive behavioral patterns.

The Empowering Statements support Bach's healing strategy. These short statements are meant to be said consecutively to help you experience the energy of the positive potential and to amplify and strengthen this potential while you take the Flower.

The accompanying Kirlian photograph of each Flower shows the subtle energy radiation from one drop of the Flower Essence. This technique was developed by the German researcher Dr. Dieter Knapp.

Typical Characteristics of Negative Bach Flower Behavior Patterns

There are two basic variants of each negative pattern. The first variant refers to patterns we use in a particular moment to deal with short-term situations (see Present Situation Questionnaire on page 290), and the second variant refers to patterns that are long-term, deeply rooted character traits (see Character Questionnaire on page 292).

Here's an example of the short-term, or acute variant: "I've been undecided for days whether or not to dye my hair—though I have no problem with indecisiveness at other times, with other decisions." To address this short-term negative behavior pattern you would take Scleranthus, even though the Flower has no general long-term relevance to you.

Next is an example of the long-term, or chronic variant: "When I'm given a choice between two possibilities, I'm always trying to decide which I should choose—I'm always going back and forth between them." In this case, the behavior pattern may illustrate an ingrained character trait. However, while the descriptions of reactions for Scleranthus will resonate with you, it's important to take the Essence only when a problem is acute at a particular moment.

Each negative behavior pattern can manifest at different levels of intensity.

The intensity may vary according to the kind of person you are, your level of awareness, or how deeply the behavior pattern is entrenched (see the following examples).

Flower Essence		**Behavior Pattern**
Holly		• irritated, easily upset
		• vengeful, full of hate
		• full of raging aggression
Vine		• very goal-oriented, authoritarian
		• compulsively needs to be right
		• tyrannical, obsessive need for control
Cerato		• obsessively prepared (collects endless articles and books with advice and information on many subjects to be ready for any contingency)
		• distrustful of own ideas (discards them and looks to others for answers
		• completely uncertain (never knows what to think)

In most situations more than one pattern is involved and they interact to form an energetic constellation in which each may color the others. Vine is used in the following examples to show how this interaction takes place. Both cases are Vine states but they are very different in makeup and color.

Vine with Pine and Centaury

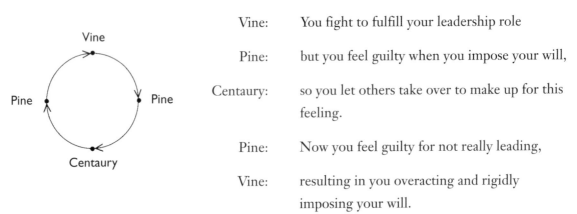

Vine:	You fight to fulfill your leadership role
Pine:	but you feel guilty when you impose your will,
Centaury:	so you let others take over to make up for this feeling.
Pine:	Now you feel guilty for not really leading,
Vine:	resulting in you overacting and rigidly imposing your will.

Vine with Rock Water and Star of Bethlehem

Vine:

Rock Water ● ● Rock Water

Star of Bethlehem

Vine:	You're a sensitive artist and have set an ambitious goal—say, to become an instrumental soloist.
Rock Water:	You practice with tremendous discipline and deny your personal needs.
Star of Bethlehem:	Shocking emotional events are ignored to avoid jeopardizing your goal
Rock Water:	In order to be less vulnerable, you deny your needs even more
Vine:	by mobilizing your willpower to concentrate exclusively on your goal.

Each individual Flower combination is thus a "new creation" and its effect is greater than the sum of its parts.

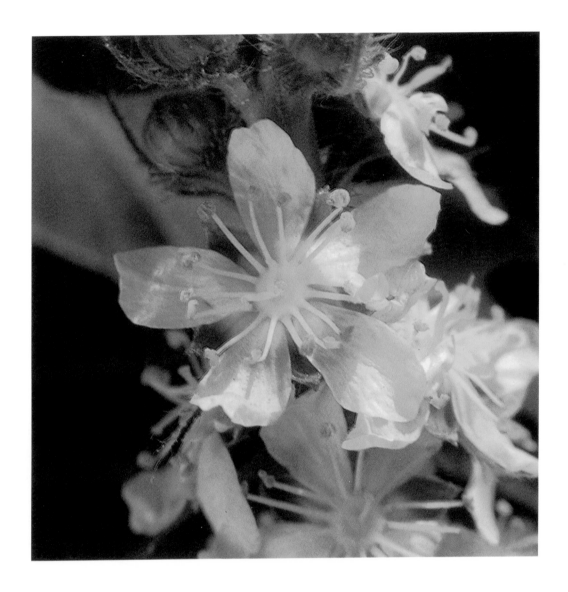

1. Agrimony: The Honesty Flower
From Pretended Harmony to Inner Peace

The jovial, cheerful, humorous people who love peace and are distressed by argument or quarrel, to avoid which they will agree to give up much.

Though generally they have troubles and are tormented and restless and worried in mind or body, they hide their cares behind their humor and jesting and are considered very good friends to know. They often take alcohol or drugs in excess, to stimulate themselves and help themselves bear their trials with cheerfulness. *

Edward Bach

Agrimony relates to the Soul's positive potentials for honesty and the ability to confront others. Unrealized potential (negative Agrimony state) is manifested in efforts made to ignore the dark side of life and to avoid any negative encounters. If you call someone who has just lost a court case and ask, "How's it going?" you'd normally expect to hear some form of despondency in the response. The Agrimony subject in the negative state, however, will respond with a routine "Great, thanks," and you'll have to know her very well indeed to sense the underlying disappointment.

Those who need Agrimony always present a cheerfully sweet and carefree face to the world. In the beginning, therefore, it can be difficult to diagnose the negative Agrimony state.

People in need of Agrimony are inwardly troubled by anxieties and fears—often material worries such as illness, financial losses, and problems at work. Yet they would rather do anything than show their feelings; what's going on in private is "nobody's business." Under no circumstances is a person in an Agrimony state willing to lose face; like an actor, she will remain cool and collected and will grin and bear it, no matter what nastiness is lurking behind the scenes. Agrimony characters are quite sensitive by nature and have a great desire for harmony. Discord and tension among those around them cause them such distress that they often soft-pedal for the sake of peace, and sometimes even make sacrifices. They're very kind to those around them in the hope that others will in turn be kind to them. Spreading cheerfulness all around, they're popular among friends and colleagues, at the club, and at the bar. They're the life and soul of the party. When ill, Agrimony people are still popular; they play down their problems and even cheer up the nurses with their jokes.

If Agrimony types with its negative manifestations ever sit quietly by themselves, their repressed problems will seek a way into their consciousness. Yet it isn't in their nature to acknowledge the presence of problems, particularly any relating to their own personality, so they make every effort to avoid spending time alone. They will throw themselves into activities, enterprises, and social functions, be it local athletic teams, community theater, or charitable organizations. Many people with an emphasis on Agrimony's negative behavior patterns may also drown their sorrows in a glass of wine, or may smoke a lot, or try to cover up unwelcome feelings with drugs. The extreme negative Agrimony state resembles the euphoria produced by alcohol: You appear relaxed, even high, on the outside, yet there's tension within.

* The original text for this and the following thirty-seven Bach Flowers can be found in Edward Bach's *The Twelve Healers and Other Remedies* (Saffron Walden, Essex, England: C. W. Daniel Company, 1996).

Because they are very receptive and susceptible to outside influence while also having a strong outer focus, Agrimony people have little staying power. A woman in a negative Agrimony state, for instance, may be very unhappy because she's unable to stick to her diet; she's driven by her inner restlessness and secretly keeps raiding the fridge at night; this will happen particularly when unpleasant thoughts eat at her.

In the negative Agrimony state people will grieve over little things they failed to do, minor failures—perhaps having forgotten to make a telephone call or mail a letter, or having an unsuccessful sexual encounter. Many such Agrimony types have small hidden vices.

The negative Agrimony state often develops in early childhood. Consider the following example: A three-year-old is standing in front of a birthday cake and many presents. Mom, Dad, Grandma, Grandpa, Aunt Erica, and Uncle Henry are all gathered around the table, observing every move the child makes, hoping the child will be especially pleased with their gifts. Telepathic communication, or the acute receptivity of Agrimony types, makes the child pick up on these expectations, and he tries to fulfill each and every one of them. There are some presents he doesn't like much, but he already senses that the idea is to keep smiling because "it's nobody's business what I really feel."

Compared with others, people with marked Agrimony traits are more focused on outer aspects of the personality, not daring to show or even be aware of what goes on inside. The surface has to be well polished, even if chaos may reign beneath.

The ancient symbol of the theater—the double mask, one crying and one laughing—seems an appropriate illustration of this dual existence: in the negative Agrimony state you present only your cheerful mask, refusing to acknowledge your somber side. Attempts are made to pretend—even to yourself—that the less pleasant side simply doesn't exist. In other words, the communication between your thinking self and your feeling self is disrupted. Often a chronic state of war is being waged between these two levels of experience.

A personality in the negative Agrimony state is subject to a dual error. Refusing to recognize a large part of itself, it's unable to make full contact with its Higher Self and therefore doesn't recognize the Soul's Life Plan. Instead, it acts according to its own limited maxims, and these tend to have a material emphasis. Yet like every living being, it's still striving to attain an ideal state and, unable to find this within, looks for it in external circumstances that have a certain lightness and spirituality. The euphoria resulting from too much wine or unencumbered dance appears to come closest to the desired state of mind for those with Agrimony's negative behavior pattern, though in reality it is a false euphoria reinforced and expanded by the artificial world that has been created.

As soon as the personality in such a negative

state acknowledges its wholeness and accepts the guidance of its Higher Self, the stabilizing forces of its own Soul will come streaming in. It will gain inner strength and sufficient stability to better face the emotional irritations of everyday life. The awareness of negative experiences will no longer need to be suppressed, but can be consciously integrated.

In the positive Agrimony state, you're aware of the relative nature of all problems, finding within yourself the radiant, joyful state you previously sought outside. Being true to yourself and honest with others will have an effect such that the people you know well become true friends. You'll be able to discuss everything, including problems, openly and with diplomatic skill.

In Bach Flower Therapy practice, Agrimony is one of the Flower Remedies often indicated with children. Agrimony children are normally cheerful and sociable, and their tears dry quickly. When they go through developmental phases of internal loneliness and sadness, like all children, Agrimony can help them communicate more easily. Even in puberty, when adolescents are dealing with many conflicting thoughts and emotions, Agrimony can be very helpful. Additionally Agrimony has been shown to be helpful in treating addictions.

In a Bach Flower interview it's best not to delve too deeply with Agrimony subjects, but to aim more for a relaxed, casual dialogue.

Agrimony patients are very sensitive to physical pain because suppressed emotional pain is pushing for recognition by way of the physical body. Internal restlessness may express itself physically in self-destructive habits such as biting fingernails, pulling hair, and pinching, or in nervous skin rashes. Many Agrimony patients grind their teeth at night.

Together with Scleranthus, Agrimony is stabilizing in situations that require adaptation in the workplace. Those who work shifts and those who fly and deal with different time zones and jet lag can benefit.

Agrimony Key Symptoms

Attempts are made to conceal disturbing thoughts and inner restlessness behind a cheerful face and a life free of worry.

Behavior Pattern in the Blocked State

- ❀ You like to live in a peaceful, harmonious atmosphere; any discord or dispute around you causes distress

- ❀ You try to please all the people all the time

- ❀ You do a great deal to keep the peace

- ❀ You give in, invent little white lies, make almost any sacrifice to maintain peace of mind and to avoid confrontation

- ❀ You hide inner turbulence and restlessness behind a mask of humor and cheerfulness

- ❀ Your motto is: No problem, keep smiling, be happy

- You minimize problems and won't discuss them, even when the subject is brought up by others

- You escape nagging thoughts by looking for excitement and variety—movies, parties, action of any kind

- You don't want to accept unpleasant situations; you look through rose-colored glasses

- You're always the good friend, the peace-maker, the life and soul of every party

- You resort to alcohol or drugs to get through difficult times and to soften unpleasant feelings and thoughts

- You're always on the move to stop yourself from thinking

- You play down discomfort when ill, even joking to entertain the hospital staff or your caregivers

- You want to live in an ideal world so you intentionally ignore flaws in a partner

- You unconsciously fear you're unable to handle painful news from others so you cut conversations short

- Children who normally quickly forget their troubles experience secret inner pain and feelings of loneliness

Even if only one or two of these patterns precisely match your present situation, you need Agrimony.

Positive Potential

- Honesty, openness, ability to deal with confrontation

- You're able to deal with both positive and negative situations and grow from them

- You feel genuine inner joyfulness

- You experience true harmony and inner peace

- You're a true optimist, a skillful diplomat, a talented peacemaker

Empowering Statements

- "I feel peaceful."

- "I am honest."

- "I reveal myself."

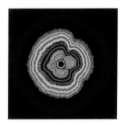

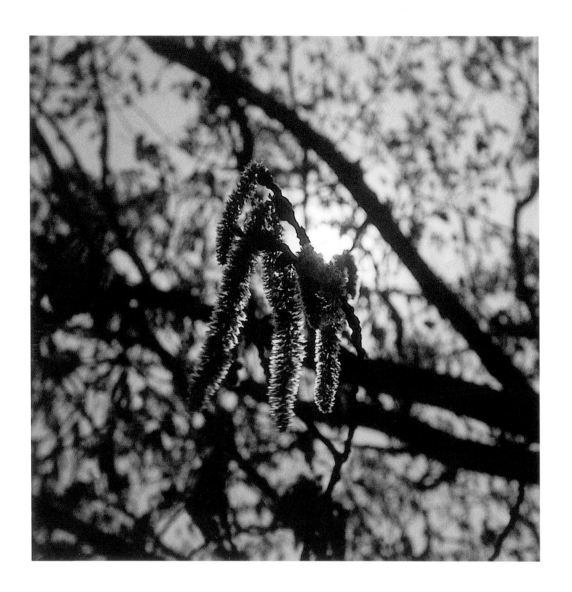

2. Aspen: The Psychic Flower
From Dark Premonitions to Conscious Sensitivity

Vague unknown fears, for which there can be given no explanation, no reason.
Yet the patient may be terrified of something terrible going to happen, he knows not what.
These vague unexplainable fears may haunt by night or day.
Sufferers are often afraid to tell their trouble to others.

Edward Bach

Aspen is related to the Soul's potential for sensitivity. People in the negative Aspen state are caught up in unconscious anxieties. It might be said that they've been born missing one protective skin layer. The boundaries of their personal physical awareness of reality in relation to all other planes of consciousness are very finely tuned. These planes hold not only the everyday experiences of the masses, but also collective concepts such as fairy tales and symbolic ideas, archetypes, superstition, images of heaven and hell, and much more.

These are the planes through which we must pass every night in our dreams to reach the transpersonal level of existence. It's through them that we are able to contact our Higher Selves, which allows constructive and healing forces to come to us while we are asleep.

People who need Aspen, much more than others, are flooded day and night with thoughts and images from these collective planes without being aware of them. Unknowingly they receive impulses and their waking consciousness is unable to make sense of them because the source of the impulse is unclear. This gives rise to fear, an eerie kind of fear that slowly creeps up the back, a goose-bumps and hair-raising fear.

"I'm so afraid, but I don't know why. I'm afraid that something terrible will happen, but I can't think what it might be." These are typical statements from those with a negative Aspen state. In extreme cases they suffer what seems to be the tortures of hell, with body trembling,

bouts of sweating, and a fluttery sensation in the stomach. But such people are without recourse and there's nothing they can do. This powerlessness is frustrating and leads to still more fear.

Aspen people in the negative behavior state temporarily lose themselves in fearful realms of collective memories where they are unable to make contact with their Higher Self. Such a state often results in sleepwalking or nightmares. They wake up panic-stricken and are afraid to go back to sleep. The supposedly comforting response that it's all in their imagination is of no assistance here.

Children, who are more susceptible to these kinds of experiences than are adults, often demand that the bedroom door be left open at night when in the negative Aspen state, or that a light be kept on in the room. They're unconsciously afraid of a monster in the closet, a crocodile under the bed, or creatures they know from television coming in through the window.

Many Aspen people in the negative state develop a strong fear of the dark for which they have no explanation. Some have a nervous, superstitious fascination with the occult and magical concepts. These people need Aspen because they may place themselves in the role of the victim in their imagination. They may be convinced that a spell has been cast on their house, for instance, resulting in "bad vibrations" that make them feel sick.

The outward appearance of the Aspen tree is a perfect symbol of the extreme sensitivity of the

Aspen state. A breath of wind and the leaves are set rustling. Aspen people in the negative state tremble like aspen leaves. They react readily to the atmosphere in their visible and invisible environment. They have an unconscious radar for a developing conflict and for psychic currents in others. It can happen that while in cheerful company they suddenly feel so bad that they have to retire.

Aspen people unconsciously register simply everything—an office atmosphere full of conflict, the morning rush and exhaustion on a crowded bus, the imminent threat and fear of inflation and war—which causes them to use up a tremendous amount of energy. These fears remain vague and indefinite in contrast to those of the negative Mimulus state, for which the fears are clearly defined and issues can be discussed with others. No name can be put on Aspen fears; thus it's difficult to talk about them with others.

Anyone taking Aspen will find that the fear and apprehension lessen while internal confidence grows. They will become aware that behind the fear lies something greater and more meaningful of which they are ultimately a part and within which they are held secure. They will become aware that above everything is the great divine law, the divine power of love, making all fear unnecessary. Such trust, once developed, makes it possible to consciously use the positive side of the Aspen energy, the ability to tune in to more subtle, nonmaterial planes of consciousness, to explore these planes without fear and use the knowledge gained for the benefit of others. These are the abilities, for example, of good teachers, psychotherapists, and artists.

Some practitioners especially recommend Aspen in the treatment of alcoholics caught up in obsessive thinking, for women who have been raped, and for children who have been abused. Such situations will certainly leave behind very specific fears of the situation itself, but can also cause a person to feel threatened in general.

People who have become very open through the practice of certain techniques that widen the consciousness may need Aspen in order to integrate their new perceptions. Anyone who has been through a drug "horror trip" will also benefit. Supported by Aspen, sensitive children will grasp that their sensitivity is a beautiful thing, something to be cherished as a gift.

Aspen Key Symptoms

There are inexplicable, vague fears, apprehensions, or secret fears of impending danger.

Behavior Pattern in the Blocked State

- ❀ You experience unfounded sensations of fear and danger

- ❀ You have sudden anxiety attacks whether alone or with others

- ❀ You wish you were less sensitive

- ❀ You feel creepy sensations of fear, as if bewitched

- ⊛ Your imagination runs wild; you can't tell the difference between fantasy and reality

- ⊛ You are fascinated with the occult and are superstitious

- ⊛ You fear persecution and punishment; you fear an invisible force or power

- ⊛ You have nightmares, waking in fear and panic and not daring to go back to sleep

- ⊛ You are afraid of your fear, but you dare not talk about it with anyone

- ⊛ You experience specific fears such as those of physical attack, rape, abuse, snakes, and ghosts

- ⊛ You wish you could protect yourself from outside influences and be less open

- ⊛ Children are afraid of the dark or of monsters under the bed

- ⊛ The atmosphere in some places is unbearable to you

- ⊛ After reading in the paper of a flu epidemic (or some similar physical scourge), you immediately develop symptoms

Even if only one or two of these patterns precisely match your present situation, you need Aspen.

Positive Potential

- You have a great capacity for conscious perception

- You are aware of your sensitivity and know how to use it well

- You proceed fearlessly and with confidence

- You are able to enter into more subtle planes of consciousness and gain deeper understanding of complex phenomena

Empowering Statements

- "I am protected."

- "I am centered."

- "I am strong."

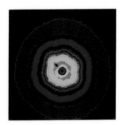

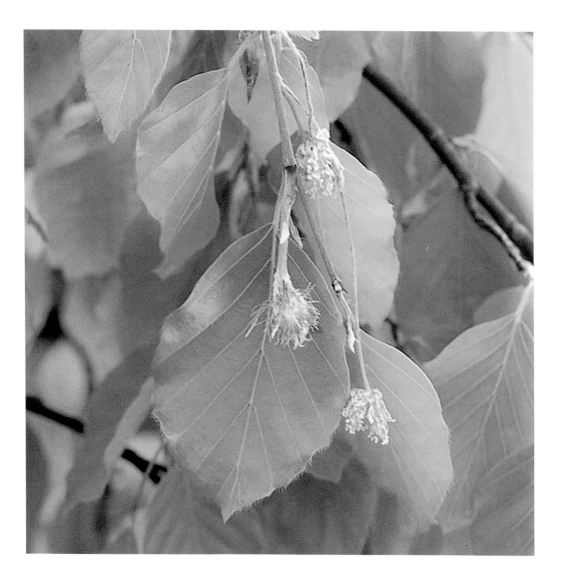

3. Beech: The Tolerance Flower
From Know-it-all to Better Understanding

For those who feel the need to see more good and beauty in all that surrounds them. And, although much appears to be wrong, to have the ability to see the good growing within. So as to be able to be more tolerant, lenient and understanding of the different way each individual and all things are working to their own final perfection.

Edward Bach

Beech relates to the Soul's potential to see and understand differences and its potential for tolerance. If you're in the negative Beech state, you'll either be overly critical and intolerant or go to the other extreme by exhibiting a false or exaggerated tolerance and understanding.

We all find ourselves, from time to time, in this negative Beech state, a state in which we tend to be arrogant and highly critical, judging others by perceived, often very narrow standards. Later we usually realize that we were mistaken because we hadn't taken into account or were unaware of certain circumstances.

In the negative Beech state you'll be very critical and judge according to narrow guidelines or intellectual premises. Other people become the subjects of your scrutiny and you classify them and make final judgments without complete understanding of their circumstances or their feelings: "I will not sit at the dinner table with a person who uses poor language!" "It's enough to simply hear the word *environmentalist!*" You polish your prejudices and inwardly draw down the corners of your mouth. Rarely will anyone appear more arrogant than the person in the negative Beech state. The people around you find it hard to imagine that originally, behind your appearance, is the wish to improve this world.

The rather snobbish Professor Higgins in George Bernard Shaw's *Pygmalion*, who wanted to transform the natural, uneducated flower girl Eliza into a "lady" for the sake of a bet, is a humorous example of the type. Totally lacking in experience, having not the least understanding of the feelings of a woman, he helplessly asks his friend Pickering, "Why can't a woman be more like a man?" Having completely suppressed his own feelings, he is unable to empathize with Eliza's situation. He hurts her feelings by employing irony in an unconscious attempt to conceal his own insecurity.

Another facet of the negative Beech state may be seen in the old-fashioned caricature of the strict, pedantic schoolmistress, dressed in gray and standing erect, always demanding absolute tidiness, accuracy, and discipline. She has completely lost sight of the fact that not everybody is born with the same nature or gifts, and not all students begin life with the same social background or opportunities.

The negative Beech state is aptly described by the saying, "She sees the speck in another's eye, but not the log in her own." In this state you tend to project too much outside, and have extreme difficulty focusing inward and digesting your experiences. In order to avoid admitting this weakness, you frequently project your undigested emotional problems onto other people. You despise other people's tendency to criticize, for example, without recognizing your own addiction to being critical. Some Beech people, therefore, may even develop gastrointestinal problems as a result of this "poor digestion."

The negative Beech state is often seen in people from families belonging to an oppressed minority. They have had to swallow much hatred, humiliation, disappointment, and injured self-esteem. To compensate for this, some of these families may deliberately withdraw from society and build their own value systems in which they are superior to others. In this way feelings of denied recognition and humiliation have a lesser impact; they're projected onto the outside world in the form of criticism and arrogance. This kind of self-defense suppresses feelings as much as possible but along with them eliminates the possibility of empathizing with anyone.

What is the "mental error" here? In the negative Beech state the personality has misunderstood and refused the learning experiences of its Life Plan and refuses to recognize the negativity it itself has been subjected to. To continue with the above scenario, the family has not begun to cope with its perceived status as "outsider" and with the painful experiences of discrimination that this perception has led to. Instead, the personalities of its members have developed their own code of ethics, incorporating certain defense mechanisms that help them shut off the voice of their Higher Self. In our example the family members have developed critical and arrogant attitudes, using them to project unwanted, humiliating feelings onto the outside world.

Such negative projections are harmful not only to the people concerned, but also to the greater unity of their immediate society. The negative thoughts that irritate those who surround people in the negative Beech state are reflected back onto the personality of the Beech individual, causing a wide variety of symptoms—often allergies. The Beech personality becomes rigid and hardened, because it is disconnected not only from its own Higher Self but from the world around it as well.

As soon as this personality lets go of its limited value judgments and opens up to its Higher Self, higher standards and greater potential for self-knowledge are revealed. Restrictive criticism is transformed into understanding; hypersensitive reactions to others become receptivity toward the impulses of the Higher Self; arrogance becomes genuine love and tolerance, the kind of tolerance, as Bach put it, that made Jesus plead for those who had tortured and crucified him, "Father, forgive them, for they know not what they do."

If you're leaning toward the negative Beech state, there are a number of principles you might well take to heart. One is the knowledge that you are but a small cell within a much larger being, and as such are able to truly live only by harmonizing with the breathing rhythm and consciousness of this larger being—not by separating from it. It's also important to realize that as a small cell, you can only partly understand the laws of the greater being, and therefore it is foolhardy to believe that your own standards are absolute.

And it's essential to know that in the final analysis we are all only reflections of mutual projections. Therefore, you should concentrate on letting the positive projections of others find resonance within yourself, rather than projecting your own negative apprehensions and defense mechanisms onto other people. Instead of feeling apart from others, you'll feel a sense of unity, a fellowship of souls, which is really what your heart was seeking through the criticism used in the negative Beech state. Being aware of this feeling of unity within will make the outside world seem suddenly more harmonious. Little things will cease to irritate because you'll be more and more able to recognize the unity in variety.

The Beech Flower Essence helps to reestablish contact with the Self and a sense of wholeness. It loosens the rigidity of thought processes and restores humor and the sense of being human. In the positive Beech state you'll be something of a "tolerant diagnostician," able to use your human "X-ray vision" and excellent judgment constructively, for yourself and for the community.

Children in the negative Beech state tend to chew their nails. On an unconscious level they criticize the behavior of those to whom they are particularly close (parents, relatives, friends) and although they would like to do something about it, they know that such an action would be too risky. Instead, they hold back, and bite off their own "claws."

Beech Key Symptoms

There is a tendency to be critical, prejudiced, intolerant, and judgmental, along with an inability to see things through another's eyes.

Behavior Pattern in the Blocked State

- ❀ The mistakes of others are readily apparent to you

- ❀ You always see only what's wrong in a situation

- ❀ You're unable to accept that no one is perfect

- ❀ You sit in judgment of others

- ❀ You are overly critical of yourself

- ❀ You become upset at the "stupidity" of others

- ❀ You have petty reactions; you lack tact and sensitivity

- ❀ You become irritated easily by small gestures and speech habits of others; your reactions are out of proportion to the situation

- ❀ You cling firmly to prejudices

- ❀ You're very touchy about personal criticism, avoiding any discussion of the issue at hand

- ❀ You habitually seek out the flaws in any situation, overlooking advantages and potentials that could develop

- You're disliked by others because of your intense criticism of them

- You're determined not to appear intolerant by showing exaggerated understanding and refraining from any criticism, even when constructive criticism would be helpful; whatever happens, "it's okay."

Even if only one or two of these patterns precisely match your present situation, you need Beech.

Positive Potential

- You have good mental acuity and the ability to differentiate and show good judgment

- You see the positive possibilities for growth behind less-than-perfect situations

- You show understanding, criticize constructively, and are able to accept criticism yourself

- You are tolerant of personality types that are totally different from yours and respect their strengths and weaknesses

Empowering Statements

- "I accept."

- "I'll meet you halfway."

- "I see the possibilities."

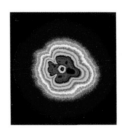

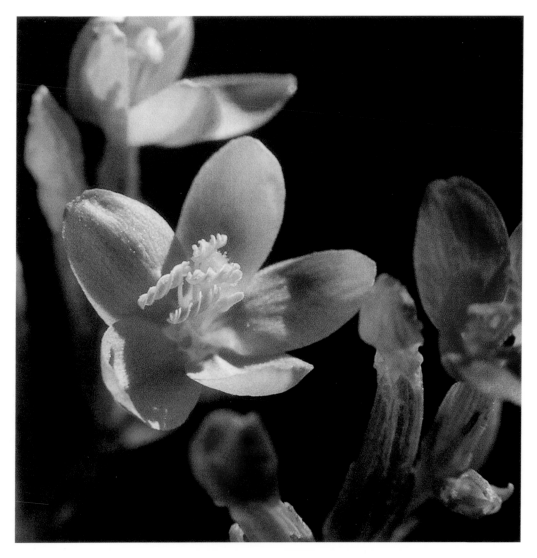

4. Centaury: The Service Flower
From Passive Service to Active Service

Kind, quiet, gentle people who are over-anxious to serve others. They overtax their strength in their endeavors.

Their wish so grows upon them that they become more servants than willing helpers. Their good nature leads them to do more than their own share of work, and in so doing they may neglect their own particular mission in life.

Edward Bach

Centaury relates to the Soul's potential for self-determination. In the negative Centaury state your own will is not sufficiently developed.

Centaury people sometimes appear to have spent all of their willpower during the birth process; they seem happy to simply enjoy being a part of any group or activity. Children with marked Centaury traits, so-called "easy kids," are good-natured and pleasant, and are responsive to praise and criticism. They are hardly ever a problem to their parents, except perhaps insofar as their peers easily take advantage of them because they're so ready to please. As adults they're easily influenced by stronger personalities who will take advantage of their innately helpful nature for egotistical purposes. One example of a person in need of Centaury might be the oldest daughter who does not marry so she can look after her ailing mother. Another is the son who would have liked to become a teacher but allowed himself to be talked into taking over the family construction firm to honor his father's wish that it remain in the family. Centaury is also warranted for the young wife who mistakes slavery for love, readily fulfilling all her spoiled husband's wishes, suppressing her own real needs for his every whim.

People in the negative Centaury state often say, while helplessly shrugging their shoulders, "I simply can't refuse," or "I'm just unable to say no." Outsiders often shake their heads at the way a Centaury type makes himself a doormat.

Strong Centaury types often complain of tiredness and being overworked, a result of taking on too much in their desire to help. Apart from this, however, they don't consider their state a painful one, failing to recognize its full implications, and therefore also failing to notice that with all their service to others, they aren't fulfilling their own purpose in life. The motive behind their helpfulness is nothing but the very human desire for recognition and validation.

In the negative Centaury state the magnificent virtues of wishing to help others, of service and sincere devotion to a cause, have become distorted. You erroneously and uncritically, like an immature child, continue to make yourself subservient to other people, giving in to their human weaknesses instead of holding to your own personality and higher principles.

To be able to serve these higher principles it is a primary necessity to develop your own personality, to make it the instrument of the Soul. In this context you must realize that the personality can only be built, supported, and preserved by your own will. Thus, a condition that is too strong in most negative states (your personality is strongly separated from others) is too weak in the negative Centaury state (your personality is not separated enough from others).

Some practitioners consider Centaury the most sensitive of all thirty-eight states. Frequently people with emerging psychic faculties initially experience a negative Centaury state. An imbalance arises if the psychic faculties are more strongly developed than the will. In this negative state Centaury people are extremely sensitive, particularly to disharmonious energies. They're insecure, easily upset, and easily hurt. They'll often become ill out of the blue, not knowing that their sickness is due to this particular state.

When paired with the negative Walnut state, Centaury people may easily become victims of powerful spiritual influences. They might fall under the spell of "enlightened" teachers or religious sects. In extreme cases they will submissively subject themselves to apparently necessary laws and group rituals, running the risk of completely losing their personalities and diminishing their own chances for personal development.

The Centaury Essence will help you restore contact with the powers of your own will, concentrating the energy potentials in the personality and stabilizing them. A sensitive person described the powerful sensation arising after the first dose of Centaury as a straightening out of the left and right sides of the body, with the sensation most intensely concentrated in the solar plexus and thyroid chakras.

In the positive Centaury state people are able to make good use of their virtues of devotion and service. They can consciously decide to serve a good cause while recognizing destructive situations that they should say no to. They're well integrated into groups, participating fully without giving up their own personalities. At times they may intentionally become the instrument that allows the entrance of divine powers for the benefit of major causes.

In the course of the therapeutic interview, patients in the negative Centaury state should come to realize that they are not always helping others by rushing to meet their desires. On the contrary, they are hindering the learning process for both themselves and those around them. It's also valuable to examine the extent to which the negative Centaury state is an escape into another person in order to evade the process of your own development, which among other things involves learning to discriminate and make decisions.

If your will has grown weak after a prolonged illness, you may be unable to do anything for yourself; Centaury could then give new vitality to your mind and body.

There are two recommendations to develop the positive Centaury potential. Question yourself before every activity: "Do I really want to do this?" And when somebody asks you for a favor, ask yourself "What are this person's real motives for asking?"

To counter the self-destructive behavior observed among people in the negative Centaury state, it can also be helpful to adjust your posture. Instead of pulling your shoulders in and bending your neck forward, consciously straighten your shoulders, stand erect, and look forward.

Centaury Key Symptoms

These are weakness of will, hypersensitivity to the wishes of others, and the inability to say no.

Behavior Pattern in the Blocked State

❀ You can't stand on your own; you give in too easily

- You don't stand up for your own interests and don't express your own wishes

- You are passive, weak-willed, and easily led by others

- You go along with others willingly, obediently, and even subserviently

- You're more sensitive to the wishes of others than you are to your own

- You sense immediately what others expect and automatically do it

- You're easily led astray by your desire to please—in extreme cases, to the point of self-denial

- You're easily taken to the cleaners during negotiations

- You let others speak for you; your time or services are often volunteered without your consent

- You let others dictate what to do

- You're easily persuaded to do things you didn't plan to do

- You're good-natured and easily exploited

- You dance to the tune of a self-centered personality who may be a parent, significant other, or superior

- You unconsciously adopt gestures, phrases, and opinions of a stronger personality

- Children are strongly influenced by praise and criticism

- You prefer to take on additional work because rejecting it would take more energy

- You often take on more than you can do and tend to give more than you have

Even if only one or two of these patterns precisely match your present situation, you need Centaury.

Positive Potential

- You are aware of your personal needs and live your own life

- You know when and why to say yes; when necessary, you are able to say no

- You're able to fit in well with groups but are always able to stay true to yourself

- You serve wisely while staying true to your own inner purpose

Positive Statements for Practice

- "I stand up straight."

- "I am who I am."

- "I do what I want."

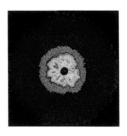

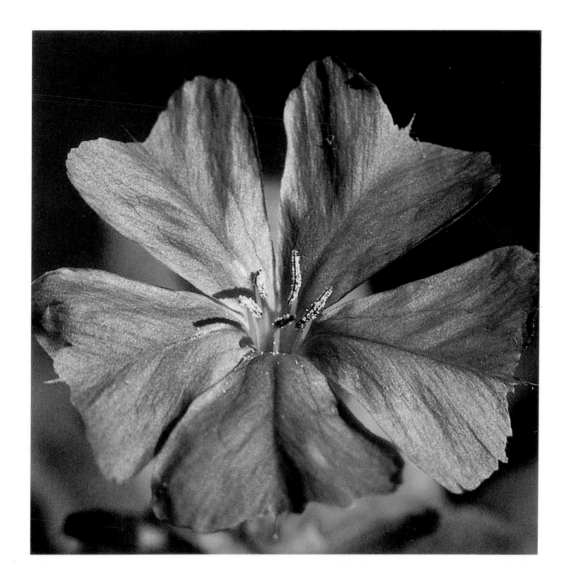

5. Cerato: The Intuition Flower
From Indecisiveness to Inner Certainty

Those who have not sufficient confidence in themselves to make their own decisions.
They constantly seek advice from others, and are often misguided.

Edward Bach

Cerato relates to the Soul's potential for inner certainty, trust in the inner voice, and intuition. In a negative Cerato state a person has great difficulty accepting his own perceptions and acting on them. When a decision has to be made the answer comes intuitively, but the head, the rational mind, doesn't accept this intuitive response. Instead, it rapidly employs various routine arguments and adopted patterns to push aside the intuitive solution. Therefore, a person may intuitively know something to be right but cannot put this knowledge into practice with conviction, and as a result an inner conflict arises. The person doubts the correctness of his own decisions and fails to trust his intuition.

For those in the negative Cerato state, the misunderstanding consists of the personality refusing to perceive and acknowledge the role of the Higher Self. Instead of realizing that only the Higher Self is able to guide to what is best, they seek an answer in the outside world, often in popular theories, doctrines, and the experiences of people who are quite different from themselves.

People needing Cerato are constantly getting on the nerves of others with their questions concerning personal problems and minor issues. "What would you do if you were in my place?"; "I know perfectly well, of course, but somehow I don't feel I can rely on my own sense of things"; "The answer can't be as simple as what I think it is"—these are typical Cerato questions.

Many people who are in the negative Cerato state are not at all aware that, in fact, they know

a great deal. They will therefore gather more and more information, hoarding it like money in a savings account instead of working with it. Because of this behavior, their knowledge doesn't help them gain experiences of their own. Yet, ironically, confidence and trust in your own ability to make decisions arises only from genuine personal experience.

People who again and again follow certain diet fads unquestioningly, despite the fact that they already know the diet doesn't do them any good, are in the negative Cerato state. "I know onions don't agree with me, but surely if the diet plan recommends them, they *have* to be good for me." Cerato patients may harm themselves against their better judgment and so appear foolish, even stupid, to others.

Cerato people pay much attention to what they are convinced are unwritten laws: "Should people wear shorts at my age?" or "Should people wear a short or long skirt to this occasion?"

People in a negative Cerato state are like millipedes that ask, "In which order do you use your legs?" The insect starts thinking and out of confusion becomes unable to move. Instead of following their gut feeling telling them whether or not to do a certain thing, these people spend too much time pondering the situation, in the process spoiling their opportunities and stifling their energy. For them it helps to realize that mistakes are a necessary aspect of learning and will be made and recovered from just as surely as one step automatically follows another.

The groundwork for developing a negative Cerato state is often laid in childhood, particularly if parents are strong personalities who look down on the impressions and ideas of their children, or ask them to do things they themselves won't do.

If you use Cerato, you'll find your inner voice growing stronger, and the more you trust in it, the more clearly it will speak. You're happy when you discover that suddenly all necessary knowledge is at your fingertips at precisely the right moment, so that you're able to quickly put your judgments and decisions to use. A great desire then often arises to use such knowledge for the sake of others.

The positive potential of Cerato is an attitude of calm certitude. No argument, however convincing it may appear, will deflect you from a decision you've recognized to be the right one. Practitioners also report that dream life is often greatly stimulated by Cerato, and that dreams are more clearly remembered.

Cerato Key Symptoms
There is a lack of confidence in your own intuition.

Behavior Pattern in the Blocked State

- ❀ You distrust your own judgment

- ❀ You constantly ask others for advice, hoping they'll make the decisions instead

- ❀ You're too scared to act spontaneously

- ❀ You talk a great deal and get on the nerves of others by butting in with questions

- ❀ You give too much weight to others' opinions

- ❀ You hunger for information

- ❀ You accumulate knowledge without using it

- ❀ You cover all the bases in order to avoid making mistakes

- ❀ You seek confirmation from authority figures

- ❀ You're led astray based on the advice of others rather than your own better judgment

- ❀ You question a decison you make the moment after making it

- ❀ You have many advisers and hope each will provide the perfect solution

- ❀ Others describe you as lacking good instincts and common sense

- ❀ You appear to lack self-reliance, to be simple or even stupid

- ❀ You tend to imitate the choices of others

- ❀ Students tend to cross out the right answer they gave at first on a test and replace it with something wrong

> **Even if only one or two of these patterns precisely match your present situation, you need Cerato.**

Positive Potential

- ❀ You're intuitive, interested, and eager to learn

- ❀ You're able to quickly form your own opinion

- ❀ You accept your Inner Guidance, trust yourself, and stand by your own decisions

Empowering Statements

- ❀ "I trust myself."

- ❀ "I pay attention to my first impressions."

- ❀ "I decide for myself."

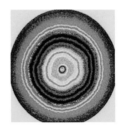

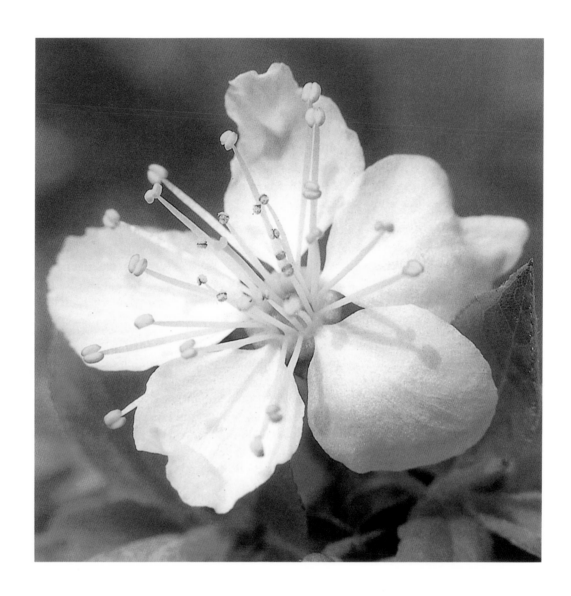

6. Cherry Plum: The Openness Flower
From Overload to Relaxation

Fear of the mind being over-strained, of reason giving way, of doing fearful and dreaded things, not wished and known wrong, yet there comes the thought and impulse to do them.

Edward Bach

Cherry Plum relates to the Soul's potential for composure. In the negative Cherry Plum state you go to extremes to repress your emotional impressions because you're afraid of them. As a child you may have experienced that the emotions you expressed were unwanted or unacceptable, so you trained yourself to suppress them. Subsequently you barely allow yourself to feel your own emotions.

The negative Cherry Plum state is not easily recognized. People in this behavior pattern often appear congested, with a runny nose; or they complain of constipation. More intense states manifest in a kind of forced calmness—the eyes are wide open and staring, and blinking is infrequent.

People who are consciously aware of their extreme Cherry Plum state may say, for example, "I'm sitting on a powder keg—I'm afraid it'll blow up at any moment" or "To my absolute horror, I find myself having such brutal thoughts as wanting to take a kitchen knife and stick it in my kid's back."

In the extremely negative Cherry Plum state people are afraid they may be heading for a breakdown, losing their self-control or even their minds. Their nerves are stretched to the breaking point; they feel as though there's a time bomb ticking away inside their bodies; they fear that they'll do something terrible at any moment that they'll regret for the rest of their lives. They feel that destructive forces they can no longer control are rising within them.

Men who have fought in wars describe negative Cherry Plum states developing after days of continuous shelling in the trenches, or after weeks of vicious interrogations in a prison camp. These circumstances so reduce a personality that there comes a point when it just wants to give up. In the extreme Cherry Plum state there is a real danger of suicide. A symbolic representation of the negative Cherry Plum State might be the medieval painting *The Temptation of St. Anthony*, which depicts the powers of hell doing everything possible to force the saint to capitulate.

From a psychological point of view, the negative Cherry Plum state is caused by an internal fear of letting go. Efforts are made by an individual to keep subconscious pictures from surfacing because he doesn't think he'll be able to cope with them.

It is interesting to consider the increased incidence of negative Cherry plum states in our society from a spiritual point of view. More and more, tender souls are being born into an atmosphere of increasing chaos, toxicity, and exploitation. A stark contrast between people's internal structure and what's happening in their environment produces a chronic Cherry Plum state on a refined level. On the surface this phenomenon shows up in young people as a kind of tense absentmindedness.

As a person's spiritual growth progresses, a negative Cherry Plum state may develop just before an important decision must be made; blocked and ambivalent emotions push to enter consciousness at such times. A person may feel unable to escape the resulting chaos.

When a person is in the negative Cherry Plum state, the personality has completely turned away from the guidance of the Higher Self. It is therefore unable to integrate the powerful forces it feels arising within itself. It reacts with fear, failing to understand the law that every mental and spiritual development is accompanied by activation not only of bright, constructive, positive forces, but also those that are dark, destructive, and negative. The personality makes an anxious effort to hold those dark forces beneath the surface—but again, every pressure results in counterpressure. This is why people who need Cherry Plum should be encouraged to immediately name and talk about all the feelings that arise in them as soon as they're noted.

As soon as the personality submits to the guidance of its Higher Self, it can be led through chaos and darkness to the light of its true destiny, and hence to ever-greater knowledge. Tremendous energy reserves become accessible, enough for the personality to endure powerful external and internal adversity.

In the positive Cherry Plum state it's possible to enter deeply into the unconscious and gain insights that can then be expressed and realized. After this you're able to handle great forces spontaneously and composedly, making enormous strides in development.

In therapy settings Cherry Plum will sometimes be needed in an individual's first combination of Flowers—it reveals the fundamental fear of the personality to further open up to the developmental process. Cherry Plum sends soothing impulses that ready a person for the leap when the time comes.

Cherry Plum has often been helpful in the treatment of bed-wetting children. These children control themselves so thoroughly during the day that at night, when there is no conscious control, they freely express their internal anxieties by spontaneously passing urine.

In cases of marriage crisis, when tension builds up for days with no solution or clarifying talk in sight, Cherry Plum will help the partners open up to each other before the china plates go flying. Generally, Cherry Plum helps to bring feelings of discord into the open before they become volcanic. Cherry Plum can also be employed to cope with everyday stress situations—for instance, problems in the workplace.

This Essence is indicated for people who think about committing suicide and those who suffer from obsessions, delusions, or a threatening psychosis for which they were once institutionalized and which they fear may reoccur. Before recommending Cherry Plum to these people, however, make sure that they are also under a specialist's observation and treatment.

Some specialists have reported that Cherry Plum has provided good support in the treatment of Parkinson's disease and similar neurological problems. Finally, it can also play a supportive role in the rehabilitation of drug addicts.

Cherry Plum Key Symptoms

There may be present a fear of losing control or going crazy, a fear of rash actions, and sudden bursts of rage.

Behavior Pattern in the Blocked State

Note: People with any of the behavior patterns followed by an asterisk (*) are strongly advised to consult a specialist.

- ❀ You're afraid to talk about your feelings

- ❀ You can barely control yourself *

- ❀ You feel blocked or congested inside

- ❀ You're in turmoil and try desperately to control yourself *

- ❀ You're in such emotional chaos that you can't even express your feelings *

- ❀ You have the feeling that a time bomb is ticking away inside you *

- ❀ You're afraid of having a nervous breakdown *

- ❀ Contrary to your normal disposition, violent impulses surface; you're afraid of needing to do something you'd normally never do *

- ❀ You have sudden uncontrolled outbreaks of rage—children may throw themselves on the ground or hit their heads against the wall; grownups might destroy a malfunctioning electrical appliance in their anger, or throw things around the room *

- ❀ Parents worry that they might hit their children *

- ❀ Children are afraid of bed-wetting

- ❀ You suffer from obsessions and crazy ideas; you're afraid of "uncontrollable spiritual powers" within you *

- ❀ You're afraid of going mad, breaking down, having to go to an institution *

- ❀ You suffer from extreme inner tension and cramps, compulsive pacing, self-monitoring, or trembling *

- ❀ You toy with the idea of suicide so that finally you can be "released" *

Even if only one or two of these patterns precisely match your present situation, you need Cherry Plum.

Positive Potential

- ❀ You possess courage, strength, and composure

- ❀ You're able to deal with emotions and express them in an appropriate manner

- ❀ You're able to deeply penetrate your subconscious, integrate the insights you gain there, and use them in your daily life

- ❀ You have access to a powerful reservoir of spiritual strength

Empowering Statements

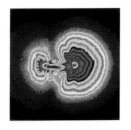

⚜ "I am courageous."

⚜ "I open myself."

⚜ "I let flow what wants to flow."

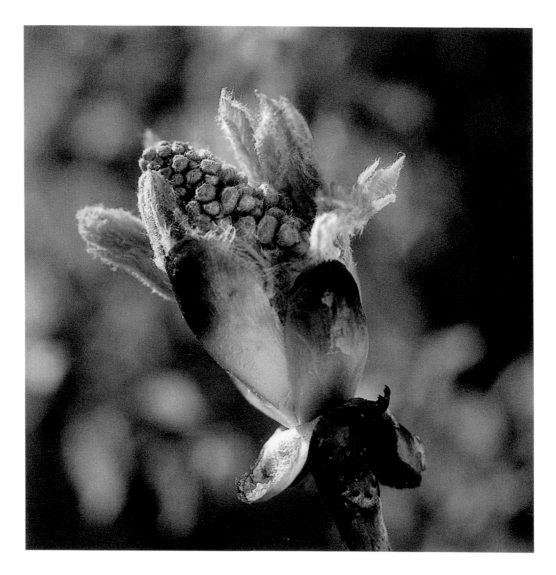

7. Chestnut Bud: The Learning Flower
From Superficiality to Experience

For those who do not take full advantage of observation and experience, and who take a longer time than others to learn the lessons of daily life.

Whereas one experience would be enough for some, such people find it necessary to have more, sometimes several, before the lesson is learnt.

Therefore, to their regret, they find themselves having to make the same error on different occasions

when once would have been enough, or observa-
tion of others could have spared them even that
one fault.

Edward Bach

Chestnut Bud relates to the Soul's potential for learning. If you're in the negative Chestnut Bud state you have a problem finding the right means to coordinate your internal world of thought with the physical reality around you. You tend to repeat the same mistakes over and over and never seem to learn from experience. A woman, for instance, will keep buying blouses in a certain shade of pink, even though she knows the color doesn't suit her and she knows that in her closet she has five almost identical blouses that she never wears. Asked why she does it, she might say, somewhat awkwardly, "Yes, it's funny really— I keep falling for this color."

Her neighbor, a bachelor who has had a long string of girlfriends, has a similar problem. The women in his life are all of the same type: assertive, outgoing, very direct. They aren't the best match for his temperate personality. "Why," his friends wonder, "doesn't he try another type?" "That's what I ask myself," he'll naively say. "All my relationships end in failure." It's a guarantee, however, that he'll flirt with the next such woman he meets.

People in the negative Chestnut Bud state hardly progress on the outside, but it's as if a rocket has been built inside them, so constantly driven are they. In their minds they're two steps ahead of reality, like an author pondering the content of his next two books while she hasn't even finished a chapter of the one she's currently working on.

The negative Chestnut Bud state can be seen in people who find it difficult to assess how they are progressing in their experiences so they can work with and profit from them in the future. On the contrary, they repeatedly throw themselves into new enterprises and ignore the ones that fail. Surprisingly, perhaps, these people aren't particularly depressed about the state of their affairs.

Chestnut Bud problems may also arise in people who are highly intelligent and can grasp information rapidly. With their thoughts racing ahead, they fail to explore the depth of the issues at hand, and in turn cannot experience the learning process.

It may happen, however, that chronic illness develops in the course of the lives of such people—migraine attacks, for instance, may always occur after the same argument on the same subject with the same person, or a duodenal ulcer will pop up like clockwork during times of exceptional stress at work. "Never mind," people in the negative Chestnut Bud state will say as they take more drugs instead of making the connection between the duodenal ulcer and their attitude toward the situation at work. The idea of consulting colleagues or family members in order to gain a better understanding of the situation is very far from their minds.

In the negative Chestnut Bud state you're like an equestrian riding a show horse up to the same fence and again and again failing to clear it because the horse refuses to jump. From the outside it looks as if the same film sequence is being repeated over and over. There is no progress in action, no development. Only if the rider got off the horse and started to reflect upon the situation would the film stop repeating. If he were to ask himself where he might change his actions, he'd be able to take the next step and the film might proceed. After he corrects the mistake, he and his horse will be able to take the hurdle with ease.

Outsiders often feel that Chestnut Bud people are trying to escape from themselves, refusing to face their past or look deeply into their life. Unable to profit from past experience, they find themselves empty-handed again and again; no foundation of solid experience has been accumulated upon which to build a future.

Such a personality assumes a childish defiance in the face of the Higher Self, refusing to be guided by it and instead behaving like a truant from the school of life. Utterly self-willed, it cuts itself off from the energy of what is actually happening. It insists on doing its own thing instead of opening up and letting itself be carried by life's greater energy.

Those in the negative Chestnut Bud state need to learn to move with the flow of life, to swim within a school of fish, so to speak, rather than swimming around anywhere in the river, or as though they had a personal aquarium all to themselves. They need to grasp that they cannot escape to the future, for the future is always the mirror of the past. The only true development is what's taking place now, right here in this moment. Nobody can escape the task of learning from experience. The past will always catch up to us, always repeat itself in new versions of the same story.

Chestnut Bud seems to be a state of very youthful energy. Its pattern is common in the young—and indeed, Chestnut Bud is frequently indicated in the treatment of children. These children characteristically appear rather absent-minded and inattentive, although not because they dwell on dreams and fantasies the way Clematis children may. They simply don't appear to be able to pay attention. Despite reminders, for instance, they'll keep forgetting to take their lunch to school. Over and over they'll make the same mistakes in spelling words and risk being held back in school by failing to keep up with their peers.

The parents may say, "My child is behind," not realizing he's operating on a different frequency and is unable to coordinate it with that of his environment. If the parents try to apply force to get the child to perform, they may achieve the opposite result—the child may appear clumsy and stop performing altogether. On the other hand, if the parents try to reach their child on his level, he'll feel accepted and develop at his own pace, making surprisingly quick progress.

Chestnut Bud helps you to better coordinate your internal thought process with the outer circumstances. Slowly but surely you learn to consider things quietly, without pressure. You'll begin to learn for the future from your own experiences and from those of others. You'll gain some perspective on yourself, enabling you to see things from others' viewpoints as well. A base will be created from which you can learn new things and enjoy life in its variety.

Chestnut Bud is an important Flower in treating learning disabilities. It also aids people who find it difficult to focus on a partner during a conversation because their thoughts race ahead, looking for solutions beyond what is being discussed.

Chestnut Bud can also be a great help and support in breaking or changing habits.

Chestnut Bud Key Symptoms

There is the tendency to repeat the same mistakes over and over. Experiences are not really digested and not enough is learned from them.

Behavior Pattern in the Blocked State

- ❂ You keep getting into the same problems—arguments with the same people, the same kind of accidents, and so on

- ❂ You're always two steps ahead of yourself in your thoughts; you are inattentive or uninterested in the problems at hand

- ❂ You prefer to start new activities rather than take some time to quietly digest past experiences

- ❂ You seem to learn very slowly from life, whether from lack of interest, inner haste, or lack of observation

- ❂ You don't draw enough from experience; you don't evaluate events in sufficient depth

- ❂ You never consider that you could learn from the experience of others

- ❂ You don't pay attention during conversations, instead planning your next question while your partner speaks

- ❂ When you solve a problem in your imagination, you lose interest in implementing the solution, or may do it superficially

- ❂ When a machine isn't working (such as a fax machine), you tend to simply push buttons instead of consulting the manual

- ❂ You seem to be careless or naive

- ❂ You appear mentally clumsy and are slow to show any progress

- ❂ You have learning disabilities, blocks, or delayed development

- ❂ Chronic physical illness—perhaps migraine, acne, or some more acute problems—may also belong to this pattern

Even if only one or two of these patterns precisely match your present situation, you need Chestnut Bud.

Positive Potential

⚘ You're mentally dexterous and enjoy learning

⚘ You're always interested in learning more and are able to make the time and peace you need to do so

⚘ You regularly observe your own behavior patterns and reactions in daily life

⚘ You learn by observing the experiences of others

⚘ You're able to comprehend complex situations more quickly; you foresee possible mistakes early on

⚘ You make the best use of your daily experience for ongoing development

Empowering Statements

⚘ "I am paying attention."

⚘ "I listen carefully."

⚘ "I am learning."

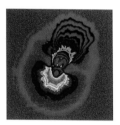

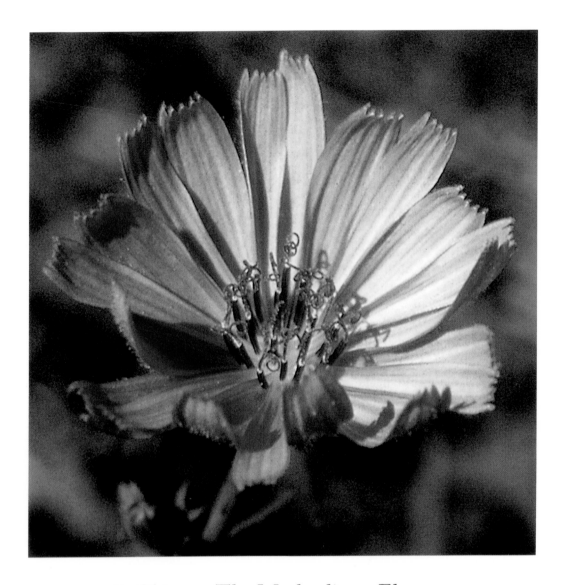

8. Chicory: The Motherliness Flower
From Demanding Love to Giving Love Freely

Those who are very mindful of the needs of others they tend to be over-full of care for children, relatives, friends, always finding something that should be put right. They are continually correcting what they consider wrong, and enjoy doing so. They desire that those for whom they care should be near them.

Edward Bach

Chicory relates to the Soul's potential for motherly and unselfish love. In the negative Chicory state, these qualities become distorted and self-centered.

The negative Chicory state often begins in childhood. Following is an example of a typical behavior pattern: At a party in her home, nine-year-old Jenny is answering the door for her parents. She looks sweet, with long curls and her first long dress, and her behavior is charming. Jenny basks in the attention she receives from the guests, acting like a gracious young film star. Gradually, however, the guests begin to discuss more adult topics, which doesn't seem to suit Jenny. Pretending to be collecting empty glasses, she moves playfully from group to group, trying to join in conversation. When midnight arrives and her mother tells her it's time she went to bed, Jenny replies smartly, "Not now, Mom—Uncle Pete just started to tell me something important about school." Her mother doesn't give in and Jenny starts to cry, once again attracting general attention.

While in the cradle infants, of course, demand attention and cry when left alone. As they grow older, however, and find that tears no longer get them what they want, they resort to new strategies. They may flatter, become overeager to help, become sick, or even use minor blackmail: "I'll do my homework, but only if I don't have to go to gymnastics tomorrow."

The negative Chicory state is very noticeable and everybody around is affected. It occurs in both sexes and at all ages. It focuses above all on gaining influence; making demands; or refusing to let go of ideas, things, and feelings. If you were to observe a couple of famous tenors at a reception, for instance, you might notice that they greet each other with much friendly and professional fanfare. At the same time, however, you might sense their lurking egos as each wonders whether the other will be clever enough to get more attention. This scenario demonstrates a typical negative Chicory sentiment.

All of us experience negative Chicory states now and then—for instance, when thinking, "I gave him a book for his birthday and all I get in return is a card" or "I've listened to her troubles on the telephone for hours and what do I get when I need a sounding board?"

People in the negative Chicory state expect a great deal of others. When they knock on the door, you tend to know already what they might want. One classic example is the "supermother" who holds on to her children with invisible tentacles, sometimes suffocating or traumatizing the weaker-willed ones. She is constantly concerned with the affairs of her family and her large circle of friends, always wanting to be part of their activities in whatever way she can. She organizes, criticizes, marshals, and directs, and she will always find something to put right, to suggest, or to find fault with. Her motto is: "I'm only telling you because I want to help."

Such behavior can also be observed among men. People influenced by Chicory display a kind of pride of ownership concerning the emotions and the lives of those close to them. A father in the negative Chicory state may be incredibly helpful, pushing his good deeds onto everybody, but he will react angrily if his involvement is not accepted with gratitude. Both fathers and mothers in the negative Chicory behavior pattern will be at ease only in the company of their loved ones. Grown children are expected to spend holidays at home, even when this accommodation requires them to make long trips. Should they try to suggest an alternative, such parents will keep calling and maneuvering until the children agree to show up.

Not every child finds it easy to free himself from such possessive parental love. Some sons, for instance, remain under such a mother's thumb for years, failing to achieve important stages in the development of their own marriages or relationships. When a child finally does find the strength to free himself, the negative Chicory mother or father will clearly voice disappointment, colored distinctly with self-pity: "How can you do this to me after everything I've done for you?"

In the business world Chicory states might be observed among salespeople dreaming up better tricks to outdo their competition, and among lawyers looking for strategies to make the other party behave to the advantage of their clients.

People in the negative Chicory state apparently have it all, but the reality is quite the contrary. Behind every negative Chicory state lies a deep lack of fulfillment, an internal emptiness, often a feeling of never having been properly loved. It's not uncommon for such people to have had childhoods without the experience of true love. They were expected early on to perform tasks far beyond what their peers had to shoulder. For instance, if one parent died prematurely, the eldest child might have been expected to assume responsibility for younger siblings, leading to the loss of much age-appropriate experience for this child as she struggled to master tasks and behaviors beyond her years. If too much was demanded of her, and too little appreciation was received, a negative Chicory state was the result.

Some describe the negative Chicory state as a black hole or a bottomless pit that constantly has to be filled with affection, recognition, and assurance. You will use the whole of your powerful will and manipulative skill to meet this need. At the same time, because of this inner sense of emptiness you are unable to give or receive love and there is a constant fear of loss. The few emotions and feelings that do emerge are then "invested" carefully: "I love you, on the condition that . . ." An English Bach practitioner aptly described the negative Chicory state as "the needy mother."

Chicory people have the potential for great inner strength and possess a true ability to love. This can be brought to life if they are prepared to acknowledge that the black hole can only be filled from the fountain of love welling up in their own hearts. As soon as the call of the Higher Self is heard and activity is selflessly devoted to the service of others and the greater whole, the spiritual fountain will begin to flow, and tremendous power and security will arise within. Affection and love will no longer have to be gained by force; they will come of their own accord. Nor will it be necessary any longer to fear the loss of affection, for the inner fountain fed by universal love never ceases to flow.

Bach himself compared the positive Chicory state with the archetype of the "universal mother," the motherly Soul potential that lies latent in every human being, both man and woman. If this hypothesis is carried further, it may be said that many people today experience the negative Chicory because too many facets of the archetypal feminine energy have been suppressed—especially in the West. In addition, while people's attention is focused on those aspects of the feminine that are considered most acceptable—the concept of the virginal woman, for instance—the creative side of womanhood still lacks sufficient recognized outlets. Another theory suggests that people who have lived under the influence of a "mother church" that has required obedience may be particularly destined for negative Chicory states.

In the positive Chicory state your great maternal energy can be fully expressed as you actively pursue your goals, drawing on rich resources, giving selflessly, and expecting nothing in return, not even in your heart. You're truly dedicated to the interests of others. You spread wings of warmth, kindness, and security, providing shelter for others.

In psychological practice Chicory problems often arise in connection with mothers. They can manifest physically in the form of blockages in the lower part of the body, or in heart problems or types of emotional poisoning. It was not without reason that the ancient Egyptians called Chicory "the liver's friend." Psychological practice also indicates that both parties affected in a Chicory-related conflict need to be treated because the behavior pattern created is one of dependency.

Chicory Key Symptoms

These are characterized by a possessive attitude, tendency to interfere and manipulate, and a feeling of receiving insufficient love and appreciation.

Behavior Pattern in the Blocked State

❁ You are emotionally demanding; you immediately try to build intense, close relationships

❁ Like a mother hen you watch over the needs, wishes, and progress of family and friends

❁ You're always ready to comment to, correct, or advise others

❁ You're overly caring and subtly controlling, which makes others dependent without them even being aware of it

❁ You make yourself indispensable

❁ You force your good deeds onto others

- You do few things without calculating your own potential rewards

- You expect gratitude for doing things for others even if you weren't asked to help

- You give conditional love: "I'll love you, if . . ."

- You try to fulfill your desires indirectly

- You manipulate or play the diplomat, cleverly managing to impose your own will or retain influence

- You use emotional blackmail

- You want to hold on to relationship roles or rituals that have had their day—for instance, you try to make your partner guilty for not saying "I love you" as often as when your relationship began; parents may still regularly perform chores for children who have long since moved out on their own

- You find it hard to forgive and forget

- You fear losing your friends, relationships, or possessions

- You feel easily offended, passed over, or hurt

- You react with self-pity if you don't get what you expect

- You may escape into illness to gain sympathy from others or influence over them

- The ingratitude of others can cause you to break into tears

- You speak about what others owe you

Even if only one or two of these patterns precisely match your present situation, you need Chicory.

Positive Potential

- You give without expecting anything in return

- You respect that everyone has to follow his or her own Life Plan

- You deal with your own emotional needs and keep an appropriate distance from others

- You know your personal needs and take care of them yourself

- You draw on your inner fullness and are able to care for others with true love and devotion

- You express the energy of the "great mother"

Empowering Statements

- "I give freely."

- "I am drawing from the well."

- "I am loved."

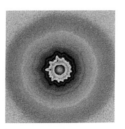

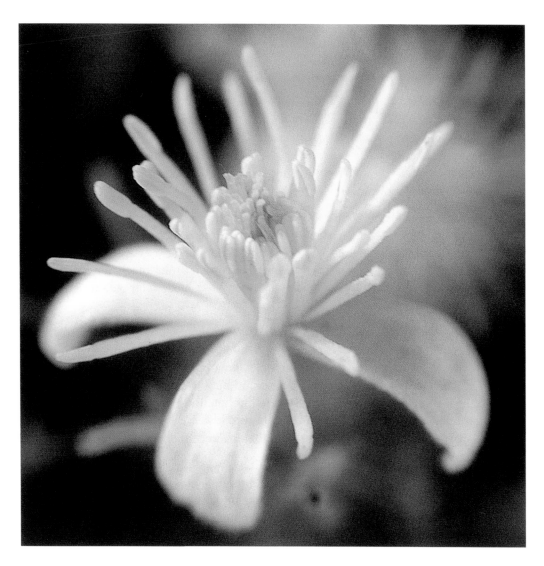

9. Clematis: The Reality Flower
From Escaping Reality to Living in Reality

Those who are dreamy, drowsy, not fully awake, no great interest in life. Quiet people, not really happy in their present circumstances, living more in the future than in the present; living in hopes of happier times, when their ideals may come true. In illness some make little or no effort to get well, and in certain cases may even look forward to death, in the hope of better times; or maybe, meeting again some beloved one whom they have lost.

Edward Bach

Clematis relates to the Soul's potential for inspired creativity. In the negative Clematis state the personality tries to take part as little as possible in real-life activities, and instead lives in a world of rich imagination withdrawn from reality.

Your neighbor's little daughter, whom you meet on the sidewalk every so often, looks at you with dreamy, faraway eyes that show no recognition of you; or, a nine-year-old is physically present at lunch, but in his thoughts he's traveling through space as commander of a spaceship —both exhibit Clematis traits. The well-known artist next door who's enormously creative but a little helpless in everyday life is also a Clematis person. "Really? You don't say!" This is the kind of reaction often absently uttered by Clematis people—because their thoughts are somewhere else entirely, they aren't really interested in what anyone wants to tell them. It's as though they are newborns who don't know that they must open their eyes and instead want to go on dwelling in their embryonic water world.

People in the negative Clematis state are wanderers between the worlds. Reality doesn't hold much attraction for them; whenever possible they'll withdraw from the bothersome present to their castles in the air. When things seem to be getting unpleasant, or even difficult, they'll often make highly unrealistic suggestions for the solution of problems or, to the horror of the people around them, give themselves up to idealistic illusions.

In the negative Clematis state the personality apparently attaches little importance to physical reality. If you're much in need of Clematis, you'll frequently lack physical energy. You may have a fairly high threshold for pain, but you tend to suffer from cold hands and feet. Your head sometimes feels completely empty. Your memory can be weak, and details in particular are recalled only with difficulty. You'll dash for the kitchen, bump into the doorpost because of poor body orientation, and once there no longer remember what it was you wanted.

Much preferring to watch your own "movies" playing at your internal theater to taking a part on the great stage of the real world, sooner or later a Clematis person in the negative state may develop visual or hearing problems. Your dreaminess might also tend to lead you to traffic accidents. People in the negative Clematis state prefer to sleep deeply, for long periods of time. Sometimes they may inadvertently or deliberately fall asleep while watching television, attending a lecture, or sitting through a sermon. Their active inner life doesn't leave much concentration for the external subjects at hand. Clematis people in the negative behavioral state nearly always seem a bit drowsy and are seldom fully awake.

With most of their emotional energy being used internally, Clematis people show little aggression or anxiety. They often receive good news with the same irritating indifference as news of devastating events.

When Clematis people get sick, physicians really have their work cut out for them. Clematis people's instinct for self-preservation is weak and so is their desire to get well. It may seem that Clematis patients have no great objection to departing from this earth, perhaps wishing to be united again with someone they love. Edward Bach called the negative Clematis state a polite form of suicide. The romantic longing-for-death movement toward the end of the nineteenth century was a perfect example of the negative Clematis state.

Clematis people often prove to have great creative potential. Therefore they often have occupations where dreams are made real, such as in the fashion trade, film industry, and print media. If their creative potential cannot be brought to realization, a negative Clematis state will almost automatically arise, with creative energy then taking such forms as exaggerated romanticism, eccentricity, and all kinds of delusions.

Many people in the negative Clematis state like to express hopes for a future in which true human ideals have been realized at last and the golden era has begun. They've failed to see that the future is always shaped in the present, and that according to higher principles, every hand, head, and heart is planned for and needed; those who simply refuse to participate, waiting for a certain moment to come, not only harm the greater whole but also have misunderstood the intention of their own Souls and the meaning of their lives on earth.

The real life of the personality will become more interesting and fulfilled on a daily basis when it finally opens up to its true purpose and is ready to live in the here and now.

Positive Clematis energy shows itself in people who apply their fertile imagination very specifically in the material world. Their surroundings are enriched due to the beauty and sensitivity of their thoughts and actions, through their work as artists, for example, or as therapists.

Clematis Essence may be used as a long-term remedy. It can also be helpful as a short-term remedy in cases of passing mental or physical trauma accompanied by a feeling of dizziness and an out-of-body sensation.

Typical Clematis people are even less likely than the average person to tolerate psychotropic drugs, recreational drugs, or sleep deprivation.

Together with other flowers, Clematis has helped married couples conceive children when there was no organic reason for their childlessness. It has also helped drivers who frequently get lost or can never remember where they left their keys.

Clematis Key Symptoms

These include daydreaming, always being somewhere else with your thoughts, and giving little attention to what's going on around you.

Behavior Pattern in the Blocked State

❀ You are lost in thought, absentminded, or rarely fully present

- You are inattentive and scatterbrained—a daydreamer

- You have little interest in the present situation and live more in your own fantasy world

- You're a "wanderer between the worlds"; often you don't feel at home in reality

- You're constantly searching for misplaced articles

- You easily lose your way

- You have trouble keeping order in your workspace; your surroundings often look chaotic

- You escape into unrealistic and illusory speculations when facing problems

- You have a far-off gaze and dreamy eyes

- You appear lost in dreams, never entirely awake, or a bit confused

- You react with the same indifference to good news and bad

- You have hardly any aggression or fear because you're not really here

- You lack vitality and often appear remarkably pale

- You often have cold hands and feet, or an empty feeling in your head

- You experience floating sensations; sometimes you feel dopey, as though lightly anesthetized

- You need a lot of sleep—you like to doze and may nod off at odd moments

- You tend to faint easily

- Sometimes you romanticize dying, though without any active suicidal intentions

- You have little sense of pain, are often out of touch with your body, and tend to bump into things

- You have a poor memory, especially for details, and don't take the trouble to listen carefully

- You are liable to develop visual or hearing problems, your eyes and ears being more attuned to the inside than the outside

- You have little motivation to get well quickly when ill; your instinct for self-preservation is weak

- You frequently tell little white lies without even realizing it

- You are sometimes unable to differentiate between fantasy and reality and can make up lies about life that you eventually believe

- When asked simple concrete questions, you invent full-blown stories (*pseudologia phantastica*)

⊗ Your creative talents often go untapped; despite artistic gifts, you end up taking pedestrian jobs just to earn a living.

Even if only one or two of these patterns precisely match your present situation, you need Clematis.

Positive Potential

⊗ You have realistic perceptions and a concrete perspective on life; you concentrate on things that can be done

⊗ You're able to dream up visions and put them into action

⊗ Your creative lifestyle enriches your daily routines to make them interesting

⊗ You're purposeful in bringing creativity to physical realization

⊗ You have excellent perception of shape, color, sound, and aroma

Empowering Statements

⊗ "I am awake."

⊗ "I see clearly."

⊗ "I create."

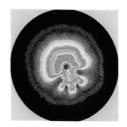

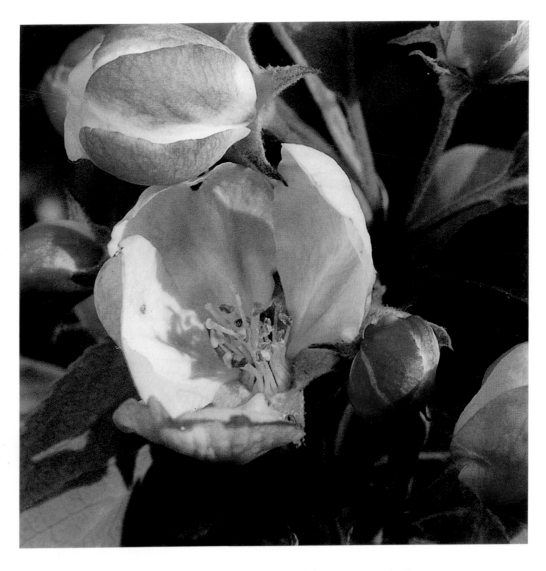

10. Crab Apple—The Cleansing Flower
From Compulsive Order to Inner Order

This is the remedy of cleansing.

For those who feel as if they had something not quite clean about themselves.

Often it is something of apparently little importance; in others there may be more serious disease which is almost disregarded compared to the one thing on which they concentrate.

In both types they are anxious to be free from the one particular thing which is greatest in their minds and which seems so essential to them that it should be cured.

They become despondent if treatment fails.

Being a cleanser, this remedy purifies wounds if the patient has reason to believe that some poison has entered which must be drawn out.

Edward Bach

Crab Apple relates to the Soul's potential for order, purity, and perfection. People can get into a negative Crab Apple state when they have very definite ideas that the world around them, their bodies, and their inner lives need to be flawless.

Anything that doesn't hold up to this ideal of personal purity will confuse and burden them. It can make them sad, sometimes desperate, and in the extreme case fill them with self-disgust. An uninvited negative thought, a sharp remark that slipped out against their real nature, or a single harmless blemish on their face may cause a great deal of upset. If the wallpaper in a newly decorated room is an inch too short in one corner, they may be able to think of nothing but rushing out to buy another roll of paper to finish the job perfectly. Whatever the flaw may be, it's usually relatively minor compared with the mental energy expended on it.

A typical negative Crap Apple trait is a need for the workplace to be tidy and clean before a new task can be started. In the extreme, the measures taken equal surgical procedures in a hospital.

In the negative Crab Apple state you err by taking the wrong perspective. Small parts of real life are placed under the magnifying glass of your own limited mental concepts. You get stuck and lost in detail, and eventually no longer see the forest for the trees. If you were able to look at things from a different angle, letting your Higher Self open the view to higher principles of order, you'd automatically step back, see things in their right perspective, and soon be at peace again.

Yet this is easier said than done with people in need of Crab Apple. They tend to be unusually sensitive, taking in much more, at subtler levels, than their general constitution allows them to cope with. This unconscious stress often gives them the feeling of being unclean, constipated, or in need of cleansing. If they have not been introduced to other means of purification besides the purely physical, they'll try to get rid of these things by physical means. This may take the form of constant hand-washing or showering. Negative-state Crab Apple people may refuse to kiss unless they first use a mouth spray. They often have a poor body image and the relationship with their own physical body is disturbed.

People who need Crab Apple are often so sensitive that a tiny detail will make a huge impression and they will spend all their energy dealing with it until no reserves remain for the interpretation of these actions or to see them in a greater context. Housewives who have the cleaning bug often have a Crab Apple type of problem. Their children's wet feet worry them primarily because of the marks they leave behind on the new carpet. The more important issue, that wet feet could play a part in a child's cold or flu, only comes to her mind once the stains have been removed.

Their great inner desire for purity will cause those in a negative Crab Apple state to be unusually nervous about insects, bacteria, food that may have gone bad, and all kinds of infection risks. The moment the newspapers report a flu epidemic, Crab Apple characters will take every possible precaution to avoid contracting the disease. This behavior is not as unreasonable as it may seem to others, since Crab Apple people appear to have a special capacity for attracting impurities and "dark" energies from their environment. Some of them are able to heal and transform such dark forces when in the positive Crab Apple state. A Bach practitioner has aptly called these people "spiritual vacuum cleaners." An extreme example of the positive Crab Apple state can be seen in a famous yoga master. In his group exercises he can absorb the blocked energies of 150 or more people and transform them like a filter before letting them flow back to the group fresh and clean.

Such unusual positive Crab Apple energy may be expressed in only a very few people, yet some faint glow of this phenomenon is experienced by everybody in the positive Crab Apple state. They will realize that external disharmony is ultimately always just a reflection of an internal imbalance—therefore it's preferable to begin cleaning up inside before establishing order outside. They come to understand that perfect harmony is hardly possible in real life. Everything is constantly changing, on the move, flowing.

Crab Apple Essence will dissolve feelings of being soiled. Its effects are double because purification can be achieved at both the psychological and the physical level. For this reason Crab Apple is used together with other Bach Flowers in the treatment of skin impurities of all kinds. It is one of the ingredients in Rescue Remedy Creme. Some practitioners recommend Crab Apple be used when fasting or to overcome the effects of a hangover more quickly. Some prescribe Crab Apple for an incipient cold, or to help ease the side effects of powerful drug treatments such as antibiotics, anesthetics, and chemotherapy. It is also recommended for people who spend a large part of their day among many other people who are sick or burdened. After a day of work these people may feel as if they've been living in a "sticky" atmosphere. Crab Apple Essence in a glass of water will help purify their energy fields from what they've picked up from others.

Crab Apple is also used successfully in combination with Rescue Remedy to treat pest-infested or transplanted plants.

Crab Apple Key Symptoms
You feel unclean inside and out; you get stuck on trivialities and have an exaggerated need for order.

Behavior Patterns in the Blocked State

- ⚙ You overemphasize the principle of purity on all levels

- ⚙ You are very aware of your mental and emotional hygiene

- ⚙ You feel self-disgust when you do something that doesn't live up to your own standards of purity and order

- ⚙ You feel you need to cleanse yourself of impure thoughts

- ⚙ You feel sinful, stained, and dirty

- ⚙ You're mired in details, allowing yourself to be tyrannized by minor things and losing sight of the big picture

- ⚙ You find it difficult to let things be when they aren't perfect

- ⚙ You're unable to start working unless everything is in perfect order

- ⚙ You become very irritated when life's circumstances are disorganized

- ⚙ You're a perfect housekeeper—everything always has to be neat as a pin; thus your surroundings appear somewhat sterile

- ⚙ You complain about both personal and public uncleanliness

- ⚙ You have problems with very earthy, physical actions such as breast-feeding and kissing

- ⚙ You're disgusted by your own skin eruptions, sweaty feet, pimples, warts, and so forth

- ⚙ You have an intense, even phobic response to all forms of dust, insects, bacteria, and the like

- ⚙ You have a greater than normal need to clear your throat, blow your nose, pass gas, and so on

- ⚙ You feel a great need to clean yourself, even to the point of compulsive washing

- ⚙ You fear spoiled food, dirty toilets, incorrect prescriptions, environmental pollution, and so on

- ⚙ You take too seriously the symptoms of illness and want to rid yourself of even minor signs of sickness without delay; when the treatment doesn't show the desired effect immediately, you become overly concerned

- ⚙ Parents raise their children with exaggerated requirements for cleanliness

Even if only one or two of these patterns precisely match your present situation, you need Crab Apple.

Positive Potential

⊛ You know that order cannot be permanent, that it is only a temporary state

⊛ You create order and care for things inside and outside

⊛ You have a sense of the overall picture and you see details in their proper perspective

⊛ You have a sense for higher systems of order and how everything fits together

Empowering Statements

⊛ "I feel good."

⊛ "I accept myself as I am."

⊛ "I see what's really important."

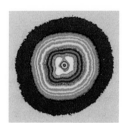

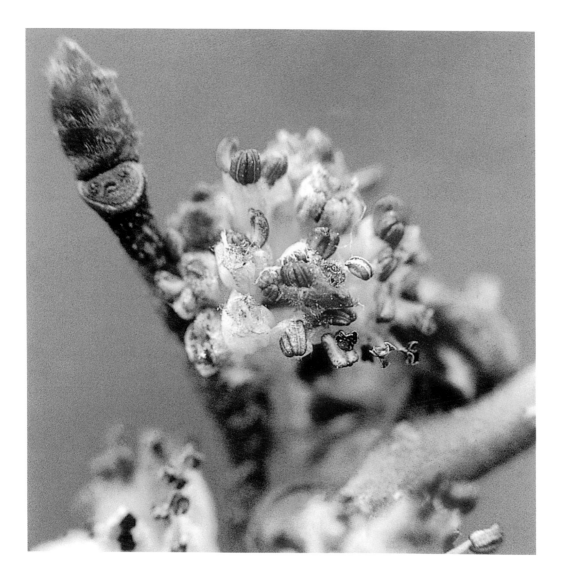

11. Elm: The Responsibility Flower
From Self-Worth Crisis to Inner Confidence

Those who are doing good work, are following the calling of their life and who hope to do something of importance, and this often for the benefit of humanity.

At times there may be periods of depression when they feel that the task they have undertaken is too difficult, and not within the power of a human being.

Edward Bach

Elm relates to the Soul's potential for responsibility. Its negative form is revealed as weak moments in the lives of the strong, at times when people of above-average ability and responsibility suddenly become so exhausted that they no longer feel up to their task.

The successful owner of a factory employing many people may suddenly feel afraid that she's unable to make a simple business decision, which could have harmful consequences for the whole workforce. The much admired mother who usually splendidly manages her large brood may suddenly feel she won't be able to cope with her youngest daughter's sweet sixteen party. While packing his suitcase for his first term away, a talented student who has received a college scholarship might become convinced that the academic challenge ahead is too big to manage, despite his extensive preparation. A capable mayor no longer feels able to sort out internal party squabbles and considers resigning her office, although she knows that the consequences for her town would be disastrous.

The negative Elm state is always only temporary. The person involved is under too much stress to handle a problem that she perceives in a distorted way. The people around this person then become nervous because their much admired and normally unshakable hero suddenly appears small and weak.

People who tend to experience the negative Elm state usually enjoy working hard and are often inherently altruistic. In the workplace they're predestined for positions of responsibility, which they normally have the strength to cope with. But—particularly these days—this often means that more and more responsibility is placed on their shoulders.

People with negative Elm behavior fully identify with their task, to the great benefit of everyone else. They do, however, sometimes forget that they too are only human with particular personal needs and physical limits. Sudden exhaustion and crises of the negative Elm state frequently occur when increasing professional pressure coincides with a normal, constitutionally determined passive physical phase—for instance, the onset of menopause or a negative biorhythm phase. At some time or other even the most powerful motivation will no longer be enough, and the body will demand its due. The weakness then causes a temporary breakdown in self-esteem.

The problem that defines these moments is that the person is identifying too strongly with the current role of the personality. The Higher Self is calling for moderation but the thinking self is not inclined to follow this guidance. It has forgotten that everybody's first responsibility is to fulfill his own personal needs in order to meet the demands of his Inner Guidance, and only after this to fulfill the expectations or needs of others.

The weak moments of Elm types may thus be regarded as warnings to them not to let themselves be carried away by the personality's performance standards. The link to the Higher Self must not be weakened by the workload. Human beings are able to stretch the limits of their capacities but cannot transcend their physical limits as long as they are in a physical body.

In England, Elm has been aptly called "psychological smelling salts." It will support the strong in moments of weakness. It will rouse them from their dream of impotent inadequacy, making sure they firmly plant both feet back on the ground of reality. It provides vision clear enough to see problems in the proper perspective and to be aware of personal capabilities. Those in the negative Elm state regain hold of themselves and grow confident that they will succeed again, either on their own or with the help that will arrive at the right time from an appropriate source.

What is the psychological key to the development of the Elm pattern? As children these people often get plenty of positive feedback for what they've done. On top of this, they place greater pressures on themselves and their own performance. In an attempt to fulfill and not disappoint the expectations of others around them, they take on too many responsibilities and realize too late that their energy reserves are already exhausted.

Elm Key Symptoms

There is a sense of being overwhelmed by responsibilities; there are temporary feelings of inadequacy.

Behavior Pattern in the Blocked State

❀ You suddenly feel overwhelmed by a task

❀ You're brought to a sudden halt by the one minor task that is "the straw that breaks the camel's back"

❀ You feel that your responsibilities are getting to be too much

❀ You feel you don't have the stamina to accomplish everything you want or need to

❀ Although normally strong and self-confident, you're temporarily exhausted and despondent

❀ You experience passing feelings of inadequacy due to exhaustion

❀ You temporarily doubt if you're really cut out for what you're doing

❀ You can't decide what to tackle first; you waste a great deal of time trying to do everything yourself instead of delegating responsibilities

❀ You've maneuvered yourself into a place where you've become indispensable and now believe it's impossible to let go of any responsibility

❀ You're afraid to stay in bed with the flu because you don't want to let down the people at work

> **Even if only one or two of these patterns precisely match your present situation, you need Elm.**

Positive Potential

❀ You're capable, responsible, and confident

❀ You know how much work you can handle and know when to delegate

❀ You're confident that if you do your best, help will arrive when you need it

❀ You take responsibility for your own needs

Empowering Statements

❀ "I do what I can."

❀ "I receive help."

❀ "I make it."

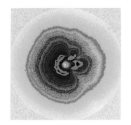

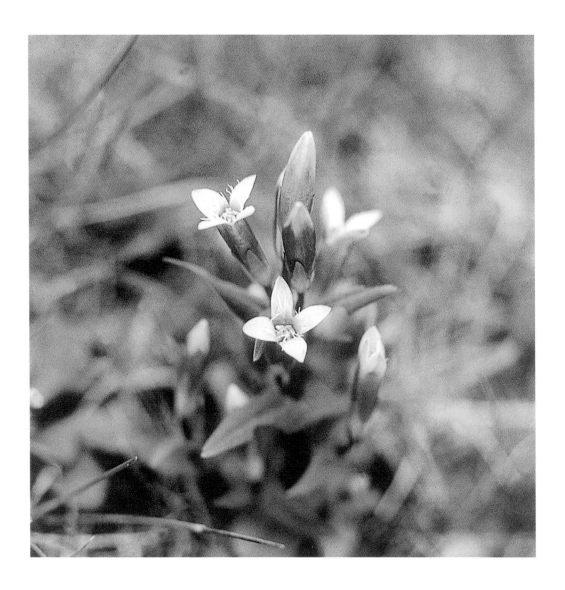

12. Gentian: The Belief Flower
From Doubt to Trust

Those who are easily discouraged. They may be progressing well in illness or in the affairs of their daily life, but any small delay or hindrance to progress causes doubt and soon disheartens them.

Edward Bach

Gentian is the Bach Flower that is connected with the Soul's potential for trust and faith, though the term *faith* should not be interpreted only in the religious sense. It can also be trust and belief in the positive in life, in the existence of Inner Guidance and a higher order, or in your own inner strength.

A small child who doesn't receive proper backing and support when learning to walk because his parents merely comment on the times he falls instead of encouraging him in the next attempt is experiencing the foundation for a negative Gentian state.

If you're in need of Gentian, you'd very much like to believe in a positive outcome, but you're just not able to do so. You always see a glass that's half empty, not half full. What is the error behind this interpretation? You unconsciously refuse to be guided by your Higher Self and you don't see yourself as part of the greater whole. Your perceptions are restricted by your own limited personality cutting you off from the "inner well" that is the only source of faith. You think you need to grasp everything by intellect alone. You analyze, brood over, and question, and this ceaseless mental activity often leaves you with a depressed view of things.

Unfortunately, in the Gentian state you don't understand that with such doubtful expectations, events can't help but take a doubtful course. This pattern causes harm not only to yourself but also to the larger whole, a concept that is even more difficult for you to grasp.

The eternal pessimist taking a certain satisfaction in how badly things are going for him and the world, the persistent doubting Thomas, who doesn't feel comfortable unless he has something to worry about—these are representatives of the extreme negative Gentian state.

As a temporary state, Gentian often takes the form of discouragement or lack of faith—for example, during convalescence. When you've made good progress but suddenly have a relapse, your world collapses and you think your illness will start all over again.

Typically, even for a therapist, you'll also harbor doubt in a corner of your heart as to the efficacy of Bach Flower Remedies, even when you experience their effectiveness.

Gentian is very helpful in cases of depressed feelings evoked by a specific incident. Examples are the death of a marriage partner, loss of a long-term job, divorce (especially as it affects children), and relocation to a nursing home.

Psychologically, the negative Gentian state may be seen as a kind of weakness of faith in which the mental process falls into a negative rut. A healthy skepticism turns into a compulsive need to question everything. People struggling with philosophical issues and those fighting for religious faith are in the negative Gentian state. "O Lord, help thou my disbelief!"—this prayer of a Christian mystic aptly describes the negative Gentian state.

Gentian Essence helps strengthen faith—not blind faith, but the conviction of a positive skeptic. If with the help of Gentian you've been re-connected with your Higher Self, you'll be able to face difficulties without falling into pessimism. You'll be able to live with conflict, realizing, at least unconsciously, that for the purpose of the greater whole, conflicts have a necessary, energizing function. You'll no longer despair upon meeting obstacles, because you can recognize them as catalysts for something better to come.

In practice Gentian has proved very useful for children who have become nervous and discouraged over minor setbacks in class and, as a result, don't want to go back to school or take another test. Above all, however, Gentian has been shown to be effective with those who couldn't get help through psychotherapy. It is also a helpful tool in a crisis between marital partners if they're too skeptical to give their relationship another try.

Gentian Key Symptoms

You are easily discouraged, skeptical, doubting, and pessimistic.

Behavior Pattern in the Blocked State

- ❀ Even small setbacks have a devastating effect
- ❀ You're easily discouraged and simply give up when you meet unexpected difficulties
- ❀ Disappointments cause feelings of dejection and depression
- ❀ You react quickly with skepticism so you won't be disappointed later
- ❀ In every new situation you're the member of the group who'll doubt the positive outcome, who'll play the doubting Thomas
- ❀ Sometimes you almost appear to enjoy your pessimism
- ❀ Your lack of faith makes you insecure
- ❀ You need plenty of positive feedback and encouragement, even during times of minor crisis
- ❀ Even in a situation where things turn out all right, you imagine what could have gone wrong
- ❀ You don't understand that the reason for some misfortunes may be your own lack of confidence

Even if only one or two of these patterns precisely match your present situation, you need Gentian.

Positive Potential

- ❀ You understand that resistance and setbacks are learning steps, and you make new attempts with confidence
- ❀ You have unshakable faith; despite difficult circumstances you know that everything will happen as it's meant to be

- You know there are solutions for all problems

- You're able to encourage and build confidence in other people

Empowering Statements

- "I am confident."

- "I expect the positive."

- "I know everything works out right."

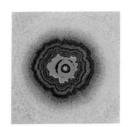

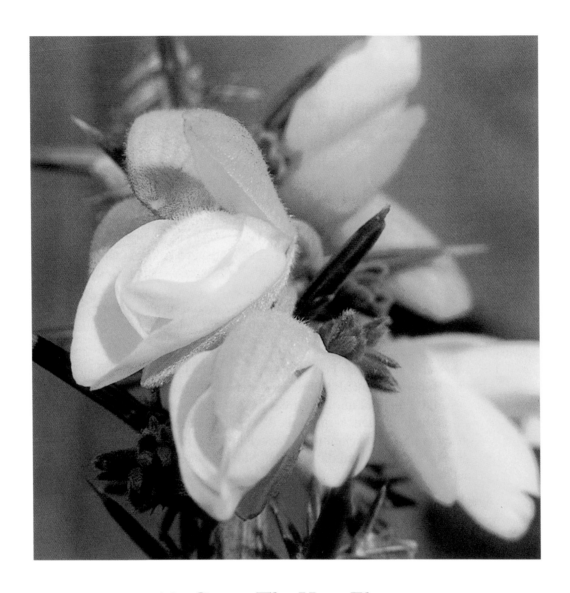

13. Gorse: *The Hope Flower*
From Giving Up to Going Forth

Very great hopelessness, they have given up belief that more can be done for them.

Under persuasion or to please others they may try different treatments, at the same time assuring those around that there is so little hope of relief.

Edward Bach

Gorse embodies the Soul quality of hope. If you're in the negative Gorse state, you have sunk within yourself, have let go of your aspirations, have become resigned, and have given up hope. One example might be a person who has been without work for three years, has had more than fifty interviews, and still has no job prospects. Another might be an individual who has courageously but futilely fought to rid herself of debt and has no ideas what to do next.

Many people in the negative Gorse state are suffering from chronic diseases. They've tried many treatments without success, and their doctors have made it clear to them that they will probably never be wholly well again. In their minds they now have come to the end of the road and thus want to give up. For the sake of their families they may try this or that additional treatment, but in their hearts they have long since become convinced that it will be of no use.

This psychological state is dangerous for two reasons. First, the patient's negative expectations will continue to reinforce the illness, thus anchoring it more firmly in the body, and the symptoms will only get worse. Second, passive resistance by the personality blocks off positive impulses from the Higher Self. People in the negative Gorse state have allowed themselves to drop out of active life. They sometimes look like they've been living in a basement and haven't seen the sun for a long time. Their faces are yellowish or waxy pale, and their eyes have dark shadows. A sensitive woman once described her negative Gorse state as one in which there seemed to be a thick piece of glass between her and her Inner Guidance; she was able to see it but not hear it.

The unconscious error again lies in the personality's refusal to acknowledge and accept the guidance of the Higher Self. Instead of leaving the responsibility for everything to the Higher Self and faithfully going along with the process, the personality stagnates in hopelessness. You're unable to imagine alternative solutions and resign from further attempts. Because you can't imagine other possibilities you never consider that things might have a meaning or that there could be something positive in all negative situations.

Like children, many Gorse patients expect that by some outside miracle everything will turn out right after all, instead of realizing that recovery can, in the end, come only from inside. People in the negative Gorse state must learn to recognize their long unused developmental possibilities, pull themselves up, and seize their opportunities.

Very often the negative Gorse state does not appear in the extreme form described above. Sometimes the whole process takes place on a psychological level without physical involvement. People who in a more subtle negative state will say things like, "I've tried everything, but . . ." In this case, taking Gorse will mark a significant turning point, with the person entering a new cycle of development.

Many people who are afflicted with the negative Gorse state grew up in circumstances of great psychological limitation. There may have been economic difficulties, a long-lasting illness in childhood, or a parent or sibling suffering from psychological or physical disabilities. Gorse can be given as a supportive measure to everyone involved in such difficult circumstances.

Some people begin to understand or just have a sense that it's the experience of suffering that constitutes the driving force behind change and bears the additional benefit of strengthening the character. Those who become aware of this principle or unconsciously understand and embrace it experience a sudden shift so that their inner psychological orientation becomes positive.

In the positive Gorse state you gather new strength and hope from deep inside, ready to actively take part again in your own destiny. This does not mean that you expect the impossible; you know that certain circumstances cannot be changed, but you'll firmly hope that everything will come together in a positive way. And so you move on, despite all that besets you. You learn to bear your sufferings without complaint, having realized that often profound learning comes from trials and painful experience. In the early stages of chronic disease, this profound inner change is often the initial spark that will set the process of real healing into motion.

Gorse Key Symptoms

Among these are hopelessness, resignation, and an "Oh, what's the use?" attitude.

Behavior Pattern in the Blocked State

✿ You're unable to imagine a change for the better

✿ You don't dare hope for a change in circumstances

✿ You're resigned; you're tired inside

✿ You no longer have the energy to give it another try

✿ You don't recognize any further possibilities; you've given up inside

✿ You say you've come to terms with a prolonged chronic illness

✿ You allow relatives to persuade you to try other treatments against your own inner conviction, and are again resigned with the least setback

✿ You've given up fighting for your destiny; stagnation has taken hold deep inside

✿ As a child you had to overcome an extended or chronic illness

✿ You grew up with a chronically sick person, someone, for example, with heart problems, alcoholism, or psychological problems

Even if only one or two of these patterns precisely match your present situation, you need Gorse.

Positive Potential

❇ You never give up hope and are convinced that all will come out right in the end

❇ You know it's never too late for a new start

❇ You recognize positive opportunities in difficult situations

❇ You're able to inspire others with your own confidence

❇ You're a bearer of hope to others

Empowering Statements

❇ "I stand tall."

❇ "I am filled with hope."

❇ "I see new opportunities."

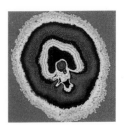

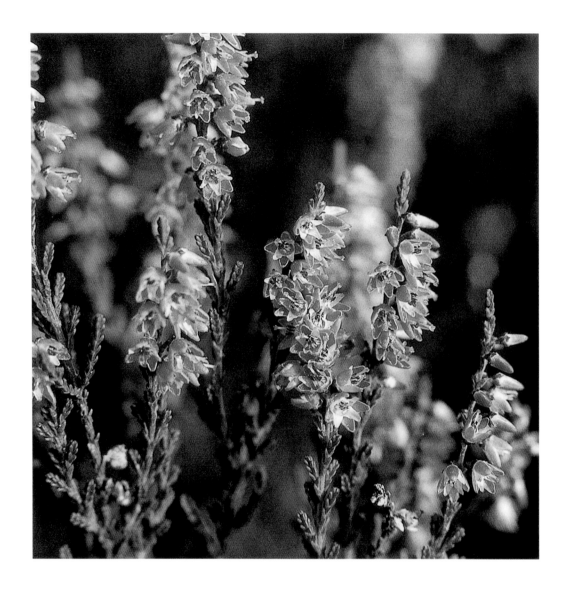

14. Heather: The Identity Flower
From Needy Child to Understanding Adult

Those who are always seeking the companionship of anyone who may be available, as they find it necessary to discuss their own affairs with others, no matter whom it may be. They are very unhappy if they have to be alone for any length of time.

Edward Bach

Heather relates to the Soul's potential for self-identification and empathy. If you're in the negative Heather state, all your thoughts and feelings revolve exclusively around yourself and your problems. This state can be seen in extroverted and introverted forms. As is true with most Bach Flower states, at one time or another almost everyone will experience the negative Heather state.

A chronic extroverted negative Heather state makes for a good cartoon character. One phrase says it all: "He came, he saw—and he kept talking!" Others politely call people of this type exhausting because they absorb your attention by talking ceaselessly. In extreme cases they possess an almost compulsive need to present themselves. They always need an audience to hear about their terribly important problems or the great things they have done. People in the negative Heather state have the irresistible urge to unload everything that happens to them by telling others about it. During a party it takes them less than five minutes to monopolize the conversation by cleverly bringing the topic around to themselves.

Strong methods are necessary to escape their intense desire to communicate; people in the negative Heather state won't easily let go once they've trapped you. They will come oppressively close to you physically when they talk to you, following you as you back away. If necessary, they will even hold on to your sleeve to detain you. Two Bach Flower characters are particularly susceptible to the negative Heather type: Centaury

often lacks the willpower to escape from such an intense influence, and Mimulus can lack the courage to get up and walk away.

Extroverted Heather types in the extreme case won't even care whom they talk to, as long as they're able to talk. They will offer their entire medical history, down to the last detail, to a complete stranger in the doctor's waiting room. If there's no one they can talk to at home, they'll talk on the phone for hours, with most of their sentences starting with *I*.

The *I* is the focus of all thought and aspirations in the negative Heather state. It never occurs to someone in this state to take any real interest in the needs of another person.

How does such an extreme form of self-centeredness come about? A Bach expert from England aptly described those in the negative Heather state as needy children, dependent upon the attentions and affection of those around them. Often it's found that people who need Heather were frequently left alone as babies. From earliest childhood they were emotionally underfed. Lacking the necessary affection and appreciation, these young egos had to fend for themselves emotionally, and learned to constantly work to draw attention to themselves. This unconscious behavior pattern is carried into adulthood. The incessant talk of a negative Heather type is really a desperate attempt by the personality to confirm that it actually exists—if it can hear itself and others can hear it, it therefore must exist.

In the first stages of ego development, children usually go through a temporary negative Heather phase and exuberantly tell you all about themselves, but sometimes this pattern is carried into adulthood, together with a tendency to exaggerate emotions and make mountains out of molehills. What could be worse for a needy child than to be left alone by those who should care for him and provide him with attention and energy? Because the adult in the negative Heather state desperately seeks the energy and focus of others, being deserted is the worst thing that can happen.

The sad thing is that others rarely recognize this emotional child in another person. This is particularly so because many negative Heather types work hard not to appear needy by acting purposefully and assertively. As a result, their intense efforts to gain contact and acknowledgment usually achieve the exact opposite. They come on so strong that the people whom they approach automatically shrink away from them. The affection that they are longing for is being repelled by their own behavior and thus, despite having an audience, they remain lonely inside.

In the negative Heather state the error results from the personality completely turning away from its Higher Self and the greater unity. It's unable to recognize that there's no need to take by force what will come naturally if you allow yourself to be guided by the laws of the Higher Self. People in the negative Heather state must develop from being needy children who want only to receive to being adults who are also able to give. Once they turn their attention and energies away from themselves and toward the world around them and the greater whole, cosmic laws will come into operation, and energy, attention, affection, and love will be returned to them many times over.

The negative Heather state can also take an introverted form. People in this behavior pattern may not talk a great deal, but their excessive concern over their own affairs takes total control over their attention to life in general.

There are times when all of us may have a normal, healthy experience of the negative Heather state. A problem may create such concern that we simply have to let off steam and talk to someone about it. Or we may become seriously ill and dependent upon others to take care of all our needs.

People in the positive Heather state are found to be good listeners. They develop great empathy and, if the situation demands it, are able to be wholly attentive to another person. They create an atmosphere of trust and confidence in which others feel completely at ease.

Those who have chosen careers as social workers, who care for the mentally challenged, and who help the needy are all representatives of the positive Heather potential.

People who wish to develop their positive Heather potential need to:

❀ Realize that other people are not "emotional gas stations," existing solely to fill an emotionally empty tank; everyone has his own problems and needs

❂ Practice listening to others; try to be patient

❂ Become active on behalf of others, perhaps volunteering a few hours each week at a nursing home, offering youth counseling, or working with the disadvantaged

Heather Key Symptoms

These are self-centeredness, preoccupation with your own troubles and affairs, and a constant need for an audience, much like a needy child.

Behavior Pattern in the Blocked State

❂ Your thoughts are entirely centered on personal problems; you take yourself too seriously

❂ You are driven to talk to everyone about yourself

❂ You're unable to be alone, feeling somehow lost when you are solitary

❂ You tend to exaggerate emotionally, making mountains out of molehills

❂ You find it difficult to listen to others

❂ You're absorbed completely in yourself and therefore have no awareness of others' concerns

❂ You try to appear stronger and more competent than you really are, and as a result you don't get the sympathy you want

❂ You take over social conversations and immediately turn them to yourself

❂ You trap others by cornering them or holding on to their sleeves when you want to make a point

❂ You were emotionally neglected or not accepted as a child and as a result still feel undernourished and in need of recognition from those around you

❂ Children regress into infantile behavior

Even if only one or two of these patterns precisely match your present situation, you need Heather.

Positive Potential

❂ You know your Inner Guidance cares for you

❂ You know you'll receive everything necessary for your personal development

❂ You're able to listen to the concerns of others

❂ You're a sympathetic adult with a great capacity for empathy

❂ You create an atmosphere of trust and comfort

Empowering Statements

• "I feel safe."

• "I receive all that I need."

• "I nurture others."

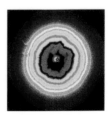

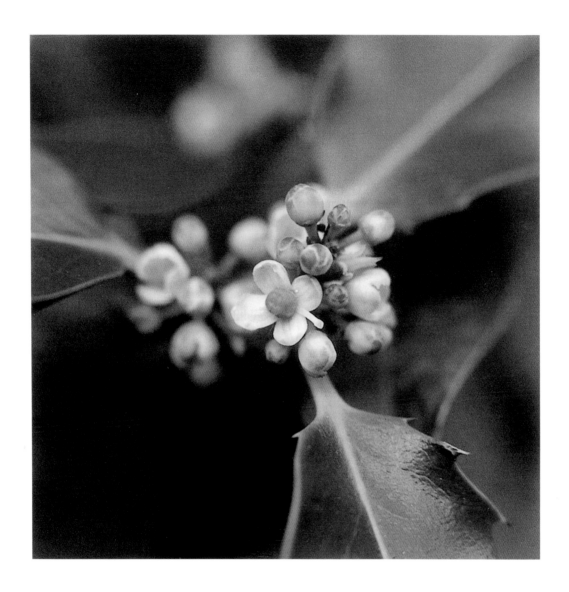

15. Holly: The Heart-Opening Flower
From Hard-Heartedness to Generosity

For those who are sometimes attacked by thoughts of such kind as jealousy, envy, revenge, suspicion.
For the different forms of vexation.
Within themselves they may suffer much, often when there is no real cause for their unhappiness.

Edward Bach

Holly's branches are often part of the Christmas decorations in English-speaking countries. With a name nearly a homophone of *holy*, this is no coincidence—Holly is connected to the principle of divine, all-encompassing love, the love that maintains the world and surpasses human reason. This love, this highest quality of energy through and in which we all live, is our true life elixir. It is the greatest healing power, the strongest motivational force, eternal truth, and joyful awareness of unity.

If this great power of love is misunderstood or not accepted, it will become a force of the opposite: one of separation, wounded feelings, or hate. This principle is the most profound cause of all negative events in life. Sooner or later, consciously or unconsciously, everyone living on this earth must face this central issue.

When you live in the stream of love, existing in a state of grace, the heart is open and all people are seen as brothers and sisters. Once you've dropped out of the stream of love, the heart hardens, and you find yourself painfully isolated, cut off from others, and hurt. Because the desire for this love is programmed into each cell, those in the negative Holly state seem to be fighting for their very emotional existence. When we come into the world, all of us want to give and receive love. If this exchange is denied, we experience unbelievable disappointment and hurt, which leads us to build barriers against the very love that we most want but now are certain that we can't have.

Because love is such a tremendous power, its dark side also engenders enormously powerful feelings, among them anger, aggression, hatred, malice, resentment, jealousy, vengefulness, and envy. These feelings, which none of us is entirely free of, either come out into the open or live at more unconscious levels, where they may form the emotional base from which severe diseases such as cancer develop. It's therefore invaluable that we recognize and acknowledge these profoundly human negative feelings in ourselves, for they mirror the distortion of our innermost needs. They show us what we are lacking and would dearly love to have and in so doing offer us an opportunity to consciously strive for it.

The negative Holly state often begins when your feelings are hurt during early childhood. Perhaps a nursing baby witnessed many angry outbursts, or maybe an infant had to endure poisoned thoughts from a mother and father, for example, who felt overburdened by the birth of the child.

Another facet of the negative Holly state is envy. The little boy who is envious of his brother's new bicycle, the accountant who is envious of her colleague's advancement, the solitary man who envies his friend's great girlfriend are all examples of people in the negative Holly state. This kind of envy is found not only in our private lives and the business world, but also in various spiritual circles. One person undertaking a big project at work, for instance, may wonder how far a colleague has progressed on a similar project; someone may envy her friend's particularly valued ability; and for those on the spiritual path who often focus intensely on love and unfoldment, such feelings would naturally arise out of polarity to the extreme positive focus until they take the step from separation to unity and find God in their own hearts.

The pathological jealousy that looks for anything that will cause suffering is the classic, tragic example of the desire for love gone wrong. If you feel lonely inside and have turned away from love, and then find a person toward whom you can direct your desire for love, you'll feel constantly in danger of losing this love. Having no knowledge of love yourself, you're unable to give it freely and end up radiating your insecurity and fears, which only leads to pain.

Not only the jealous need to recognize that love is not fulfilled when it is directed exclusively to another human being unless, at the same time, this love is striving for divine unity.

In the case of jealousy, a distinction needs to be made between normal and morbid forms of its expression. The former will temporarily arise in any relationship. When the highest feelings of love are present, their counterparts will also inevitably be activated in order to give the impetus to further development. Pay careful attention, though, to people who say they're so tolerant that they know no jealousy. It's improbable that you're talking to someone with truly sublime wisdom. More likely the person is paralyzed inside to such an extent that he's no longer able to suffer and to love.

From this point of view it's always reason for joy when Holly comes up in the diagnosis, for it shows that there is a potential—which could be developed—that the person is longing for love and has the means to give it.

Edward Bach said, "Holly protects us from everything that is not universal love. Holly opens the heart and unites us with divine love." We develop a feeling for where we've come from and where we belong. We realize that we are all children of love. Holly helps us to live in the state of love again, in that state of beauty, solemnity, and fulfillment in which we share one heart and one soul with the world. Here we are able to recognize and acknowledge everything as part of the natural order and to wholeheartedly share the pleasure of other people's success without envy, even at times when we may have some problem of our own.

The Soul potential of Holly is the ideal human state, the goal we are striving for as long as we live. Sri Aurobindo wrote, "To experience and love the god of beauty and goodness, even in what is ugly and in what is evil, and to long with all our love to heal it of its ugliness and its evil, that is a true virtue."

In real life, the negative Holly state is often not apparent. We would hardly expect anything else in cultures where for generations it has not been considered good manners to speak about personal feelings. It's necessary in an interview, therefore, to try to sense the negative Holly state of another person. A first sign of this state is often your own personal irritation and tendency to seem stressed and unfriendly.

Holly people in a negative behavior pattern tend to give in to anger and rage. They will put up a destructive defense in the presence of positive emotional expressions because they have been hurt too early and too often. Sometimes a negative Holly state has created a pervasive, poisonous pattern through an entire family, which can be passed on from one generation to the next. Ill feelings may even go as far as prompting something like the boycott of the funeral of a much disliked father or sister-in-law.

A common negative Holly experience occurs when a second child is born and the first shows his jealousy in the form of moodiness, rebelliousness, and so on. Holly has proved very useful in such cases, as it has with dogs that show jealousy when suddenly confronted with a baby in the family. In addition, at times of conflict during puberty and in the beginning of treating relationship problems, Holly has always been a helpful tool.

Holly Key Symptoms

These may include anger, rage, feelings of hatred and envy, jealousy.

Behavior Pattern in the Blocked State

- ✼ You're easily annoyed; you react in an unfriendly or aggressive way

- ✼ You're bad-tempered, discontented, and frustrated but you don't always know why

- ✼ You're envious; you think about revenge and gloat over another's misfortune

- ✼ You're jealous and distrustful

- ✼ Your heart is hardened and your feelings seem poisoned

- ✼ You react explosively, becoming overheated, enraged, or violent

- ✼ You feel that others are insensitive to you and you fear their moods

- ✼ You have fears of being deceived

- ✼ You feel that others misunderstand your feelings

- ✼ You often suspect something negative behind what people say or do

- ✼ You easily grow suspicious of others

- ✼ You frequently feel offended or hurt

- ✼ You belittle others; you create enemies

- ✼ Your reactions irritate people who share emotional information—for instance, you laugh upon hearing of someone's death

- You feel a stab of pain when you hear about someone else's luck or happiness

- Children exhibit rage, anger, sudden outbursts, and even physical violence

Even if only one or two of these patterns precisely match your present situation, you need Holly.

Positive Potential

- You think with your heart

- You approach others openly and with good will

- You have a profound understanding of human emotions

- You take wholehearted pleasure in the achievements and successes of others

- You live in a state of inner harmony, radiating goodwill and warmheartedness

Empowering Statements

- "I am full of joy."

- "I am connected."

- "I am loving."

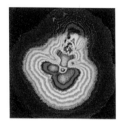

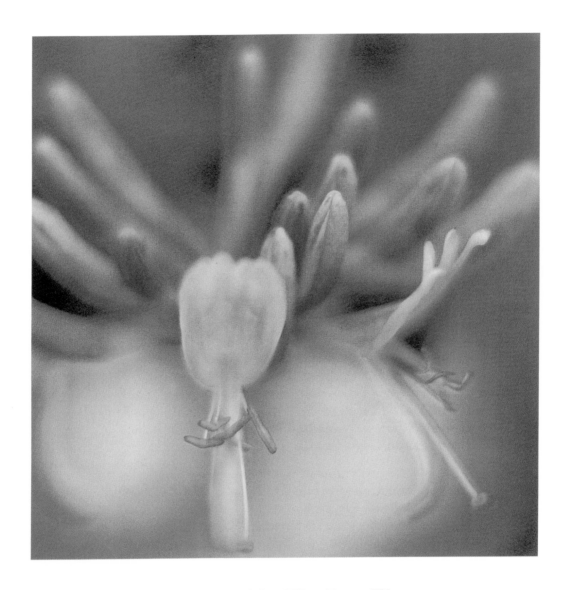

16. Honeysuckle: The Past Flower
From Then to Now

Those who live much in the past, perhaps a time of great happiness, or memories of a lost friend, or ambitions which have not come true. They do not expect further happiness such as they have had.

Edward Bach

Honeysuckle relates to the Soul's ability to adapt. If you're in the negative Honeysuckle state, you strive to hold on to things in the past and are out of touch with the flow of life. Imagine visiting a zoo with your family at the age of four. You're in front of the primate exhibit and a little chimpanzee extends its hand toward you. You're just about to return the gesture when your father pulls you along on the sidewalk in order to catch up with the others. While you follow your dad you wonder how close you and the little chimp might have come to touching each other. In the next moment you find yourself together with your family by the sea lions. There's a great deal of commotion because they have just been fed and they're dashing out of the water now to catch the fish. You, however, are not touched by the scene, because your mind lingers with the chimp and how close you might have come to it.

The problem in the negative Honeysuckle state is a lack of inner movement. There's a certain inertia; you're mentally lingering in the wrong place at the wrong time, and you are unable to act. The classic example is Lot's wife, who in the Bible story was turned into a pillar of salt. She chose to disregard the advice of her guardian angel, allowed herself to be drawn to the past, and turned around to look back at Sodom instead of concentrating all her energies on the imminent tasks of her escape and rescue.

If you're in the negative Honeysuckle state you're physically in the present but mentally stuck in the past. To be in two places at the same time and to bridge the gulf between past and present require a great deal of psychic energy. This energy goes up in smoke and becomes painfully unavailable in the present—where the course is set for the future.

In the negative Honeysuckle state the personality refuses to be guided by its Higher Self according to its Life Plan. It ignores the fact that one of the most important life principles is continuous change, that everything is in a state of flux. Instead it wants to determine its own destiny, particularly in emotional situations, and the standards it applies are narrow and self-centered.

A widow who for years keeps her dead husband's study untouched so that it appears as if he only just now left his desk is in the negative Honeysuckle state. An even more extreme example is a movie star who has not budged mentally from her days of greatness. At sixty-five she still wears the clothing, hairstyle, and makeup that she wore in her youthful days of success. Others who need Honeysuckle are: a Peace Corps engineer working for a long period of time in Africa, far from his home in the United States; a young man who stays away from new relationships after his young wife dies; and a couple who have had to move to another part of town but cannot stop talking about how much they miss their old neighborhood— it's no wonder they're failing to settle down properly or make new friends.

Such people unconsciously refuse to see and accept new developments. Honeysuckle types in the negative state, more often than other people, will start their sentences with "I used to . . ." or "When I was still . . . ," showing that they're still clinging to the past. They're unable to build a fluid connection between the past and their present situation because they can't or won't consider the past from all angles. They fix their minds on only one aspect of it—usually one that is pleasant. For instance, a man might recall: "When our father was still alive everything was a lot nicer. We would go on great trips together during the summer." The fact that every year the father took out loans that could not be paid off to finance the trips is the dark detail that's no longer mentioned. The result is that negative experiences are not integrated and cannot be used for the development of the personality.

The negative Honeysuckle state is an escape from facing the difficulties of today. Frequently recalling the feelings we experienced in the past that are no longer appropriate is merely a sentimental attempt to compensate for present moods. This state is a normal phenomenon at class reunions or at anniversary celebrations, and it makes sense that it's prevalent among the elderly who are in the process of assessing their lives. While it does not involve guilt feelings, it encompasses regret for missed opportunities and unfulfilled hopes—all those things we wished we'd done differently. The negative Honeysuckle state has usually built up over a long period of time, though it may also be of short duration.

About Honeysuckle, Bach wrote: "This is the remedy to remove from the mind the regrets and sorrows of the past, to counteract all influences, all wishes and desires of the past and to bring us back to the present."

In the transformed, positive Honeysuckle state, however, we have a living connection to the past, learning from it but not clinging to it unnecessarily. We are able to work with our yesterdays, keeping the things that are worth keeping. Archaeologists, historians, and dealers in antiquities are in a positive Honeysuckle state from this point of view. In reincarnation therapy Honeysuckle can help establish the link between past and present and make sure that the past is not overvalued but instead is given its proper place.

Honeysuckle has often helped those who are homesick—whether they're attending boarding school, working away from home, or traveling—to integrate more easily with their new place. A few drops of Honeysuckle in a glass of water can also help us part, during spring cleaning, with old items that, though they may be dear to us, have no more real use.

Interestingly, some people who select Honeysuckle during a spontaneous choice are barely able to remember the first three or four years of their life, largely because they have unconsciously avoided a confrontation with some aspect of the past. This circumstance may now be introduced with the support of Honeysuckle Essence.

Honeysuckle Key Symptoms

You may experience a longing for time gone by and regrets over the past, which prevent you from living in the present.

Behavior in the Blocked State

- A pleasant or unpleasant past situation is as clear in your mind as though it happened yesterday

- You constantly refer to the past in your thoughts and in conversation with others

- You glorify the past, wanting to have things as they were

- You wistfully think back to the good old days

- You can't get over the loss of a loved one, a pet that died, or a lost item

- There is something you don't want to make peace with

- You're stuck in memories of beautiful moments—for example, the first ride on your very own motorcycle

- You're homesick

- You regret not having taken advantage of a unique opportunity in a personal or job-related situation

- You have little interest in current affairs because you're mentally living in the past

- You have no expectations for the future

- You feel an unfulfillable longing to start all over again

- You're unable to give up old memorabilia—shoes or souvenirs, for instance—even after many years

- You have a very poor memory of your early childhood

- The picture of a past situation comes up again and again in your mind's eye, so clearly that you're able to paint it

- You constantly remember a particular person

- Others become tired in your company

Even if only one or two of these patterns precisely match your present situation, you need Honeysuckle.

Positive Potential

- You know that life is taking place in the here and now

- You have a living relationship with the past and realize its bearing on the present

- You take from the past what had true value and awaken it to new life

Empowering Statements

- "I live today."

- "I look to the future."

- "I take the next step."

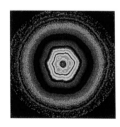

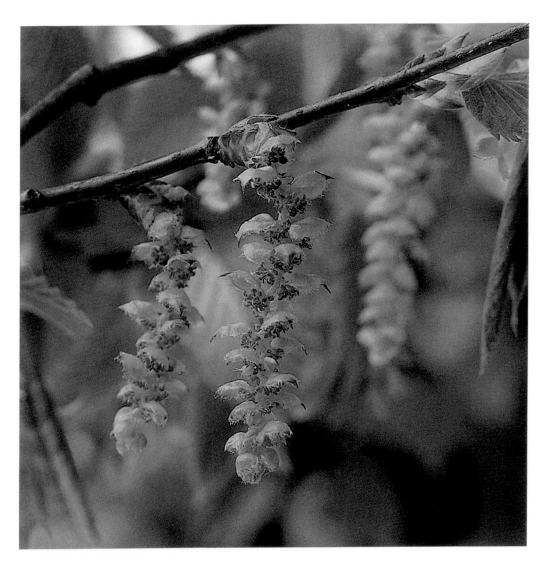

17. Hornbeam: The Vitality Flower
From Listlessness to Mental Freshness

For those who feel that they have not sufficient strength, mentally or physically, to carry the burden of life placed upon them; the affairs of every day seem too much for them to accomplish, though they generally succeed in fulfilling their task.

For those who believe that some part, of mind or body, needs to be strengthened before they can easily fulfill their work.

Edward Bach

Hornbeam embodies the Soul's potential for mental vitality. In the negative Hornbeam state you feel tired and worn out, like an old rubber band gone limp. However, this fatigue largely takes place only in your mind. Every office worker knows the feeling when the alarm clock rings on Monday morning and your routine once again beckons. What lies ahead is a largely familiar, monotonous work week offering little variety or genuine responsibility but many tedious demands—a thousand little things to keep track of, routines to be maintained, unfinished projects to be completed, guidelines to be followed. All this looms like a dark mountain, and you believe you don't have the strength to cope. Funny enough, though, by the afternoon you find that you have satisfactorily completed nearly everything that you had to do, only to wake up the next morning with the same weary feeling. People who need Hornbeam often grew up in an environment where everyday life was directed by stark routine. Many things that were done simply *had* to be done. Now you look subjectively at your least favorite activities and find them more exhausting than they really are because you so often have to muster fresh motivation to perform them.

The Hornbeam weariness is a state of exhaustion arising from one-sided demands on the mental level with no way to balance things physically. It may begin as a temporary state, but it can become chronic. It's temporary, for instance, when a student has been studying for months for an examination and has neglected his exercise routine. Or when a patient spends a long time in bed with a complicated fracture, doing a lot of reading, thinking, and planning but never getting out to catch some fresh air. A kind of heavy-headed weariness leads this patient to think that she's not yet ready for physical rehabilitation.

The more long-term Hornbeam weariness is characteristic of the modern city dweller who eats too much, watches too much TV, and produces or creates too little. People who take in many more impressions than they're able to digest mentally find it hard to get up in the morning because they have such heavy heads. They may feel as though they're semi-automated members of society who live a standardized life. Even leisure and holidays follow a set pattern, often more resembling duties than relaxation. While such people may have a great deal going on around them, there is very little activity going on inside them. Their spiritual vitality has gone flat.

Interestingly, the Hornbeam weariness disappears instantly when something out of the ordinary happens, something challenging enough at another level to pull you out of your mental rut. The phone rings while you're watching TV at night—an old friend is in town and suggests meeting at the train station. Even if you were just about to go to bed, her offer has awakened you and you're eager to head out the door.

The error of the negative Hornbeam state lies in the personality's materialistic, self-imposed limits against what you like and have fun doing. You are "shortsighted" and "hard of hearing" where the impulses of the Higher Self are concerned, preferring to accept comfortable, automatic patterns. You deprive yourself of spontaneous opportunities for development and much that makes life enjoyable and worth living. In the negative Hornbeam state there is a one-sidedness that does not include the alternation between times of tension and times of relaxation. This one-sidedness upsets the balance of your energy system—your different energy levels don't communicate well, energy exchange is disturbed, and overall energy production is reduced. The only possible outcome is an energy deficit.

Sensitive people describe Hornbeam impulses as akin to a refreshing, cool shower equalizing and toning individual energy levels. It has been said that Hornbeam gives "backbone." It clears your head, vitalizes your perceptions, and allows the impulses of your Higher Self to be heard again. The right way to alternate between activity and relaxation is rediscovered, life and work become a pleasure again, and you know you have the energy you need to achieve what you wish.

Hornbeam and White Chestnut are frequently needed at the same time. When added to a moist pad, Hornbeam has been found to relieve tired eyes, particularly for people who spend long hours in front of the computer. Another external benefit is the tightening of weak connective tissue around varicose veins. Finally, Hornbeam belongs among the Flower Essences that can return energy to drooping plants.

Hornbeam Key Symptoms

You feel mental exhaustion, temporary or prolonged weariness, or that "Monday-morning feeling."

Behavior Pattern in the Blocked State

- You feel that you lack enough energy to master the demands of everyday life

- You feel heavy-headed, tired, and exhausted

- You experience mental hangovers, that "Monday-morning feeling."

- Your head buzzes after watching too much television, reading too much, studying too much, and the like

- You expect the work you need to do to be very exhausting

- You lack enthusiasm and feel mental inertia

- Upon waking you doubt that you can deal with the day's chores, but this feeling subsides after taking a shower or getting dressed

- Merely the thought of a particular task provokes debilitating fatigue

- You miss your former vitality and feel constantly overburdened with demands

- You must push yourself to fulfill daily responsibilities

- After a prolonged illness you doubt you'll have enough strength to return to work, despite evidence to the contrary

- You believe it's impossible to start work without a stimulant such as coffee, tea, or some form of tonic

- You come to life when something interesting occurs unexpectedly

- You feel exhaustion after years of performing the same disliked tasks

- You wake up in the morning more tired than when you went to bed

- You feel pressure or a burning sensation in or around your eyes

- You experience connective tissue degeneration

Even if only one or two of these patterns precisely match your present situation, you need Hornbeam.

Positive Potential

- You have a lively mind and you balance variety and routine

- You spontaneously leave routines behind to follow an unexpected impulse

- You're sure you can master the tasks ahead without fearing you'll get exhausted

- You know every day is different and can look forward to your regular work

Empowering Statements

- "I feel fresh."

- "I have energy"

- "I enjoy working."

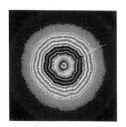

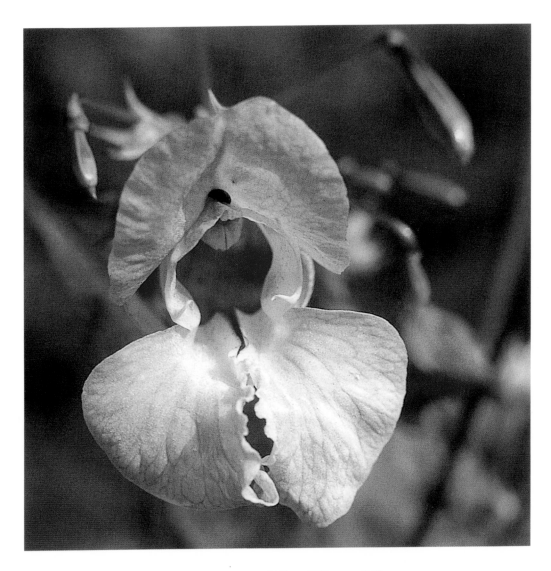

18. Impatiens: The Time Flower
From Impatience to Patience

Those who are quick in thought and action and who wish all things to be done without hesitation or delay. When ill they are anxious for a hasty recovery.

They find it very difficult to be patient with people who are slow, as they consider it wrong and a waste of time, and they will endeavor to make such people quicker in all ways.

They often prefer to work and think alone, so that they can do everything at their own speed.

Edward Bach

Impatiens relates to the Soul qualities of patience and gentleness. In the negative Impatiens state, you are impatient, with an inner tension that tends to cause irritability toward others. Because you move very quickly mentally, everybody else seems very slow. You often feel like a thoroughbred forced to pull a plow while harnessed with a farm horse. Frustrated inside, you nevertheless adapt to the work and slower pace of others. This adaptation, however, takes a great deal of energy, resulting in constant mental strain.

In positions of authority negative Impatiens people are not always popular because they know how to do everything more efficiently themselves and are not exactly diplomatic in sharing this with their employees: "Never mind—leave it. I'll have the job done myself long before I can explain the whole thing to you." Instructors who are the negative Impatiens type find it very difficult to stand by patiently while watching the awkward first attempts of their trainees. "Let me do it—it makes me nervous to watch you." They're also prone to finishing the thoughts of others before they've reached the end of their sentence.

It's unwise to make any critical comment to someone in the negative Impatiens state, however diplomatic. He is likely to flare up, though his anger passes just as quickly as it arises. Convinced that being deliberate is a waste of time, negative Impatiens bosses tend to push their staff to the point of being perceived as slave drivers. The regrettable fact is that Impatiens people do not assume leadership gladly. In fact, they have no ambition to lead—unlike Vine, for instance—and would prefer to work entirely by themselves and get things done at their own pace without outside interference. Their independence is dear to them. This is why Bach includes Impatiens in his "loneliness" group of Flowers. Negative Impatiens types are aware of their difficulties and when in a balanced state of mind are open to and grateful for good advice.

People in the negative Impatiens state are like mental sprinters. Some you can identify as babies by the way they take to their mother's breast. They see things more quickly, deliver sentences with machine-gun rapidity, react in a flash, make ad hoc decisions, and, of course, become exhausted more quickly. "I'm so hungry I could eat a horse!" would be the standard exclamation of an Impatiens person only three hours after breakfast. In next to no time, he then would wolf down enough potato chips to cause an immediate stomachache.

This quickly changing disposition is often apparent on the outside. Those in the negative Impatiens state may turn red all of a sudden and just as quickly grow quite pale. Their nervous tension can lead to sudden cramps or pains in different parts of the body. Overreactions of every kind are normal for this type. Great inner restlessness can make them impetuous and therefore accident-prone, yet in the end they have fewer accidents than you might expect because they're able to react in a flash and can get out of many critical situations.

The error of the negative Impatiens state is in doing things only your own way, thereby limiting yourself. Impatiens people forget that everyone is part of a great whole, and that in the end we all depend upon each other—even upon those who seem less capable. Nor does the personality consider that those more capable are indeed required to place their greater gifts at the service of others, to help them in their development.

Impatiens people in the negative state are asked to learn something very difficult for them: to hold back from active involvement, to let things happen, to practice patience. This would be easier to accomplish if they put aside their linear thinking and instead use different kinds of perception, which allow for more complex comprehension of a situation.

The negative Impatiens state is usually very obvious; those who exhibit it are natural extroverts. If they don't reveal their state in words, they'll frequently do so in gestures such as nervous drumming of their fingers on the table and fidgeting in a chair. When gestures don't reveal the state, it might be visible as nervous skin rashes or skin irritation.

Frequently it turns out that this state merely represents the tip of an iceberg—it won't be resolved until the other, more profound behavior patterns connected to it are addressed.

Positive Impatiens types have great empathy and angelic patience. They fully understand the different temperaments of others and are diplomatic in placing their quickness of mind, powers of decision, and intelligence at the service of others.

In practice, Impatiens Essence has proved to be very useful in daily family life. Children who squabble when they go shopping or visiting with their parents, or who get into temper tantrums, will respond well and quickly to Impatiens. So will parents who in certain situations easily run out of patience with their children.

Impatiens Key Symptoms

Among these are impatience, irritability, and a quickness to react.

Behavior Pattern in the Blocked State

⊗ You're mentally tense; you feel driven by a fast inner tempo

⊗ You feel constantly pressured by time

⊗ You expect everything to go quickly and smoothly

⊗ You find it hard to wait for things to take their natural course; you want to finish everything quickly

⊗ You talk, eat, and work faster than others

⊗ People who work more slowly than you drive you crazy—you have no patience or diplomacy for them

⊗ You cut off other people and finish their sentences before they can

- You don't finish your own sentences

- You impatiently take things into your own hands

- You make rash decisions

- You prefer to work alone at your own pace

- You have a great desire for independence

- You easily flare up and are curt and brusque, though your anger passes just as quickly

- You bring an end to jobs that aren't completely finished because you just want to get them done

- You react ungraciously if not served promptly in a restaurant

- When you're ill you feel that your symptoms are supposed to disappear immediately

- Children can't sit still; they make nervous movements and may be hyperkinetic

- Your reservoir of strength is quickly used up and you may experience sudden pains or temporary phases of exhaustion

Even if only one or two of these patterns precisely match your present situation, you need Impatiens.

Positive Potential

- You're alert, quick thinking, quick acting, and independent-minded

- You're good at initiating new developments and keeping things rolling

- You're gifted at empathizing with various temperaments

- You can wait for things to take their natural course

- You have patience and gentleness

Empowering Statements

- "I have time."

- "I am patient."

- "I am relaxed."

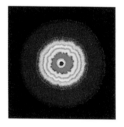

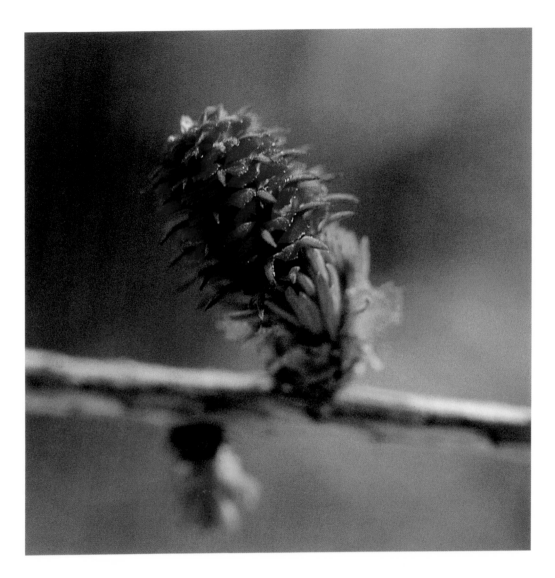

19. Larch: The Self-Confidence Flower
From Self-Restriction to Self-Unfolding

For those who do not consider themselves as good or capable as those around them, who expect failure, who feel that they will never be a success, and so do not venture or make a strong enough attempt to succeed.

Edward Bach

Larch relates to the Soul quality of self-confidence. In the negative Larch state you feel inferior to others from the start: "It's a fact that I have no musical ear"; "When it comes to computers, I have absolutely no clue—it's all lost on me"; "I just can't do math." It's not merely a question of doubting your abilities; you feel absolute conviction that you are inferior. Because you are sure that you can't do certain things, you don't even attempt them. Through this attitude you take away from yourself the most beautiful thing life has to offer: the opportunity to learn, grow, and change through new experience, and to live life to the fullest. Rather than unfolding, the personality starves. All that remains is discouragement and a trace of melancholy beneath the surface.

The error of the personality in the negative Larch state is that it holds on to bad experiences and then uses them to measure itself against all situations in life. Instead, it must allow itself to be guided by its Higher Self, to learn to use all of its experiences and to assess them only in terms of its own nature and abilities.

Many people find it difficult to recognize their own limits. If you're in the negative Larch state, however, you suffer from exactly the opposite problem. From the start in approaching a problem, you assume there are limitations, which then become the cornerstones to a wall blocking your development.

Negative Larch types usually appear quite sensible to those around them; their explanations for why they can't or won't do certain things seem to make perfect sense. They may argue, "As a woman, I don't really have a chance" or "I don't have the high test scores that other people have" or "I'd really like to do this, but I know already that my abilities don't match those of my competition."

The foundations for such genuine feelings of inferiority are as a rule laid in early childhood. The child's progress, for example, may be constantly compared to that of others: "You aren't as smart as your sister." Frequently the child has literally absorbed his parent's feelings of inferiority as he has his mother's milk. Negative Larch reactions may also be the result of growing up in an environment that doesn't match your own nature—for example, a musical child growing up among athletes, or an immigrant from a different culture attending a school in the school system of her new country. In all these situations the certainty of failure can become an automatic response reinforced by each new "failed" attempt. A vicious circle has been set up.

Just as the larch tree is structured quite delicately, so too are people who are in frequent need of Larch. Psychologically they have a tender constitution and they react to stronger personalities. They measure themselves with other people's measuring sticks instead of their own, consequently finding themselves at a disadvantage. This is a pity—usually they're not only just as capable as others, but, in fact, they are also often more capable than those around them.

Take, for example, an assistant buyer in a chain-store company who began as a secretary. As the years progress she turns out to be more capable and efficient than her boss—but when a position as buyer becomes available in another department and her colleagues kindly advise her to apply, she declines, stating that she has been trained only as a secretary. This argument is wholly meaningless in light of her actual experience. At the same time, and with a certain underlying admiration, she will talk about a friend who dared to take a similar step and was successful. There is no envy (Holly) or bitterness (Willow) in her words, but the wrong kind of modesty, quite out of place in her colleagues' opinion—a modesty obscuring her unacknowledged longing for further development.

Larch helps you leave self-limiting concepts behind and develop those abilities that you have not yet put to use. Somehow you're suddenly able to take a more relaxed view of things, and to consider alternatives. You take action without predetermining the outcome. You calmly accept that either positive or negative results are possible, and that there's little benefit in exaggerating the possibilities of success or failure. The expression *I can't* has been eliminated from your vocabulary. You continue to assess things critically, but from a constructive point of view, so that you're able to determine your proper place in life by recognizing your individual and specific abilities.

In practice Larch is used both for long-term treatment and for dealing with temporary problems of self-confidence. It has proved useful, for instance, before taking exams, during divorce proceedings when both partners often suffer great blows to their self-esteem, and for children who won't venture out on their own but always want to have Dad or Mom go with them. Larch has also given a boost of self-confidence to people with disabilities and to those who feel discriminated against. Some practitioners have seen good results in the treatment of alcoholics who drink in order to erase their belief that they aren't as capable as others and to deal with feelings of inadequacy that stem from believing that failure is inevitable.

There are two recommendations that people in the negative Larch state might find helpful: First, observe others carefully and realize that even those who appear most capable are themselves human. Second, a personal scoreboard listing those things that you have done better than others may be a helpful tool at the beginning of Larch therapy. A habit of comparing yourself to others, however, should soon after be abandoned for good.

Larch Key Symptoms

You may have an inferiority complex or may experience expectations of failure due to lack of self-confidence.

Behavior Pattern in the Blocked State

❀ You automatically feel inferior to others

- You don't believe yourself capable of those things you admire in others

- In comparison with others, you always place yourself in an inferior position

- Firmly convinced that you cannot do something, you don't even try

- You place yourself behind others

- You react hesitantly and passively when offered a real opportunity

- You use illness as an excuse to avoid tackling a problem

- You express modesty due to a lack of self-confidence

- You feel "second class" due to your family background, language, color, or disabilities

- Children who are students feel like failures

- Second-born children experience problems with self-esteem

- You don't hold the position at work that matches your abilities.

Even if only one or two of these patterns precisely match your present situation, you need Larch.

Positive Potential

- You believe in your own ability to realize important personal goals

- You can assess and accept personal strengths and weaknesses objectively

- You've developed your own personal measures of success

- You use and develop your personal talents

- You seize opportunities with reasonable expectations

- You take your proper place in society

Empowering Statements

- "I can."

- "I want to."

- "I do."

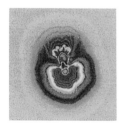

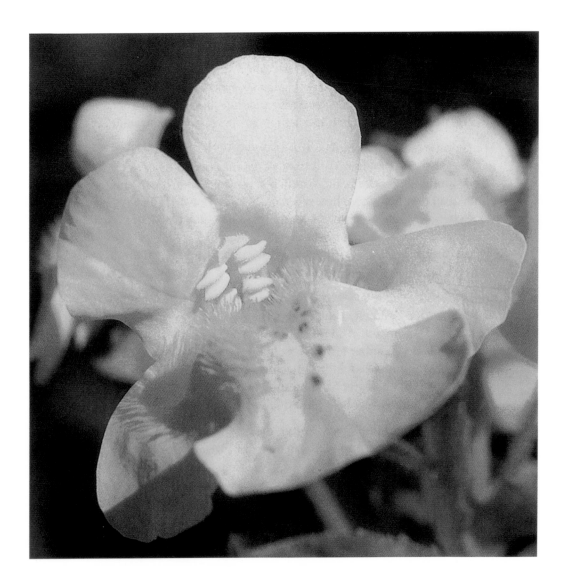

20. Mimulus: The Bravery Flower
From Fear of the World to Trust in the World

Fear of worldly things, illness, pain, accidents, poverty, of dark, of being alone, of misfortune. The fears of everyday life. These people quietly and secretly bear their dread, they do not freely speak of it to others.

Edward Bach

Mimulus relates to the Soul's potential for courage and trust. Those in the negative Mimulus state must learn to overcome their exaggerated and often childish fears. These include very specific, tangible fears that arise in everyday life, such as fear of going on escalators and of AIDS. Further examples might include being anxious about inviting people to your house, fear of the neighbor's dog, and fear of an injection at the dentist's. You never speak about your fears of your own accord, but if asked a direct question, you'll name more and more anxieties: fear of being alone, fear of quarrels over the household budget, fear of a difficult entryway to a garage . . . the list is endless. It includes practically every shade of the great archetypal fears of humans.

One could imagine that such fears represent a residue of the archetypal fear of the newborn: a fear of the harsh world and of life in the physical body. The Mimulus baby, starting to cry for no apparent reason upon waking, clearly shows how painful it must be to enter into this physical reality. People who are in the negative Mimulus state sometimes say that life on earth is like a burden on their backs. It's as if they're children who do not really wish to grow up, face life, and take care of themselves.

Some people with marked Mimulus traits tend to be of delicate build or show other external signs of fragility. Some resemble precious china dolls in human form. Others are like frightened mice, always needing a certain amount of protection. Other Mimulus types are very sensitive physically, and in the presence of others are apt to blush, stammer, or suddenly have a frog in the throat. Some will giggle nervously, talk far too much from sheer nervousness, or suffer from sweaty palms.

There are others who are good at disguising their negative Mimulus state and in everyday life appear strong and extroverted. Only at second glance will you become aware that they're really rather reserved and sensitive—in their hearts they would rather not have much to do with the world. This is a trait often seen in artists and especially in actors and musicians.

People in the negative Mimulus state find it difficult to tolerate too much of anything. They seem to have more subtle standards than others do and are less able to deal with noise, blinding lights, large amounts of food, or too many activities. Hypersensitive to many things in the environment, they often feel like "a hummingbird caught up in a colony of crows," as an English Bach specialist put it. Many Mimulus people in a negative state fall ill if the pressure becomes overwhelming. They will then develop "my headache," "my stomach cramps," "my bladder problems," and the like. Mimulus patients are also inclined to be overly careful in convalescence and thus delay the process of recovery.

Because of their sensitive constitutions, people with a Mimulus character are usually peaceful. Even if they have an occasional outburst of anger, it's never impressive; they're no more threatening to their environment than is an enraged butterfly.

If you take Mimulus a great deal, there are two crucial lessons for you to learn: One is to find a way to live with your sensitive constitution, which is something precious indeed. This includes learning to withdraw from the world at times without feeling guilty about it, in order to recharge your batteries and give your nerves a chance to recover. For this reason it's very important for Mimulus types to have a room or personal place all to themselves. Another lesson is to come to terms with the phenomenon of fear, and to realize that your fearful thoughts are forces that can actually materialize. Like all thoughts, each additional anxiety will reinforce the first, tying up further energies and increasingly tangling you.

"In the world you have tribulations; but be of good cheer because I have overcome the world." These words from the New Testament provide the key to a positive Mimulus state. As long as the personality uses only worldly standards, it will always find itself facing real fears. If, however, it allows itself to be guided by its Higher Self, it gives up its worldly limitations and turns more toward the greater whole. Then it will be able to overcome the world—that is, its fears.

By taking Mimulus you'll find the way out of your confusion of fears and anxieties and come back to your own true nature. You'll learn that fear is primarily a problem in your own mind and can be tackled from the mind. From this perspective you're able to deal with it more effectively. You'll cease to imagine something horrible that might take place in a certain situation and instead wait it out, calmly assessing the outcome realistically. In this manner you can grow beyond your anxieties and use your fine sense of humor and human understanding to help others who are in a similar situation.

When Mimulus comes up in the diagnostic interview with a person who's concerned about an introduction to the new neighbors, for instance, the concrete fear of the moment needs to be stated in very specific terms. A therapist should convey that Mimulus will help resolve this particular anxiety block. It may even be effective to recommend courageously practicing the parts that contain the scary moments in the form of a role play.

If the patient's specific anxiety has disappeared in the course of treatment, experience has shown that at the same time several other anxieties will have dissolved as well.

Mimulus Key Symptoms

There can be shyness, timidity, and specific and well-defined fears, including a general fear of the world.

Behavior Pattern in the Blocked State

- ❀ You're shy, timid, and careful

- ❀ You're physically delicate and have a sensitive nature

❀ You fear a certain situation but you don't talk about it

❀ You imagine everything to be more difficult and dangerous than it really is

❀ There's always something you're afraid of at any particular moment

❀ You suffer from specific anxieties and phobias such as fear of cold feet; dark corridors; illness and pain; horses, mice, dogs, and other animals; making telephone calls; being in new situations; having to go to the hospital; dying a painful death; losing possessions; being in crowds; having an accident; losing a relative; entering an enclosed place; beginning something new; and so on

❀ You are hypersensitive to cold, noise, bright light, loud voices, strong smells, and so forth

❀ You want to be left in peace; to be talked to by no one

❀ Your anxieties cause you inner tension

❀ You suffer from occasional speech difficulties, stammering, or nervous laughter; you talk a great deal out of nervousness

❀ You blush easily, or your palms sweat

❀ You unconsciously procrastinate because of your anxieties

❀ You're afraid of new things and always need to start slowly

❀ You hope that certain things will take care of themselves

❀ You're afraid to be alone, but are shy and nervous in company

❀ You get very anxious when met with opposition or when things don't work out right away

❀ You're overcautious during convalescence—for instance, you don't dare move your broken leg after it comes out of the cast for fear of hurting it or undoing the healing that has taken place

❀ You easily fall ill when faced with the things that you fear

❀ Babies cry for no apparent reason upon waking in the morning

❀ Children are scared by strangers and hold on tightly to Mom of Dad

❀ Children refuse to listen to fairy tales that contain violence

Even if only one or two of these patterns precisely match your present situation, you need Mimulus.

Positive Potential

⊛ You've grown beyond your anxieties, know your limits, and are able to face the world with cheerful composure

⊛ You feel up to the world's challenges and are able to bravely get involved in the next task

⊛ You have a refined, sensitive character

⊛ You have personal courage and understand others in similar situations

Empowering Statements

⊛ "I am brave."

⊛ "I dare."

⊛ "I step forward."

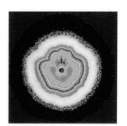

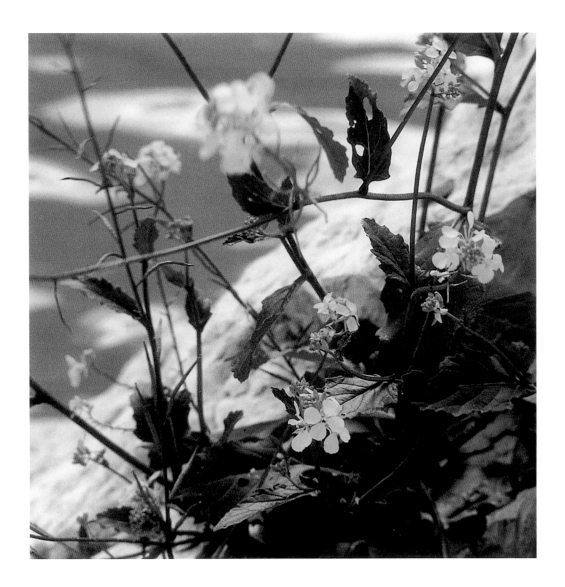

21. Mustard: The Light Flower
From Soul Pain to Soul Grandeur

Those who are liable to times of gloom, or even despair, as though a cold dark cloud overshadowed them and hid the light and the joy of life. It may not be possible to give any reason or explanation for such attacks.

Under these conditions it is almost impossible to appear happy or cheerful.

Edward Bach

Mustard relates to the Soul qualities of cheerfulness, serenity, and clarity. In the negative Mustard state you're surrounded by gloomy depression. Out of the clear blue sky, deep melancholy of an unknown origin can descend upon you. It's all around, isolating you from the rest of the world with a layer of deep sadness. You suddenly feel like a stranger in your own land—all thoughts remain held within you and all your energies are seemingly drained by an invisible channel. While this dark force lingers, you're completely at its mercy and there is no trick in the world, neither a diversion nor common sense, to help you escape from the nightmare. Nor is it possible to cover things up to the outside world the way negative Agrimony types do. The immobile dark weight is too heavy, keeping you imprisoned until it lifts of its own accord, disappearing just as suddenly as it arrived. Then you're free again and with gratitude take a deep breath of relief until the next cloud descends.

All of us have experienced such illogical and irritating attacks of unexpected gloom, though not always in the extreme form described above. The negative Mustard state can also take place on a more internal level of awareness. Extreme cases of a negative Mustard state are comparable to the beginning stages of clinical depression, which appear without specific reason, sometimes in temporary phases. Characteristic Mustard symptoms that go hand in hand with this disorder are slowed movements and perception as well as a lack of motivation.

The negative Mustard state clearly exemplifies that every negative behavior pattern is a state of reduced vibrational frequency in which all functions are depressed physically (slowness of movement), psychologically (lack of drive or motivation), and mentally (reduced perception). In this negative state it seems as if a strong, unknown, outside frequency is overtaking your personality, at times almost completely severing your connection with the outside world. It's therefore not easy to pinpoint the error involved in this state. We might try to discern it from a different point of view, though: It's possible that your spiritual separation from the greater whole has resulted in the Soul's sadness over its "lost" home.

It's interesting that many famous painters and musicians have repeatedly suffered from dark Mustard states. People like these are more open to the collective human experience and find inspiration in this reservoir. Some have compared themselves to sponges soaking up everything, then letting it all work within before finally transforming some of it into art during a creative phase.

How does overwhelming grief sometimes pervade the atmosphere of collective human experience? Because people tend to suppress the pain and mourning of major experiences such as war * and natural disasters, large amounts of unresolved grief build up around us. Those who

---

* Toward the beginning of the war in Bosnia, so many people tapped into the grief and sadness of this experience that Mustard was prescribed in above-average amounts in Germany, Austria, and Switzerland.

are open to collective planes are then "flooded" by this grief and sadness during periods of low energy. People without creative outlets for this feeling are forced to suffer passively through these phases.

According to this view the personality in a negative Mustard state seems to err in its weak orientation toward its individual Life Plan while being too open to the collective experience. It's important for Mustard personalities to make the best of this state by understanding that the dark periods are part of their own Life Plan and can be transformative in a constructive manner. Experience has shown that the Mustard state is immediately lightened once this has been accepted: You may consciously enter into the mourning state, and you may consciously pass through it. Seen in this way, every negative Mustard state then becomes a precious gift, a reopening of long-shut doors to your inner depths.

The negative Mustard state often occurs before decisive steps are taken in personal development. In the course of our spiritual development almost all of us go through negative Mustard phases so that we may experience this dark cosmic energy within ourselves, live through it in pain, and thereby become transformed.

Some people appear to have a special affinity for this energy quality and are able to transform more of it within themselves than others can. It may be a comfort to them to know that every transformation achieved in the individual has an effect on all others and on the greater whole.

With every dark Mustard day conquered, a little more light is brought to our planet. With this knowledge those in the negative Mustard state may be able to live through their melancholy with more composure.

Edward Bach wrote: "This remedy dispels gloom, and brings joy into life." Anyone taking Mustard has the feeling of slowly waking from a deep, dark dream. People in the positive Mustard state will have a feeling of joyful serenity that stays with them through gray as well as sunny days. They still see the dark clouds, but they don't allow themselves to be depressed by them.

Negative Mustard states show up often in areas such as Scandinavia, where there are long periods without sun in wintertime. Mustard is particularly helpful in fall and spring when phases of depression may set in. During menopause it can be helpful when the production of certain hormones decreases. To address the feelings of collective grief that they've absorbed without even being aware of it, children will select Mustard for themselves in a spontaneous choice.

Observation and experience have shown that depression due to a known cause (Gentian) will additionally cause a drifting toward a negative Mustard state in people with marked Mustard traits.

Mustard Key Symptoms

There are periods of deep gloom and melancholy, which suddenly appear and disappear for no apparent reason.

Behavior Pattern in the Blocked State

- You don't feel like doing anything anymore

- You cry easily and need to shed tears frequently

- You're unable to enjoy anything

- Time seems to pass more slowly

- You don't sense new outer impressions; you feel blocked and cut off from them

- You don't want to move your body

- You suddenly feel weighed down

- You suffer deep depression

- Something heavy, black, and unknown descends; your Soul is in mourning

- Gloominess comes out of the blue, enveloping you in a black cloud

- You feel excluded from normal life

- You find no logical connection between this condition and the other parts of your life

- You feel such deep melancholy that you barely notice what's going on

- You're completely within yourself and caught up in grief

- You're unable to hide this mood from others

- You're unable to overcome the mood through logical thinking, or to shake it off at will

- You're at the mercy of this feeling until it lifts of its own accord, when you feel as though you've been set free from prison

- You're afraid of these attacks because they're totally out of your control

Even if only one or two of these patterns precisely match your present situation, you need Mustard.

Positive Potential

- You feel carried by the stream of life

- You accept the ebb and flow of nature, knowing that joy always returns just as the sun comes back from behind the clouds

- You pass through even cloudy days in serenity, with clear inner confidence

- You have rich emotions and sense things deeply

Empowering Statements

- "I feel light."

- "I am happy."

- "I am in the light."

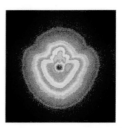

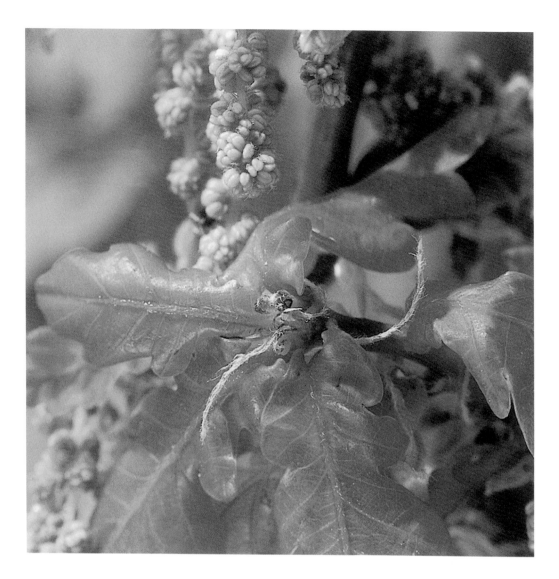

22. Oak: *The Endurance Flower*
From Unflagging Duty to Inner Commitment

For those who are struggling and fighting strongly to get well, or in connection with the affairs of their daily life. They will go on trying one thing after another, though their case may seem hopeless.

They will fight on. They are discontented with themselves if illness interferes with their duties or helping others.

*They are brave people, fighting against
great difficulties, without loss of hope or effort.*

Edward Bach

Oak, the holy tree of the Druids, relates to the Soul's potential for strength and endurance. In the negative Oak state these potentials are used in too rigid a manner. Instead of allowing itself to be guided by the Higher Self through both difficult and enjoyable periods in life, the personality becomes stuck in self-imposed high-performance stress. Life is then a constant struggle. An Oak person has all the attributes of a winner: inborn rugged strength and resistance,* almost superhuman endurance, tremendous will-power, courage, devotion to duty, unbending resolve, and high ideals.

But those in the negative Oak state may have forgotten that it's not only performance that makes life worth living, but also the more subtle, playful, or tenderhearted moments in their existence, which in turn reenergize them for new accomplishments.

If they don't allow themselves these creative, refreshing interludes, their inner lives will grow more and more austere and impoverished. They'll work on, but their hearts won't be in their efforts. Endurance will imperceptibly become a

goal in itself, making these individuals rigid high-performance engines, automatically running on and on until the wear and tear finally bring them to a stop. Then there will be a sudden attack, a nervous breakdown, a seizing up that could manifest in physical symptoms representing rigidity and loss of flexibility.

It's no coincidence that the colloquial German term *German oak* is used for people for whom doing one's duty is one of the highest virtues. Former chancellor Otto von Bismarck, for example, called *der eiserne Kanzler* (the Iron Chancellor), had many attributes of the negative Oak type. In fact, it has been said that he would stand next to the gigantic oak trees on his estate in the forest of Saxony in order to "load up on the strength of his ancestry." Interestingly, people needing Oak often have a strong and gnarled appearance, much like the oak tree itself.

"He is the mainstay of the firm, a real worker, and the only one you can really rely on," others will admiringly say of a person with marked Oak traits. "No good complaining—it's got to be done!" an Oak person herself will say, rolling up her sleeves and getting on with it. Oak people will pursue a degree in evening classes even if it takes them years. Oak mothers in the negative state are unceasing in their efforts at looking after the family. They may not have had a vacation for years, but would never admit to being overworked.

People with Oak characteristics do not take the easy way out. It's they who will keep the

---

* It's interesting to note that oak trees are so highly resistant that they can survive in places where the earth's radiation is of such intensity that other trees, for example beeches, will perish. These locations, however, attract lightning, hence the German saying: "When in a thunderstorm, seek the beech tree for shelter and avoid the oak."

whole family going through difficult times or who are able to sustain an entire nation in periods of crisis. Their enormous contribution is not always properly recognized and suitably compensated, and this is partly their own fault. The strong Oak type in a negative behavior pattern feels an inner aversion to ever appearing weak in front of others. Unjustifiably worried about being dependent, she would rather do anything than ask others for help. During an illness he will do his best to get well again quickly.

Many Oak characters have an honorable, indeed noble, mind. They help others of their own accord, and nothing makes them more discontented and unhappy than to be unable to meet the obligations they have accepted. Nothing makes them more depressed than having to disappoint what they perceive to be other people's expectations of them. It's a joy to them to feel the reflection of the pleasure they've given to those around them, pleasure they believe they have to deny themselves on their strenuous, stony path through life. Others often wonder what makes such people strive for tremendous achievement without ever losing courage in the face of adversity.

Psychologically, the roots of the negative Oak state are to be found in childhood in families where achievements are taken for granted and little feedback is given in terms of praise or disapproval. In adulthood the need to achieve becomes a purpose of its own. As soon as the personality consciously or unconsciously recognizes this and, instead of mindlessly battling on, becomes flexible in following its Inner Guidance, the sooner the journey through life will become both easier and more pleasant.

When taking Oak, you'll soon find inner pressure reducing, with energies flowing more freely and abundantly. Heart, body, and spirit are given new life. The playful elements return and, with them, joy in life. It will then be possible to meet your commitments without an overly strong effort. You'll be indeed as strong as an Oak, with new primal energies constantly arising from the very soil.

Oak has proved helpful during recovery from long-term illness when a patient, despite resolutely persisting, slowly grows tired of continued treatments such as physical therapy. It will provide new momentum and power to persevere in a more relaxed way.

Oak helps students who have a great deal of work to master their tasks without becoming overly grim.

Oak Key Symptoms
You are like the exhausted fighter who struggles on bravely, never giving up.

Behavior Pattern in the Blocked State
❁ You're overly dutiful and reliable, no matter what the costs

❁ You overwork yourself, and then grow despondent

- You work very hard but never complain

- You have almost superhuman endurance but little concern for your own needs

- You force yourself to finish any work that you've started

- Unceasing and persistent in your endeavors, you force yourself to keep going even when you have no energy

- You fight bravely against all odds, even if there's little hope left

- You often continue to work only from a sense of duty

- You think in terms such as, "I owe this to myself"

- You shoulder the burdens of others

- You ignore natural impulses to rest

- You try not to let your tiredness and weakness become obvious to others

- You're admired because you don't let things get you down

Even if only one or two of these patterns precisely match your present situation, you need Oak.

Positive Potential

- You fulfill your duty within the parameters of what is possible

- You deal creatively and skillfully with difficult, stressful tasks

- You accomplish a great deal but are also able to say, "That's enough!"

- You master life joyfully, with strength and endurance

Empowering Statements

- "I relax."

- "I finish easily."

- "I feel free."

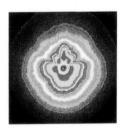

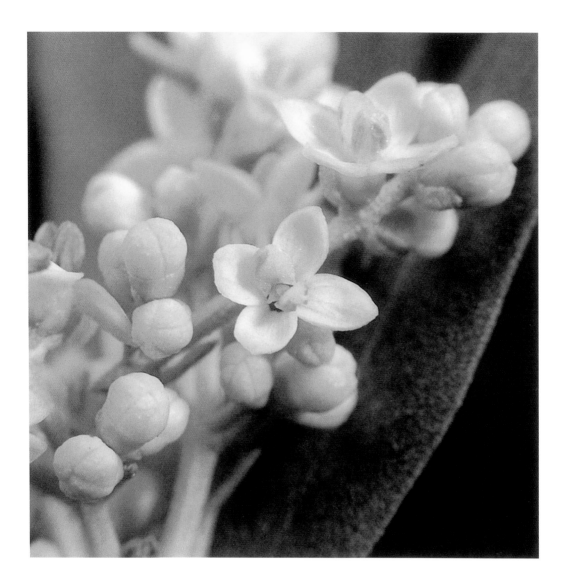

23. Olive: The Regeneration Flower
From Exhaustion to Inner Renewal

Those who have suffered much mentally or physically and are so exhausted and weary that they feel they have no more strength to make any effort. Daily life is hard work for them, without pleasure.

Edward Bach

The dove brought Noah an olive branch to indicate that the flood was over and peace and quiet had returned to the earth. In a similar way the Flower Olive relates to the principle of regeneration, to peace and order being restored. The negative Olive state is the "calm" following the storm, when your body, mind, and spirit are utterly exhausted and spent after a long period of great strain. It occurs, for instance, after a long-term physical illness; a prolonged unbalanced diet; severe lack of sleep; a period of time in which you've neglected yourself in order to nurse a family member; years of volunteer work on top of a full-time job; or a powerful inner development process that has absorbed a great deal of energy.

The negative Olive state always represents a reaction that might be best summarized as "There's nothing left." You don't want to see or hear anymore but just want to go to sleep or be allowed simply to sit. The smallest jobs—even doing the dishes and opening the mail—become insurmountable obstacles. "I'm so exhausted I could cry"; "I'm completely finished"; " I'm so tired I feel sick"; "I'm not even interested in doing my favorite hobby now"—these are typical expressions of the negative Olive state.

If you find yourself quite often in this state, you'll have to learn to manage your vital energies properly. Your error lies in completely spending yourself at the personality level, where energies are limited, rather than drawing strength from a higher source.

Especially during periods of extraordinary strain and demand, this negative state shows that we can't rely only on personal energy to keep up our performance. To survive without harm from the tasks that push us beyond our personal limits, we must learn to draw on a source higher than ourselves. This form of cosmic energy has no limits, and we can access it if we ask for it consciously, knowing that, as children of the universe, we must rely on it.

At the same time it's important to recognize and accept the needs and requirements of our own bodies. Our Inner Guidance uses signals to let us know that we are draining ourselves emotionally, mentally, or physically. People who have taken on too much for a long time find it difficult to receive and accept the warning because the signals of the physical body become very weak.

In the practice of Bach Flower Therapy it's essential to pay particular attention to the physical condition of a person in a negative Olive state. Poor physical function often serves to indicate that the flow of energy is disturbed throughout the entire system, which can manifest as abnormal oxygen levels in the blood, for instance, or as reduced kidney function, or toxic intestinal flora. The negative Olive state calls for a thorough medical checkup and follow-up treatment. Interestingly, Olive is always of great assistance in the treatment of debilitating physical conditions because it strengthens the entire human system.

When taking Olive, people usually experience a great need for sleep. Just as with all Bach Flower reactions, you need to accept and give in to this natural healing phase. In doing so your body regenerates and you finally begin to feel rested. If this surrender does not occur, the memory of the exhaustion may linger far beyond the time when the body has caught up. Olive is instrumental in relieving this sensation of "leftover" spiritual exhaustion.

Those in the positive Olive state will find that they have enough strength and positive thinking to enable them to cope with even the greatest stress. To others they appear to have inexhaustible resources and the ability to remain flexible in adapting to the energy demands made of them. Such people give themselves up completely to Inner Guidance, knowing that cosmic energy will flow to them from the universe whenever needed.

Olive Key Symptoms

You feel complete exhaustion and extreme physical and mental fatigue.

Behavior Pattern in the Blocked State

- ❁ You feel completely sapped; everything is "too much"

- ❁ You experience exhaustion following a long period of strain or physical illness

- ❁ You feel completely washed out, finished

- ❁ You want only peace and quiet

- ❁ You have no energy or motivation to do anything

- ❁ Even talking on the telephone or reading a letter requires too much effort

- ❁ You experience deep inner weariness after periods of great inner struggle and transformation that have absorbed a great deal of psychic energy

- ❁ You've recovered physically but not spiritually

- ❁ Phases of great productivity are regularly followed by those of extreme exhaustion because you've given too much of yourself

Even if only one or two of these patterns precisely match your present situation, you need Olive.

Positive Potential

- ❁ You can make economical use of your own reserves

- ❁ When needed, you're able to summon great strength and vitality

- ❁ You understand your connection with Mother Earth and draw on nature's energy reserves

- ❁ During periods of stress you rely on Inner Guidance, and are thus able to cope appropriately with even extreme demands

Empowering Statements

- ❁ "I am peaceful."

- ❁ "I am strong."

- ❁ "I am renewed."

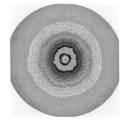

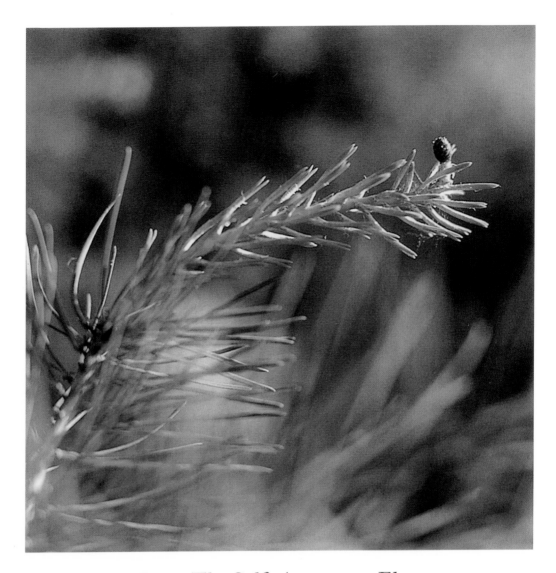

24. Pine: The Self-Acceptance Flower
From Self-Negation to Self-Respect

For those who blame themselves. Even when successful they think they could have done better, and are never content with their efforts or the results. They are hard-working and suffer much from the faults they attach to themselves.

Sometimes if there is any mistake it is due to another, but they will claim responsibility even for that.

Edward Bach

Pine relates to the Soul quality of self-acceptance. If you're in the negative Pine state, you'll put yourself down due to inappropriate feelings of guilt. The scale of self-accusations varies from minor to severe. One person upbraids himself for having neglected to greet his neighbor in a friendly enough manner, another feels remorse for consuming meat, and a third feels the remnants of the archetypal guilt of original sin. Negative Pine together with negative Holly may be one of the most profound and deeply human negative archetypal states. Taking Pine can free us from feeling tied down by feelings of unnecessary guilt. This Essence may be one of the greatest gifts Edward Bach left for us.

The negative Pine state often betrays itself in unconscious, guilt-tinged statements such as, "I'll never forgive myself for having been so careless"; "Please excuse me for taking this seat"; "I know it's my fault that my son is so noisy"; and "Well, my parents actually wanted a girl, but they had to make do with a son."

Experience from studying many cases suggests that a negative Pine state often originates in the mother's womb. A child who was not planned, for instance, may not be accepted, or a child may be considered by the parents as the "wrong" gender, or perhaps the mother became very ill during the pregnancy.

As a Pine type in the negative state, your whole feeling for life may be colored by guilt and therefore you tend to feel physically tired and worn out. Joy plays practically no role in your existence. You're never really satisfied with yourself despite many positive accomplishments, and you blame yourself for not having taken more trouble to do something. You ask more of yourself than you do of others, always focusing on the missing 2 percent, yet despite your Herculean efforts, you still have a chronically guilty conscience.

Another common trait of the negative Pine state is a readiness to assume the blame for the mistakes of others, feeling that you share responsibility for them. Those with negative Pine behavior patterns may feel guilty for asking an inconsiderate neighbor to turn down the stereo. Children in this state tend to be the scapegoats in class and will uncomplainingly take punishment for misdeeds they haven't committed. When such people are ill or overworked, they'll apologize to everyone. A Pine person shopping at the bakery will stand back if there are only four loaves of bread left and there are five people in line—he would feel guilty if another person had to go without while he walked out with the last loaf.

As a Pine type in the negative state you are always apologizing to the extent that it seems you are sorry for existing altogether, as though you lack a heartfelt conviction that you deserve to be on this earth. You unconsciously seem to await punishment for your "wrongdoing" due to a childlike anxiety characterized by a strong inner sense of right and wrong.

And when there's no punishment from

greater powers, you punish yourself. This is why many people in the negative Pine state unconsciously "take up the cross" by accepting an unnecessary burden. Some negative Pine types have an almost masochistic desire to sacrifice themselves and may punish themselves for years by, for instance, unconsciously choosing a brutal partner. They are determined to offer love though they never may be able to ask for it in return.

This is the tragic, life-destroying error of the negative Pine personality. Because, through self-designed circumstances, it shuts itself off from receiving love, no love and no divine energy can reach it, and ultimately it becomes unable to give love. It not only cuts off its own life energy but also commits a sin against Unity and, through its self-destructive guilt, irritates and damages its surroundings.

The reason for such an attitude is based on the personality looking in the wrong direction, limiting itself to live by its own concept of good and evil, claiming the right of being its own judge, rather than accepting what it learns under the guidance of its Higher Self.

If you're in the negative Pine state, you need to understand the profound meaning of being human and that the very fact that we live and breathe on this earth makes any doubt about our right to exist an utter absurdity. There is but one trespass: to disobey your Inner Guidance and ignore the needs of your Life Plan.

To differentiate between true or appropriate guilt and guilt that is uncalled for (Pine), you must face your guilt again and again throughout your life. People who have opened up to the positive potential of Pine have found self-respect after a long journey of getting to know themselves and being responsible for themselves. These people are the priests of everyday life— they can support others whose consciences are tormented by guilt.

Pine is an important remedy after abortions, or as an accompaniment to the psychotherapeutic treatment of the victims of severe child abuse.

Pine Key Symptoms
Among these are self-reproach, inappropriate guilt feelings, and a tendency to apologize frequently.

Behavior Pattern in the Blocked State
⊛ You apologize in all kind of situations

⊛ You haven't forgiven yourself for something you've done and still blame yourself after many years

⊛ Your troubled conscience is easily triggered and is then difficult to turn off

⊛ You feel responsible for other people's mistakes

⊛ You feel guilty if you're better off than others

⊛ Even if you do something successfully, you feel you could have done some part of it better and are consequently unable to enjoy the success at all

❁ You feel you must justify things you have bought for your own comfort

❁ You feel unworthy and undeserving, like a naughty child waiting to be punished

❁ You excuse yourself for being ill, depressed, or exhausted

❁ You find it difficult to accept presents, unconsciously feeling you don't deserve them

❁ You feel guilty when you need to speak firmly to others

❁ You take little for yourself and give others the first choice when supplies are low

❁ You chastise yourself for not making as much money as others

❁ You blame yourself for being part of a society that destroys the environment and takes advantage of other people

❁ You feel undeserving of love, refusing yourself the right to exist—"Forgive me for having been born"

❁ You feel like a child fearfully waiting to be criticized

❁ You feel an almost masochistic desire to sacrifice yourself; you are given to negative narcissism

❁ Any appropriate guilt you feel is blown out of proportion

Even if only one or two of these patterns precisely match your present situation, you need Pine.

Positive Potential

❁ You're aware that everybody alive has the right to exist

❁ You know that you're worthy of being loved, just as is every human being

❁ You have a deep understanding of human nature, particularly of human weaknesses

❁ You're able to accept presents and to praise yourself for a job well done

❁ You know the limits of your own responsibility and know where that of others begins

❁ You're a good listener and adviser to others who suffer from guilt feelings

Empowering Statements

❁ "I am allowed to . . ."

❁ "I am accepted."

❁ "I am freed."

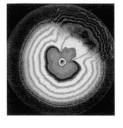

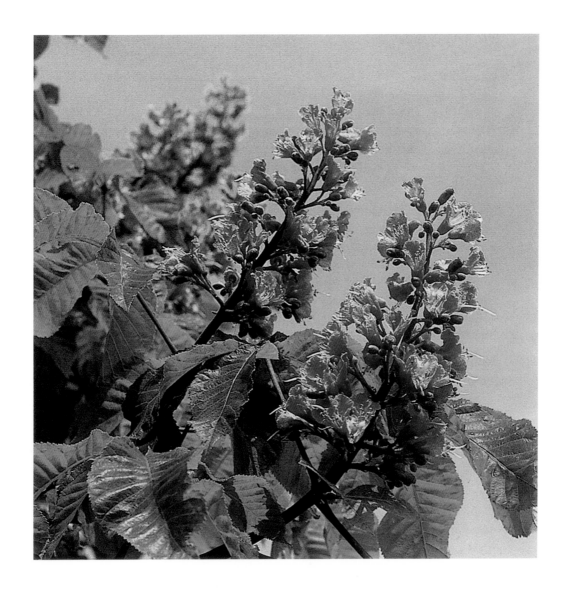

25. Red Chestnut: The Cutting-Free Flower
From Symbiosis to Autonomy

For those who find it difficult not to be anxious for other people.
  Often they have ceased to worry about themselves, but for those of whom they are fond they
may suffer much, frequently anticipating that some unfortunate thing may happen to them.

Edward Bach

Red Chestnut relates to the Soul's potential for caring and having compassion for others. The main characteristic of the Red Chestnut state is a powerful energy link between two individuals. People who frequently need Red Chestnut find it very easy to tune in to other people, to identify and empathize with them and imagine themselves in their places. Red Chestnut types are able to project their energy very strongly. From an energy point of view, they are great transmitters. People for whom they feel concerned—relatives, children, friends, and so forth—are well aware of this fact.

Red Chestnut people in the negative state are seemingly altruistic in their care for others, always watching out for them in case the worst happens. These are the fathers who can't go to sleep at night until their teenage daughters are home safe and sound after an evening at the movies. These are the mothers who can't be at peace—even late at night—until their grown children have called to report that they've safely reached their travel destinations. These are the grandmothers who choke up when they think about their grandchildren crossing a busy road on their own.

Red Chestnut people in a negative behavior pattern suffer for those they love and think the others don't notice their anxiety or concern. However, they remain unaware that they're projecting their own fears onto others, doing harm not only to themselves but also to those they care for. There is indeed a risk of actually attracting the things they dread with their negative energy. Bach described a trip he once made to an emergency room. He could feel in the form of acute physical pain the concern that his colleagues at the hospital had for him.

Those in the negative Red Chestnut state could also be said to experience a symbiotic relationship to their loved ones similar to that between mother and infant. The infant depends wholly on her mother for survival. The mother, too, is emotionally tied to the child. Mothers and fathers in the negative Red Chestnut state tend to hold on to the close bond with their children for too long. In many cases the cord is never severed, or is insufficiently severed. The disadvantage, then, for both parents and children is that their respective spiritual developments can be delayed. Neither is able to recognize their personal Life Plan because of the interference of the other. The equilibrium of an existing symbiotic state needs to be maintained in order for it to function so that when one partner attempts to sever the cord, the other will accept it.

Illustrating this is the case of a divorced mother and her depressed sixteen-year-old son, which was reported in England. In the course of psychotherapeutic treatment the mother realized that she was using her son to meet her own emotional needs. Her son, being unconsciously aware of this, started withdrawing from her and from reality into his own world of fantasy. The mother then took Red Chestnut. A few days later her son grew extremely depressed. When he came out of this phase, however, he was prepared to undergo treatment himself, something he had refused to do for years. Red Chestnut had enabled the mother to loosen the bond between them, and at that moment the son, too, was for the first time able to take steps on his own.

Similar symbiotic bonds are also common among married couples, particularly when powerful parental projections are involved. The wife may project her problematic bond with her father onto the husband, or the husband may try to maintain a relationship with his mother by projecting it onto his wife. Occasionally an unrecognized symbiotic bond may also exist between two people when one is no longer alive, as between a son and his father who was killed during a war.

In reality, the negative Red Chestnut state is nothing but a connection at the wrong level. It takes place at the subjective, emotional, and anxiety-ridden personality level rather than at the spiritual level between the Higher Self of one person and that of another. In the negative Red Chestnut state the concept of caring is misunderstood by the personality. You unconsciously use another person as an object onto whom you project your own fears, worries, and doubts. It's important for you to realize that things always work out differently from the way our minds have planned them. It's impossible, however great your effort, to prevent others from meeting their destinies.

A German proverb suggests that humans do

the thinking, but God shows the way. "I hope she does well. Let's hope the best for her. She'll find the right way"—once you begin thinking in these terms, you'll experience the positive side of Red Chestnut energy and have the pleasure of seeing things turning out better and better for yourself and those around you.

Together with Walnut, Red Chestnut is a helpful tool for people whose work involves taking care of others. It can keep them from becoming too involved on a personal, emotional level, and can help them to concentrate instead on keeping up the dialogue with their own Inner Guidance. Red Chestnut also has been helpful during weaning when given to both mother and child. Combined with White Chestnut, Red Chestnut will help those whose worries concerning another person keep returning despite efforts to make them go away. In combination with Rock Rose, Red Chestnut will help when there is extreme, acute worry about another person. Even people who feel as though they have been completely taken over or possessed by an addiction or powerful desire can often be helped with Red Chestnut.

Red Chestnut Key Symptoms

You experience fear or excessive concern for others; you are too emotionally connected to another person.

Behavior Pattern in the Blocked State

✮ Your inner bond with another person is too strong

- You experience excessive concern for the safety of others—such as children or a partner—with no fear for yourself

- You worry too much about the problems of others; your feelings are drawn too strongly into another's life

- You feel the life of another as if it were your own

- You know the feelings of another better than your own

- You're afraid something bad may have happened to another person who is late for an engagement

- You immediately feel the symptoms of an illness another person is talking about on the phone

- You're afraid that behind the harmless symptoms another person describes lurks a more serious disease

- You've been unable to "cut the cord" with someone close to you

- You constantly warn children or grandchildren to be careful

- You burden others with your worry over their well-being

Even if only one or two of these patterns precisely match your present situation, you need Red Chestnut.

Positive Potential

- You always know how to balance your concern with a respect for another's autonomy

- You're able to put yourself into another person's shoes

- You can empathize with the sorrows of others without making them your own

- You're able to radiate to others positive thoughts of security, well-being, and courage in difficult situations

Empowering Statements

- "I am myself."

- "I stay with myself."

- "I am me and you are you."

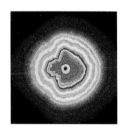

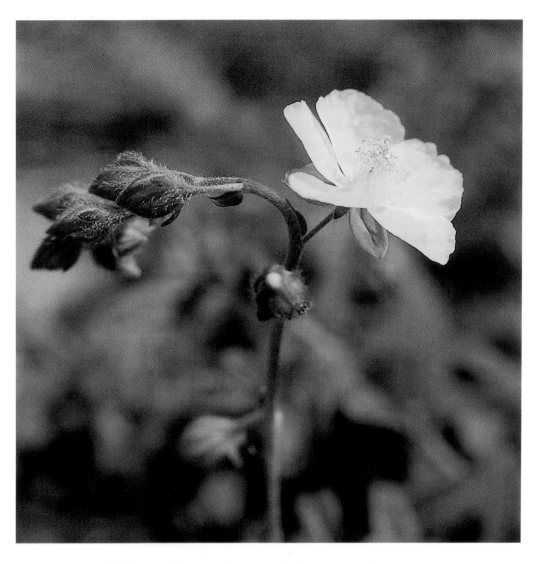

26. Rock Rose: The Liberation Flower
From Panic to Heroic Courage

The remedy of emergency for cases where there even appears no hope. In accident or sudden illness, or when the patient is very frightened or terrified, or if the condition is serious enough to cause great fear to those around. If the patient is not conscious the lips may be moistened with the remedy. Other remedies in addition may also be required, as, for example, if there is unconsciousness, which is a deep, sleepy state, Clematis; if there is torture, Agrimony, and so on.

Edward Bach

Rock Rose relates to the Soul qualities of courage and steadfastness. Within the negative Rock Rose state, Bach perceived the strongest fear a human can experience. Therefore, this Flower is one of the most important components of Rescue Remedy. The following scenario illustrates the negative Rock Rose state: A refugee escapes across the border. The ground has been mined. Searchlights are sweeping the area at regular intervals. Suddenly, the sound of barking dogs comes from behind. Has he been spotted? His heart is beating wildly. In total panic, and feeling like a hunted creature, he runs and runs for his life.

A personality in the negative Rock Rose state is under acute threat mentally and often physically, as well. These are moments of crisis—exceptional situations such as accidents, sudden illness, and natural disasters, when a human being is unable to cope with the onrush of elemental energies. Everything is happening too fast, going in the wrong direction. The personality cowers fearfully within its mortal confines, separated by worlds from its Higher Self, unable to trust in and receive the energies of its Inner Guidance, which it sorely needs in order to master the situation.

This is an extreme case of the negative Rock Rose state. Not every situation is as dramatic, but all Rock Rose states show a characteristically intense level of inner alarm. For example, you're coming home from the airport in a taxi late at night, and you get ready to take out your purse with your money and house keys—but the purse is nowhere to be found. Suddenly breaking into a sweat, you desperately try to figure out whether you left it on the nightstand in your Paris hotel or possibly packed it in the suitcase, which is in the trunk and cannot be checked now. Your mind is racing, fear grabs hold of you because you have to face the driver with no money to pay for the fare. You're totally unable to think clearly.

The Rock Rose state has been aptly described as "a punch to the stomach," for the solar plexus does indeed tense up. Too much is coming in too quickly, and the central nervous system is unable to cope. The solar plexus chakra freezes in a wide-open position. To some people in this situation, the solar plexus resembles a sore hole or a stone in the pit of the stomach. In such a state people feel helpless, exposed, and completely at the mercy of the world around them. They "sweat blood and water" and every cell in their body reacts with fear. Some sensitive people have reported that the fear spreads into every part of the aura.

Rock Rose energy liberates the personality from its state of fear, letting the pendulum swing from the negative back to the positive state.* Self-centered fear becomes courage. In extreme cases it can even become heroic courage leading to a forgetting of the self for the sake of others. This is the courage that allows a mother to stop a

---

* The flowers of the Rock Rose are a particularly brilliant yellow, which is the color of flowers capable of storing the greatest amount of the sun's energy.

rolling car with her bare hands when it threatens to run over her child who is happily at play. It's the heroism that helps people stand up against an oppressor's army of overwhelming power and win. Rock Rose is able to mobilize tremendous forces that allow us to grow beyond ourselves.

Normally the negative Rock Rose state is only temporary. It's quite often found in children, whose psyches aren't yet as stable as adults'. Among adults there are genuine Rock Rose types, although they may not always appear very nervous on the outside. Still, they are easily stricken by panic, when they lose perspective and run around almost literally like "a chicken with its head cut off." These individuals are born with a nervous system so delicate that their energy resources are easily exhausted. In medical terms they have an unstable vegetative system or are labeled chronically nervous. Frequently it's found that those in a more chronic negative Rock Rose state had a parent who experienced drug- or alcohol-related problems. Negative Rock Rose states may develop from engaging in some spiritual practices that suddenly confront you with overwhelming archetypal darkness.

Children who wake up screaming from a nightmare should be given sips of Rock Rose until they have calmed down again. Likewise, someone who has narrowly escaped a car accident and still feels the fear in his bones will benefit from Rock Rose. At times Rock Rose is recommended as additional medication in the conventional treatment of sun- and heatstroke.

It has often been proved to be helpful for fear of thunderstorms. In everyday life, if your nerves are on edge and you tend to overreact, Rock Rose—like Rescue Remedy—will help restore balance.

Rock Rose Key Symptoms
You acutely feel fear, panic, and terror.

Behavior Pattern in the Blocked State
* You tend to panic easily

* Your nerves are weak; you overreact and often feel helpless

* Your anxiety level quickly escalates in threatening situations

* You feel terror, horror, and naked fear—as though your nerves have gone haywire

* When in a panic, your senses stop working; you're unable to see, hear, or speak, and your heart nearly stops

* You panic in accidents and natural disasters, or if you experience a life-threatening illness or disease

* You can still feel the fear in your bones after barely escaping a dangerous situation

* Children easily get sweaty palms, and their hearts often beat wildly

* Your solar plexus hurts or feels rock hard

Even if only one or two of these patterns precisely match your present situation, you need Rock Rose.

Positive Potential

❁ You meet emergencies with a calm presence of mind and are able to do things for the benefit of others

❁ In serious crises you rely consciously on your Inner Guidance

❁ In crisis situations you are able to mobilize tremendous forces that allow you to do more than you are normally capable of doing

❁ You show heroic courage; you fight in the front lines

Empowering Formulas

❁ "I will survive."

❁ "I keep things in perspective."

❁ "I follow my Inner Guidance."

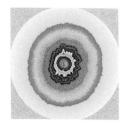

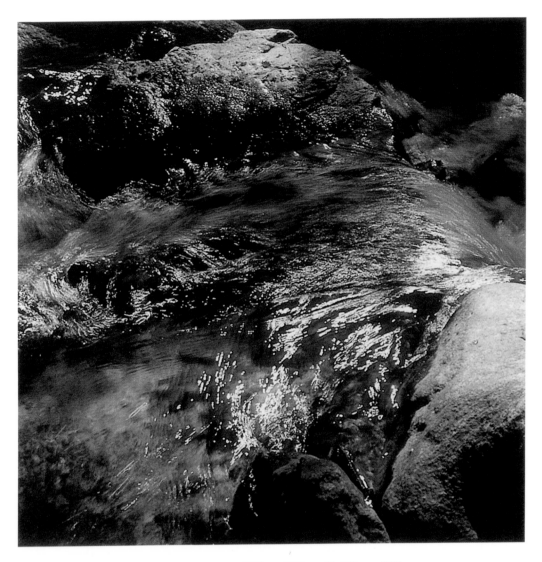

27. Rock Water: The Flexibility Flower
From Dogmatic Discipline to Attentiveness

Those who are very strict in their way of living; they deny themselves many of the joys and pleasures of life because they consider it might interfere with their work.

They are hard masters to themselves. They wish to be well and strong and active, and will do anything which they believe will keep them so. They hope to be examples which will appeal to others who may then follow their ideas and be better as a result.

Edward Bach

Rock Water relates to the Soul qualities of flexibility and inner freedom. In the negative Rock Water state you try to fulfill theoretical ideals that are out of touch with what is realistically possible. People in a negative Rock Water state erect a mental monument of high spiritual ideals, moral guidelines, and perfectionist concepts and then feel dwarfed by these and by the responsibility they impose upon themselves to live up to them.

If you're in the negative Rock Water state, you deny yourself many of the things that make everyday life pleasant and enjoyable in the belief that these don't fit in with your strict, often downright ascetic vision of life. At a silver anniversary party you'll be the only teetotaler raising your glass of mineral water to toast the happy couple, rather than a glass of champagne.

Rock Water types want to be in top shape both mentally and physically and will avidly pursue any course that might lead them to this prime condition. A classic Rock Water type is the woman who arrives at the swimming pool at seven in the morning after having jogged through the woods for half an hour. She doggedly swims her fifty laps and thereafter sits down with a serious face to eat whole-grain cereal, which she has ground herself. If you're in the extreme negative Rock Water state, you also want to be an example to others. You quietly hope to move others to take up your own ideals so that they, too, find the right path.

Many Rock Water types expect themselves to be "saints on earth." They force themselves into an iron corset of high standards and discipline, particularly through activities that are tangible and can be tracked. They will frequently overdo things, spending hours every day on yoga exercises, rigidly adhering to macrobiotic principles, or going through a specific regimen of mental exercise wherever they may be.

Often, the high theories and ideals of Rock Water people come from ancient traditions that achieved great things in their time and place but are not entirely compatible with contemporary life—and are therefore almost impossible to realize. Those in the negative Rock Water state will, however, fail to recognize this. They will torture themselves with self-reproach when the demands of everyday life make it impossible to meet their daily training quota. This, of course, can harm their development much more than hours of training, meditating, and the like are able to offset.

People in the negative Rock Water state don't make good partners in discussions. Whether the subject is politics, pollution, or philosophy, their position will always be "right" and absolute. They can't acknowledge arguments that don't fit their scheme and so simply ignore these.

Yet unlike the Vervain type, those in the negative Rock Water state won't attempt to impose their philosophy on another person because they're far too busy trying to meet their exaggerated self-imposed standards. Similar to those in the Water Violet state, there is a tendency toward conceit for those in the negative Rock Water state—a sort of spiritual pride, a shaking of the head in pity while saying, "It's a good thing I'm doing it the right way."

In the Rock Water state you don't recognize the constant inner coercion that's occurring, or the fact that you're constantly suppressing important human needs. You fail to note the extent to which you're regularly using force upon yourself, or the degree to which pleasure in life has been suffocated by your self-imposed disciplines. In many people these ceaseless, exaggerated demands are sooner or later expressed in different forms of physical inflexibility. Negative Rock Water types rarely understand or integrate physical needs.

In the negative Rock Water state you are too strongly identified with principles on the mental plane. The personality becomes frozen in the dogmas and beliefs it has decided upon while ignoring the demands of reality. It absolutely must be what it considers "good," and must not be what it has identified as "not good." Yet the things it believes to be "not good" may be precisely those things necessary for its development. The error lies in a personal drive that is too strong, limited, and self-willed, and in a misdirected, material approach to life. The personality egotistically wants to force its development, confusing external effect with inner cause. It fails to see that an external effect—say, a change in lifestyle—will come of its own accord once the inner conditions for it are met. It does not understand that certain behaviors are the consequence, not the cause, of spiritual growth. In wanting to enforce external changes that are against its Life Plan, the personality is fighting its Higher Self rather than letting itself be guided by it. It is above all failing to understand that self-mastery is achieved not by concentrating on the self but by forgetting the self in service to the greater Unity.

If you're in the negative Rock Water state, you need encouragement to bravely face your true personality in the spirit of the sentiment "nobody's perfect." If you can learn to forgo high-minded theories and trust yourself to the rhythms of real life, you'll transform from a rough rock to a smooth stone traveling without difficulty from one current in life to another. Cast off your straitjacket once and for all and stop passing up the fullness and abundance of life! Interestingly, one sensitive person who took Rock Water felt "gently caressed all over my body," experiencing at the same time a "rebirth into reality," as he put it.

People in the positive Rock Water state may be described as flexible idealists. They are able to put aside their principles and much lauded convictions when confronted with new insights and greater truths. They keep an open mind. They are alert and use discipline in constantly monitoring their ideals with respect to their real-life situation. Consequently they are able, over time, to truly bring many of their ideals to proper realization, and this, of its own accord, makes them an example to others.

Extreme negative Rock Water cases are admittedly not very common. Yet Rock Water is quite frequently indicated for many; all of us encounter life situations in which we unconsciously suppress or consciously push aside vital needs such as exercise, sex, and food. In Bach Flower practice, Rock Water has come up in interesting combinations. People who are fighting to build some sort of inner structure benefit from Clematis and Rock Water because they are trying to forcefully integrate their castles in the air with the real world and somehow keep both. Those who choose to undergo frequent elective surgery may need the combination of Rock Water and Willow.

Rock Water Key Symptoms

You're hard on yourself, have strict and rigid views, and suppress your inner needs.

Behavior Pattern in the Blocked State

- ❀ You have a strong desire for self-perfection

- ❀ Your life is ruled by dogmatic theories and high ideals

- ❀ You deny yourself many things because they are not compatible with your principles and consequently much of the pleasure in life is lost

- ❀ You do everything possible to achieve and stay in top shape; self-discipline is a primary goal

- ❀ You've set the highest standards and force yourself to live up to them, almost to the point of self-martyrdom

- ❀ You're unaware of the pressures you constantly place on yourself

- ❀ You often say "I can't afford to let myself do this"

- ❀ You have a workmanlike approach to spirituality, clinging to one particular practice (meditation technique, special diet) and turning it into dogma

- ❀ You compulsively strive for ever-higher spiritual development without challenging your rigidly fixed ideas

- ❀ You don't finish certain projects because you always think they can be improved upon

- ❀ You secretly look down at people who are playful

- ❀ You believe that worldly desires inhibit spiritual development; you endeavor to be a "saint on earth," an ascetic, or a fakir

- ❀ You fall into your own trap when meditating by wanting do it too well

- ❀ You suppress essential physical and emotional needs, such as exercise, sexuality, and food

- ❀ You reproach yourself if you're unable to maintain your self-imposed discipline

- You very strictly adhere to certain principles in your eating habits, whether vegetarian, macrobiotic, or abstinence from alcohol

- You practice the piano until your fingers go numb or ballet until your toes are bloody

- Menstruation can be very painful or disrupted

Even if only one or two of these patterns precisely match your present situation, you need Rock Water.

Positive Potential

- You're able to hold high ideals yet let go of theories and principles if confronted with new insights or deeper truths

- You allow your inner child enough room in your life

- You're respectful of both your physical and your spiritual needs, knowing when each is appropriate

- You rely on your Inner Guidance and, due to your natural discipline, are a good example to others

Empowering Statements

- "I allow myself . . ."

- "I am curious."

- "I am spontaneous."

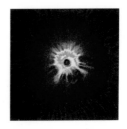

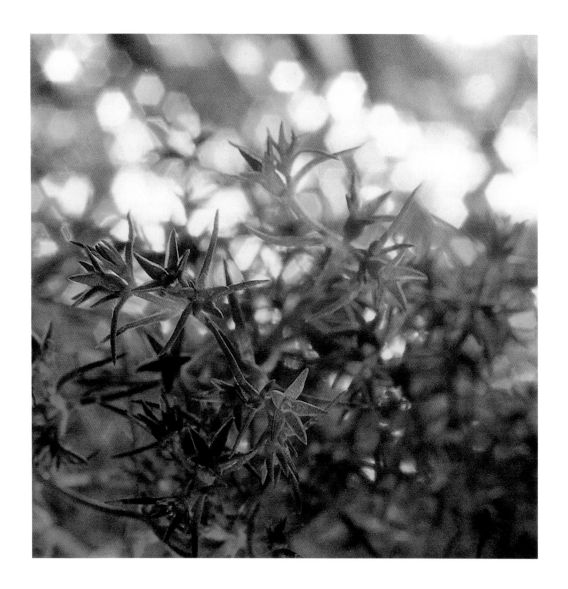

28. Scleranthus: The Balance Flower
From Inner Conflict to Inner Equilibrium

Those who suffer much from being unable to decide between two things, first one seeming right then the other.

They are usually quiet people, and bear their difficulty alone, as they are not inclined to discuss it with others.

Edward Bach

Scleranthus relates to the Soul's potential for balance and decisiveness. Those in the negative Scleranthus state vacillate between different (usually two) possibilities. If you've ever seen a grasshopper respond to the slightest movement in its vicinity by making huge leaps here and there with apparent aimlessness, you can imagine what it feels like inside to be in the negative Scleranthus state. Any outside impulse is enough to spark a reaction, first in one direction, then in another: The new neighbors are charming and you're immediately on the friendliest terms with them, but the next day they get on your nerves to such an extent that you'd really like to slam the door in their face. In the evening you definitely agree to join your friends in renting a house for a weekend vacation, but when you wake up the following morning you wonder what possessed you and you call to get out of the deal. In the course of the phone conversation, however, you allow yourself to be persuaded to reconsider. There will be further to-and-fro on your part until your friends finally find someone else more able to make up his mind.

If you're in the negative Scleranthus state, you're like a balance that's constantly in motion, swinging from one extreme to the other. You're in seventh heaven or miserable as hell; extremely active or completely apathetic; one day, enthusiastic over a new idea, the next, completely uninterested. This constant change of moods and opinions makes those in the negative Scleranthus state appear unstable and unreliable in the eyes of others.

The woman unable to decide between two men is a classic example of this state. When she's with the quiet accountant it's perfectly obvious to her that she'd have a happy, secure home with him. When she goes out with the adventurous engineer who wants to move to Mexico with her, she wonders what's really keeping her at home. When she's on her own and tries to consider what she truly wants, she's never able to come to a decision, but keeps swinging to and fro between the two possibilities for weeks, indeed for months. She doesn't share her doubts—not even with her parents or good friends; unlike Cerato, the negative Scleranthus type will always try to find her own solution, however long that it takes. In his *Handbook of the Bach Flower Remedies*, Dr. Philip Chancellor describes the case of a general who took three months to make up his mind to finally start Bach Flower Therapy.

The vacillating nature of those in this negative behavior pattern may also find expression in nervous, fidgety gestures. The body is constantly involved in one movement or another. "Stop fidgeting!" are words often heard by the child in the negative Scleranthus state. Many of those in need of Scleranthus change their clothes several times a day in reaction to their fluctuating moods.

Patients in this state are irritating to their doctors because their symptoms move around all over the body. "And where does it hurt today?" the practitioner might ask, wondering if it's even worthwhile taking the new symptoms seriously. The lack of inner balance sometimes finds expression in physical symptoms such as dizziness, motion sickness, problems of the inner ear, lateral imbalances, and thyroid problems. Changing moods are also reflected in variations between physical extremes: constipation and diarrhea, above-normal and subnormal temperatures, ravenous hunger and loss of appetite. Because many variations do occur during pregnancy, Scleranthus is often indicated at this time.

Some practitioners are of the opinion that a disposition that tends toward the negative Scleranthus state may develop during the first two or three hours of life, when the baby's environment is chaotic and so many stimuli act at once. The personality can no longer focus clearly; it reacts like a lens covered with tiny cracks from multiple impacts. In the same manner the Scleranthus personality in the negative state is unable to gather and organize thoughts and impulses and focus them to make a purposeful and unambiguous decision. At times its energy meanders aimlessly to and fro through different facets of its consciousness.

The error of the Scleranthus personality in this state lies in refusing to clearly accept the guiding role of its Higher Self. As a result it has no inner direction to give it strength and a sense of balance. As long as it fails to make a clear decision with regard to its Life Plan, it will fall under the influence of many different forces, becoming something like a ball tossed about by earthly dualities, bouncing from one extreme to the other. It therefore squanders valuable time and resources, making no headway in its personal development.

If you're in the negative Scleranthus state, you must do everything possible to find your center and an inner rhythm that's truly your own. A first step would be to consciously seek the middle ground within you, avoiding the extremes of positive and negative experiences. Your attitude should be that of a tightrope walker who starts out by carefully attuning himself to the rhythm of his own movements and then, feet firmly on the rope, eyes firmly focused ahead, lightly moves toward his goal.

This lightness, coming from great inner strength, is typical of people in a positive Scleranthus state. They make their decisions with intuitive confidence at exactly the right moment. People in the positive Scleranthus state are able to incorporate more and more new potentials into their lives without losing their balance. Their inner calm, decisiveness, and straightforward approach has a positive, calming effect on nervous or anxious people around them.

Scleranthus Key Symptoms
You are indecisive and erratic—opinions and moods change from one moment to the next; you lack inner balance.

Behavior Pattern in the Blocked State
❀ You're indecisive, with a certain inner restlessness

- In many areas you vacillate constantly between two possible options because both have advantages

- Your moods fluctuate; you're either crying or laughing, in seventh heaven or miserable

- You respond to numerous outside impulses, jumping to and fro like a grasshopper

- You appear unreliable because you frequently change your mind

- You lack equilibrium and inner balance; your reactions are unstable and nervous

- You find it stressful to reply to questions that require a yes-or-no answer

- Lacking focus, you jump from topic to topic in conversation

- Your indecisiveness costs valuable time and you may miss good opportunities both personally and professionally

- You don't ask advice of others when in inner conflict—instead you try to reach decisions by yourself

- Your gestures are quick and "jumpy"

- Physical symptoms from energy imbalances can include: extreme fluctuation between activity and apathy; body temperature that rises and falls quickly; symptoms that shift all over the body— one day an arm hurts here, the next day a leg hurts there; problems with balance; alternation between hunger and loss of appetite, constipation and diarrhea; motion sickness; and morning sickness

Even if only one or two of these patterns precisely match your present situation, you need Scleranthus.

Positive Potential

- You can focus and concentrate

- By keeping in touch with your center, you maintain your inner balance and rhythm

- You arrive at decisions without delay and with precision

- You are flexible; you have many interests and are able to integrate an increasing number of them into your life

Empowering Statements

- "I stand firm."

- "I know what I want."

- "I decide."

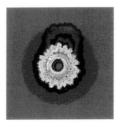

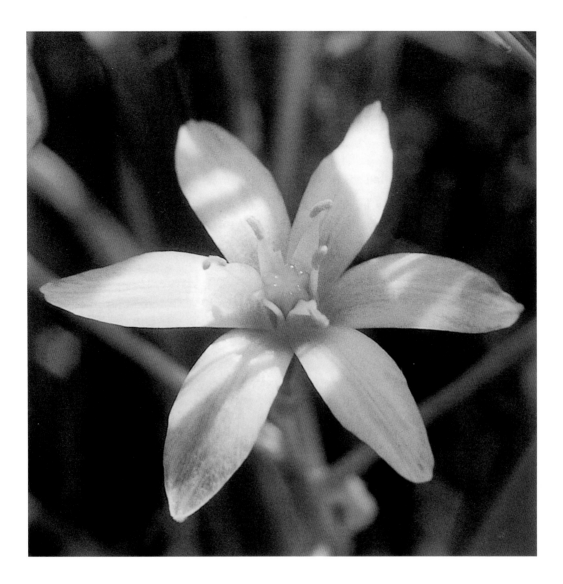

29. Star of Bethlehem: The Comfort Flower
From Shock to Reorientation

For those in great distress under conditions which for a time produce great unhappiness.

The shock of serious news, the loss of someone dear, the fright following an accident, and such like.

For those who for a time refuse to be consoled, this remedy brings comfort.

Edward Bach

Star of Bethlehem relates to the Soul potential for resurrection. Those in the negative Star of Bethlehem state have been shocked and remain in a kind of inner numbness. Star of Bethlehem is indicated for all the consequences of physically, mentally, or spiritually traumatic experiences, irrespective of whether they occurred at birth or only yesterday. It is one of the most important ingredients in Rescue Remedy—it rapidly neutralizes any form of trauma and restores the self-healing mechanisms of the body.

The word *shock*—not to be confused with the medical term—here constitutes any impact of energy on our bodies or minds that is too strong for our energetic systems to handle so that distortions result. Whether or not they have been consciously registered by the personality such shocks will live on* in our energetic systems, causing a certain degree of paralysis or frozen tension.

Practically all of us experience shocking events in the course of our lives that we are unable to cope with. Some of these result in immediate physical symptoms. One case, for instance, documents a beautician who was given notice to vacate her business premises within twenty-four hours and immediately lost full and normal hearing—until she was given Star of Bethlehem. In another case a teacher found herself compelled to run out of the room during a party whenever

someone was about to open a bottle of champagne. It was revealed that as a student she had witnessed an incident in which a flying cork had hit her friend directly in the eye. After taking Star of Bethlehem, she was able to stand by calmly as a bottle was opened.

Even traumatic experiences that occurred twenty years ago can sometimes be cleared with Star of Bethlehem. In one case, a woman who had lived through a bomb attack in a war began Bach Flower treatments because she often felt numb and suffered from chronic arthritis. After taking Star of Bethlehem for several months the memory of the bombing experience resurfaced, after which the numbness released and the arthritis disappeared.

It's important to know, however, that in some cases the cause of this kind of shock may never be identified, or may come to the surface only after studying the circumstances carefully and possibly after months of taking Star of Bethlehem.

In still another case, a mother whose son died when he was twenty-six from a disease that wasn't correctly diagnosed until long after he died was practically petrified after she received the news of the diagnosis. For weeks and months she became more and more quiet—until she took Star of Bethlehem, which brought her back to life. Dr. Bach described this remedy as "[t]he comforter and soother of pains and sorrows."

Although the negative Star of Bethlehem state is not often a character trait, in those rare

---

* Psycho-neuro-immunologists describe this phenomenon vividly by using the term *fingerprint* (in German) or *imprint* (in English) on the immune system.

cases where it is, these people are very sensitive and appear somewhat subdued. They tend to speak in a quiet voice that becomes even more inaudible toward the end of each sentence. They move slowly, often tend to retain water, and sometimes are subtly inclined toward magic and mysticism.

The error in the negative Star of Bethlehem state stems from an inner refusal on the part of the personality to allow itself to fully experience emotional impressions and take a more active part in life. Rather than playing the role on the stage of life that the Higher Self has assigned to the personality, it withdraws from everything that it doesn't want to feel. It "battens down the hatches" and plays dead. The result is that a great deal of impressions that haven't been integrated collect in and clog the more subtle pathways of the psyche. In fact, these can become poisonous psychotoxins, and as they collect it grows more and more difficult for information to be conveyed from one energy level to another. As a consequence even the smallest energy requirement will prove too much for the system to handle, paralyzing it and over time causing more and more parts of the system to cease proper functioning.

Star of Bethlehem rouses the personality from its mental numbness, reconnecting it with its Higher Self. It vitalizes energy links so that psychotoxins begin to dissolve. The personality reintegrates on all levels, becomes livelier, and regains the ability to cope with normal external energies, sensing great vitality, mental clarity, and inner strength.

Frequently (though not always) Star of Bethlehem is needed early in Bach Flower therapy. Consider this Flower when there has been no real response to treatment. It may be that an unconscious shock lodged in the system is still blocking any movement. Star of Bethlehem can act as a catalyst in such cases.

With psychosomatic conditions that prove to be resistant to treatment, Star of Bethlehem sometimes yields remarkable results, particularly after it has been taken for a number months. It has also often been shown to have relaxing effects on tension in the throat or nervous problems with swallowing (both symbolic of shocking events that "stick in the throat"). Symptoms such as being unable to see, hear, walk, or feel something when it is touched may also indicate a need for Star of Bethlehem. Those who have taken many narcotics in their life may benefit from Star of Bethlehem combined with Crab Apple. Star of Bethlehem may be given to newborns to counteract the trauma of cutting the umbilical cord—together with Walnut, it helps ease the change to a new form of existence. Some practitioners suggest adding the mixture to an infant's bathwater.

Another use for Star of Bethlehem is in the easing of some women's heavy menstrual periods; because every menstruation might be seen as a "little birth," each is a kind of mini shock. Finally, treatments designed to help people work through psychic traumas—rebirthing, for instance—can gain valuable support from Star of Bethlehem.

Star of Bethlehem Key Symptoms

These can be any of the aftereffects of physical, mental, or psychic shocks that occurred recently or long ago.

Behavior Pattern in the Blocked State

❀ The rudeness of some people leaves you speechless

❀ You're unable to accept comfort

❀ You experience physical side effects including a loss of feeling, an uncertain gait, a change of voice, and water retention

❀ Unpleasant emotional experiences reverberate inside you for a long time

❀ You're shocked and then sad because of an unpleasant experience

❀ A piece of terrible news "knocks you out"

❀ You can't get over a fight that was unfriendly and hurtful

❀ There's an old wound in your life that you don't dare remember

❀ Following an accident or a surgical procedure, you don't feel like yourself anymore

❀ You react slowly, as if sedated

❀ You let things get too close for comfort, then are unable to cope with them

❀ You repeatedly suffer from the same nightmare

❀ You're easily bruised, physically as well as mentally

Even if only one or two of these patterns precisely match your present situation, you need Star of Bethlehem.

Positive Potential

❀ You take things in deeply and can sense their subtle differences; you're able to relate to all shades of other people's feelings

❀ You've learned to deal appropriately with your emotional experiences, using them for personal development

❀ You give comfort to others

Positive Statements for Practice

❀ "I feel."

❀ "I breathe."

❀ "I am alive!"

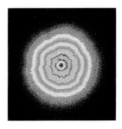

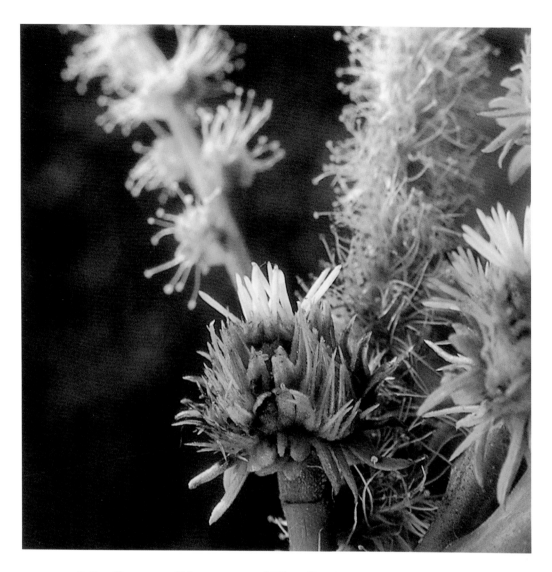

30. Sweet Chestnut: The Deliverance Flower
Through Darkness to Light

For those moments which happen to some people when the anguish is so great as to seem to be unbearable.

When the mind or body feels as if it had borne to the uttermost limit of its endurance, and that now it must give way.

When it seems there is nothing but destruction and annihilation left to face.

Edward Bach

Sweet Chestnut is related to the principle of deliverance. People in the negative Sweet Chestnut state are convinced that there is no longer hope for help. Considering the intensity of the suffering it involves, Sweet Chestnut is probably one of the most intense negative Soul states. It represents the apex of a crisis, but doesn't always present itself dramatically. It occurs more frequently on the inner planes, often without the affected person's awareness.

In the negative Sweet Chestnut state the personality is completely on its own, cornered, utterly helpless and unprotected, like a young bird that has fallen from the nest. Those in this state feel suspended in empty space, like a skydiver who has pulled the ripcord of his parachute a number of times but to no avail. They struggle uncomplainingly, with courage and hope, but ended up empty-handed. For them there is no more yesterday or tomorrow—merely an empty, desperate presence in the here and now and a sense that it's only a matter of hours before the storm-driven flood tide tops the dike.

The negative Sweet Chestnut state is the moment of truth, the extreme confrontation of the personality with itself and at the same time its last, erroneous attempt to fight and resist a crucial inner change. Night has to fall if day is to rise again. The intensity of the suffering seems to go beyond what can be endured. Indeed, endurance is pushed to its very limit so that all the old, fixed structures of the personality may be uprooted and abandoned, making room for new dimensions of consciousness. Suffering is increased to the point where the personality becomes ready to make a quantum leap in development and come up transformed—the Phoenix rising from the ashes.

Sweet Chestnut largely initiates new stages of development, such as letting go of a long-standing destructive relationship, or giving up a profession that does not suit you. The Sweet Chestnut state can also be the guardian of the threshold of genuine spiritual development. When you learn what it means to be truly lonely, left totally to your own devices, the way can open up to another level of consciousness. You realize that everything has been taken away so that you're able to step ahead with your hands free to grasp the new inspiration you meet. You must give yourself up completely in order to be totally reborn.

Typical Sweet Chestnut characters tend to be caught up by extreme, fateful situations and their lives can be very dramatic when compared with the average person. They experience things differently and more intensely. Some who are particularly daring may go beyond traditional mental limits and explore the frontiers of consciousness.

People in the negative Sweet Chestnut state—much like those in the negative Agrimony state—attempt to hide their inner despair from others. But even at times of extreme depression they would never think of wanting to put an end to it all, as negative Cherry Plum people may.

As a result it's not always easy in Bach Flower interviews to recognize a negative Sweet Chestnut state. Indicative are phrases such as "I'm at my wit's end" and "I feel as though I'm at the bottom of a deep hole."

"God's help is near when need is greatest," goes the saying, aptly describing the effect of Sweet Chestnut energy. Sweet Chestnut helps you get through difficult periods of transformation without losing yourself or breaking apart in the process. The positive Sweet Chestnut state is the ability to trust in a higher power, however great the adversity you're experiencing. It's the moment when your cry for help is heard and when miracles happen.

Sweet Chestnut Key Symptoms

You're in a state of deepest despair; you've come to your limits and it's more than you can bear.

Behavior Pattern in the Blocked State

- You've found yourself in an extremely difficult position that you just can't bear any longer

- You believe there's no way out; you don't have any idea of what to do anymore

- You know only that you can't make it any further on your own

- You need to throw in the towel but can't admit it to yourself

- You no longer see the light at the end of the tunnel

- You feel you've reached the utmost limit and your burden is about to destroy you

- You can't believe that anyone should ever have to suffer this much; you feel God has abandoned you

- You feel utterly lost inside, as if in total isolation in a helpless void

- You're experiencing extreme mental anguish, the "dark night of the Soul"

Even if only one or two of these patterns precisely match your present situation, you need Sweet Chestnut.

Positive Potential

- You know how to use crises as opportunities for transformation

- You can handle extreme situations without allowing harm to your Soul

- You know the right moment to take action and the moment to let go

- You know when to say, "Thy will be done"

Empowering Statements

- "I look up."

- "I accept."

- "I let go."

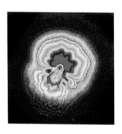

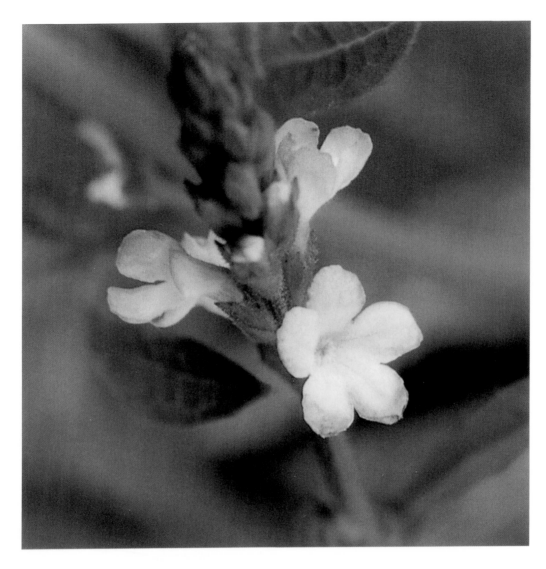

31. Vervain: The Enthusiasm Flower
From World Savior to Light Bearer

Those with fixed principles and ideas, which they are confident are right, and which they very rarely change.

They have a great wish to convert all around them to their own views of life.

They are strong of will and have much courage when they are convinced of those things that they wish to teach.

In illness they struggle on long after many would have given up their duties.

Edward Bach

Vervain relates to the Soul's potential for enthusiasm. In the negative Vervain state, your enthusiasm is exaggerated and your energy is squandered by using it in a missionary way, as can be seen in this example: During a weeklong field trip Peter has been appointed by his teacher to keep reminding her of the time so that the schedule can run smoothly. Bursting with pride at the responsibility, he sets about the task with great eagerness. He gets up in the morning thinking of the time, he goes to sleep thinking of it, and if he wakes at night, his first thought is "I wonder what time it is?" He's almost outdoing himself with his eagerness and energy; he's giving 100 percent. When his teacher looks at him by chance, he shouts out the time. If the other boys and girls are dawdling, he runs after them, almost begging them to hurry up, to remember how important it is to be on time. This field trip turns out to be stressful for Peter. He's on the job all the time and his classmates end up calling him "the clock." Peter is exhibiting an early negative Vervain state.

An inner flame burns within Vervain people in this negative state. If they have a positive idea that utterly consumes them, they are unable to rest until everybody around them has been convinced of the idea as well. Chairpeople of volunteer organizations, donating their free time and many nighttime hours to a good cause, never fearing to say what has to be said, can often be negative Vervain types. They are always on call, feeling dedicated to their role. With missionary zeal they will try to win over everybody they meet—sometimes successfully, sometimes not. The reason they sometimes fail to do so is that in their eagerness they tend to overdo things. Always passionate protagonists, they bombard others with their arguments rather than play the skilled diplomat who will let those around them have a say as well.

With such excessive use of willpower they tend to draw too heavily on their energy reserves. They can become tense and nervous inside and out and can react angrily when things don't progress as well as they expected. As a result they get even more involved, trying to give even more of themselves. They'll never allow themselves a free minute throughout the day and get only a few hours' sleep at night as they overestimate their vital energy and carry on regardless of their health. Then, all of a sudden, an illness will pull them up short—they'll catch the flu, for instance, because they have no resistance left.

Some people are so keyed up when in the negative Vervain state that even if they wanted to, they would find it difficult to relax physically. The enormous tension in their muscles is reflected in their extreme facial expressions and they perform physical activities with exaggerated efforts. They'll grip a pencil so hard, for instance, that it almost breaks, and when they come up the stairs, it sounds as though they're wearing army boots.

Vervain types pour out their energy and, unlike Rock Water types, sometimes want to force happiness onto others. They are revolutionaries at heart, often unaware that they are triggering a whole avalanche of complications. They are itinerant preachers, people conscious of their mission, people who can never keep quiet and are prepared to go to prison for their convictions. In one extreme case a student poured gasoline over himself and set himself on fire in public to draw attention to an ideal. Unfortunately, such people are often doing more harm than good for their causes—often they appear to others as silly children or are quickly written off as lunatics. This is the tragedy of the negative Vervain state.

If you're in this negative state, you've heard the calling of your Soul and want to follow it. After this you're flooded with a great deal of positive energy, but your personality is not yet ready—it still lacks knowledge of certain laws and experience in dealing with such large amounts of positive force. Because the energy is available, however, the personality tries to use it, following its own limited concepts rather than simply allowing energy to flow into it as water in a vessel. The result is the same as forcing a strong jet of water through a hose that is too narrow.

The personality needs to grasp the idea that this energy was not given to be squandered indiscriminately or as it sees fit, but to be spent wisely and economically for a higher goal. Part of this wise use includes looking after the body,

an important vessel for energies, instead of ignoring it or treating it lightly. Another concept it must realize is that pressure always produces counterpressure. A good idea needs no hard-sell pressure; a much more convincing strategy is to embody the idea and let others discover it for themselves. As Bach said, "It is by being rather than doing that great things are accomplished."

In practice, Vervain is recommended for any kind of exaggeration—for those who tend to get too carried away with a task, who can't measure their activity well, or who are so driven by their energy that they are unable to stop what they are doing whether it is work, eating, sex, sports, or anything else that is being overdone. Often it seems that in these exaggerations a person is trying to prove something to himself, or find his limits.

In a situation that takes a great deal of willpower—such as having to learn to walk again after an accident—Vervain can help a person to avoid overdoing and to learn how to use energy in a balanced way.

Those in the positive Vervain state have become the masters of their divine unrest and use their energies not eagerly, but lovingly and effectively. They're completely involved in the task at hand, but are also prepared to hear the opinions of others and review their own position if necessary. Hence, they have a broader perspective, and with this view an individual's exuberant character is able to inspire others and carry them along easily.

Vervain Key Symptoms

Your enthusiasm—even in support of a good cause—strains personal energies; you are high-strung, even messianic.

Behavior Pattern in the Blocked State

- You're enthusiastic about an idea and want to get others involved too

- You become incensed by injustice

- You're very intense and overly focused; you try to give 150 percent

- You're impulsive and idealistic to the point of being a missionary; you're wound up inside and are always on the job

- You tell others how to do things to the point of doing things for them; you try to force others to do or follow what's good for them

- You want to convert others and in this desire you absolutely drown them with your energy, eventually tiring them out and turning them away

- You hate to get sick because you don't want to lose your momentum at work

- You're sure of what's right for others

- You overdo things, get ahead of yourself, and at times become fanatical

- You accept unwarranted risks and sacrifice too often to achieve your goals

- You force yourself to keep going, even when you're physically exhausted

- You grow irritable and nervous when things don't progress the way you want

- You find it difficult to do less than too much

- You don't know when to stop, exaggerating your pursuit of eating, sex, work, or sports

- You're totally keyed up and unable to relax; you suffer from muscle tension, pain in your eyes, or headaches

- Children are hyperactive and won't go to bed at night

Even if only one or two of these patterns precisely match your present situation, you need Vervain.

Positive Potential

- You know the appropriate amount of energy to use in all activities

- Your reactions are tolerant and poised

- You stand up for your own ideas but respect those of others and discuss them objectively

- You're able to let others dance to their own drummer without having to interfere

- You use your excess energy wisely and carefully when there is a good cause

- You're able to effortlessly enthuse, inspire, and motivate others in the name of a higher ideal

Empowering Statements

- "I relax."

- "I give space to others."

- "I pace my energy."

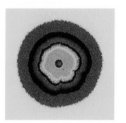

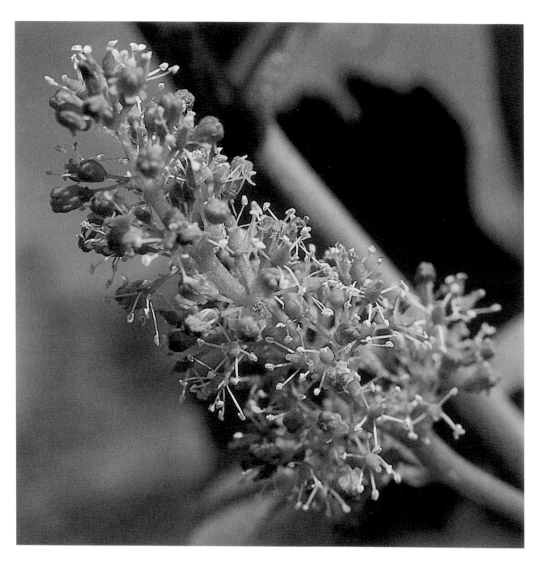

32. Vine: The Authority Flower
From Leading to Being Led

Very capable people, certain of their own ability, confident of success.

Being so assured, they think that it would be for the benefit of others if they could be per-suaded to do things as they themselves do, or as they are certain is right. Even in illness they will direct their attendants.

They may be of great value in emergency.

Edward Bach

Vine relates to the Soul's quality of authority. In the negative Vine state, you don't deal well with the principle of authority. You'll either deny it or become carried away by it. Those who deny it may easily fall victim to power plays. Those who are carried away by it need to have their way at any price—they can be ruthless and have no respect for the individuality of others.

Vine is a very powerful form of energy, giving you above-average leadership qualities while at the same time making extreme demands on your personal development. There is a constant temptation to allow yourself to be hypnotized by this volcanic force. Vine types are very capable and ambitious, and are unsurpassed when it comes to willpower and presence of mind. They find a way out of every crisis situation, always holding the reins. In the struggle for survival they seem to come out victorious every time and so become used to success. Sooner or later this may result in their conviction that they have complete infallibility. In fact, they will believe they are doing others a favor by telling them how to do things and insisting that things be done exactly so.

"I can't see what the guys are upset about. It's all done in their best interest," says the authoritarian head of the department to a colleague who is trying to suggest that his leadership style may be somewhat militaristic. "They haven't got a clue anyway," he will add, shaking his head and getting on with the day's work. The next time sales figures are assessed, his department comes out on top again and he wonders if he ought not to make use of the opportunity to take over his colleague's department as well. Human regard, fairness? That's ridiculous! Business is business! So says the person in a negative Vine state.

Many villains and tyrants in history—Nero, Catherine the Great—were representative of the negative Vine type. Open any newspaper today and the sheer number of reports of dictatorial regimes and human cruelty will tell you that negative Vine energy is still wreaking havoc on our planet. People in the negative Vine state have switched off all feeling for other people and have fallen victim to their own powerful ideas. A father, for instance, will say, "The boy needs to be disciplined!" even though he knows his son's affection for him will be replaced by fear. A strict ballet teacher will preach, while swinging her baton, "Don't think, just do exactly what I say!" though her students may have questions about a point of instruction.

Among people who need Vine, you will find a surprisingly high number of performing artists who combine high sensitivity with extreme ambition. With iron discipline, they force themselves to train every day. At the same time they may be worried about their form, panicked over their next appearance, and fearful of the intrigues of their colleagues. This fear and the obsession to be successful create a crucial conflict in many negative Vine personalities.

In the Vine state the error is in using tremendous personal forces for narrow, egotistical ends instead of making them available in service to a higher ideal. "What benefit is it to you to be a demigod if you fail to express our divine nature?" This admonition applies particularly to people with strong negative Vine attributes.

By taking Vine and opening up your Higher Self, you come to realize that you're carried by the very power you have been using to gain control over everything. You'll sense the shift in willpower now uniting with love and power uniting with wisdom. Once your actions are no longer entirely egotistical but carried out in relation to the greater whole, new strength will arrive of its own accord. As the instrument of a higher plan, these actions will automatically serve the positive interests of the people around you. Their conscious or unconscious recognition will always provide new energy to positive Vine types, lending a natural authority without the need for an imperious air.

In the positive Vine state you'll realize that strong leadership qualities are actually needed only in temporary crisis situations, and that most of the time you're merely "the first servant of the country," as the Prussian king Frederick the Great put it so aptly. Your task becomes helping others find their own way.

People born with Vine potential who don't cultivate and apply it actively will sooner or later find themselves in a situation that requires it. You may, for example, have problems with a family member, a dominant partner, in-laws who want to have too much of a say in your children's upbringing, or a tyrannical child. At work you may be asked to lead others by giving them orders and controlling them. Taking Vine will support you in developing its positive potential.

In Bach Therapy practice, the Vine state very often appears together with other, seemingly opposite Soul states such as Centaury. This conflict in the personality may, for instance, show up when a person tries to compensate for his impressionable nature (Centaury) with willpower and hardness (Vine).

Vine is indicated as part of an individual combination when illnesses develop that are of a compulsive character, such as anorexia. It has also been successful in treating people with multiple sclerosis.

Vine Key Symptoms
Among these are a tendency to be domineering and ambitious, to strive for power, and to become tyrannical.

Behavior Pattern in the Blocked State
❁ You need to have your way at any price; you're unable to give in

❁ You always want to have the last word

❁ You find it difficult to obey

❁ You gladly take up the role of the leader, of being the "savior" in a difficult situation

❁ Or the opposite may be true: It is difficult for you to lead and tell others what to do

- You run the risk of misusing your great gifts for personal power

- You ruthlessly disregard the opinion of others

- You rarely doubt your superiority and try to make everybody dance to your tune

- You constantly measure your strength or power and question established hierarchies

- You're hard, cruel, and pitiless without conscience

- You're narrow-minded and accept only your own opinion

- Your head comes before your heart

- You intentionally instill fear in others

- When hospitalized, you tell the physician what to do and keep the nurses on their toes

- You don't discuss things because you believe you're always right

- You bow to your superiors and tread on underlings underfoot

- People who will not participate in the struggle for power are ignored

- You cannot tolerate anyone contradicting you

- You accept only a selected few, and refuse to take others seriously

- Children will beat up their classmates

- Older people rigidly insist on their opinions

Even if only one or two of these patterns precisely match your present situation, you need Vine.

Positive Potential

- You accept the rights of others and pay attention to their needs

- You know how to discriminate between healthy and overweening ambition

- You understand that your task is to fill your role in the theater of life in as humane a way as possible

- You help others to help themselves find their own way

- You're the wise, understanding leader who has natural authority

Empowering Statements

- "I empathize."

- "I show respect."

- "I value and support."

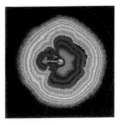

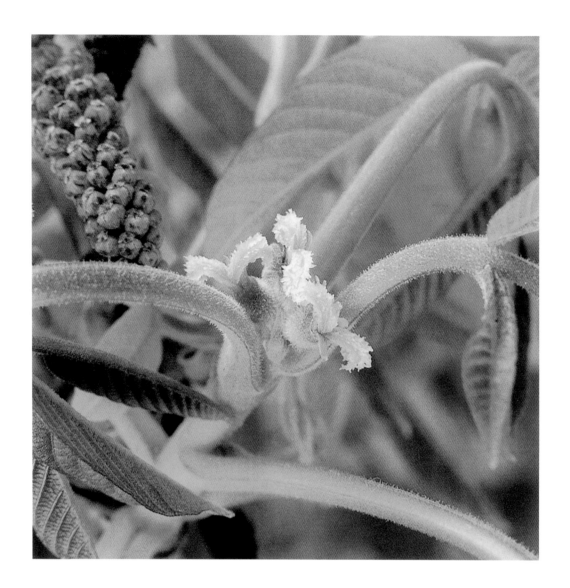

33. Walnut: The Midwife Flower
From Vacillation to Inner Steadfastness

For those who have definite ideals and ambitions in life and are fulfilling them, but on rare occasions are tempted to be led away from their own ideas, aims and work by the enthusiasm, convictions or strong opinions of others.

This remedy gives constancy and protection from outside influences.

Edward Bach

Walnut relates to the Soul's potential for following your inner call to a new beginning. If you're in the negative Walnut state, you hesitate to take the final step before a new beginning because you're constantly being diverted by outside influences.

Our ancestors revered the Walnut as a regal tree—the Romans dedicated the tree to their god Jupiter—and the Walnut Flower Remedy also holds an important position among the thirty-eight Bach Flowers. Whenever major changes are about to take place, Walnut is the Flower used to ease the way. Such situations might include conversion to another faith, entering a new relationship, changing to a completely different occupation, and emigrating to another country. While it helps mentally and spiritually with these kinds of new beginnings, Walnut also proves useful in major stages of biological change such as teething, puberty, pregnancy, menopause, and the terminal stage of a serious illness. These, too, entail vital inner alterations that completely set free new energies.

All situations involving major change are phases of increased stress, and therefore of pronounced instability. Even stable people who normally know very well what they want are inclined to vacillate between going forward and not when facing important changes. They become susceptible to the warnings and skepticism of others; fall back into old habits; and get caught up in sentimental musings, conventional ideas, or old family traditions, running the risk of abandoning their inner resolve.

In the negative Walnut state, mentally speaking, you're sitting in a boat that is about to take you across a river. You clearly see the opposite side but the boat is still partly moored. All that's missing is the decisive push, the captain giving the word for takeoff. The last invisible ties are still in place and, as if by a magical spell, keep you unconsciously tied to the past. These ties might be an unfulfilled promise, a relationship that is unclear, or an oath sworn to a professional or service organization. Because of its ability to dissolve these magical ties, Bach termed Walnut "the spell breaker." He further wrote that Walnut is "the remedy for those who have decided to take a great step forward in life, to break old conventions, to leave old limits and restrictions and start on a new way." Such a farewell to old relationships, thoughts, and feelings can be painful and frequently expresses itself physically in problems with the teeth.

True Walnut personalities are like pioneers, often ahead of others in fighting for certain ideals. These are the people with innovative ideas. They have firmly defined life goals and are likely to be rather unconventional in bringing them to realization. There is a temporary danger of being led astray, however, since those with open minds will often have to deal with being outsiders and facing the pressure of the conventional masses who most often oppose new ideas, which jeopardize the new course that is, as yet, only a possibility. Walnut people can fulfill their purpose only if they are able to stay mentally free and so must shake off any outside influences. Walnut Essence* provides the needed steadfastness to do this.

The error of the personality in the negative Walnut state is a weak or delayed reaction to the impulses of the Higher Self. While open to Inner Guidance, you allow mental influences from outside to be distracting rather than submitting fully to the guidance of the Higher Self. The personality will still at times take its lead from other people and their ideas, instead of concentrating on its own Life Plan.

People in the positive Walnut state have set themselves free inside, and are able to set sail for new horizons, making progress in fulfilling their purpose in life unaffected by outer circumstances and the opinions of others. Edward Bach himself was an example of the positive Walnut type. In the last years of his life he let go of everything: social approval, financial security, traditions of orthodox medicine, and his entire past professional life. Despite wry looks from his former colleagues and living in the most modest of financial circumstances, he followed his call.

In practice Walnut has been found to be helpful during stages of progressive change such as the kind that would occur during psychotherapy, when completely new elements of the personality become accessible and lead to new decisions. A similar time is during divorce proceedings, when physical separation has already taken place but something still ties a person to his or her former partner, whose negative thoughts are still difficult to shake. Still other experiences would be the beginning of retirement, a voluntary move to a senior citizen home, the period of time following a stroke or other illness that brings about a major change in lifestyle, the period of time following treatment for malformations of the jaw, and in times spent learning a new language.

Since Walnut has been described as "the flower that helps you to break through," some people might take it by mistake in order to find a new goal in life (which would call for Wild Oat instead). Walnut can help manifest only a goal that is already well defined.

Walnut Key Symptoms

You may be uncertain, too easily influenced, and inconsistent—particularly in transitional periods of life.

Behavior Pattern in the Blocked State

❀ You have clear goals and desires and normally know exactly what to do, but now you falter and have problems staying true to yourself

❀ You are usually very independent but are temporarily distracted by family

---

* It is interesting to note that the inside of a walnut and the cerebrum show very similar convolutions.

obligations, social conventions, or memories of old promises and commitments

- ❂ You're making a major life change but find that you can't take the last step

- ❂ You wish to leave behind all restrictions and influences but can't quite manage to do so

- ❂ When making an important life decision, you find it hard to escape the influence of an important role model, a parent, teacher, boss, or the like

- ❂ An unexpected outside event forces you to rethink the plans you have for your life

- ❂ You want finally to understand and integrate a major change in your life

- ❂ Despite new decisions, you still feel like holding on to some old habits

- ❂ You've given up a relationship, but despite physical separation, you're still under the old partner's spell

- ❂ Major changes in life are taking place: marriage, birth, a change of occupation, a move to another city, divorce, retirement, and so forth

- ❂ Major biological changes are about to occur: menopause, pregnancy, puberty, teething, terminal stages of illness

Even if only one or two of these patterns precisely match your present situation, you need Walnut.

Positive Potential

- ❂ As the pioneer, you stay true to yourself

- ❂ You dare to do what is new

- ❂ You take the final step

- ❂ You're immune to outer influences and open to inner inspiration

- ❂ You have character

- ❂ You move forward confidently following your Life Plan.

Empowering Statements

- ❂ "I am sure of myself."

- ❂ "I stay true to myself."

- ❂ "I go my own way."

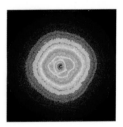

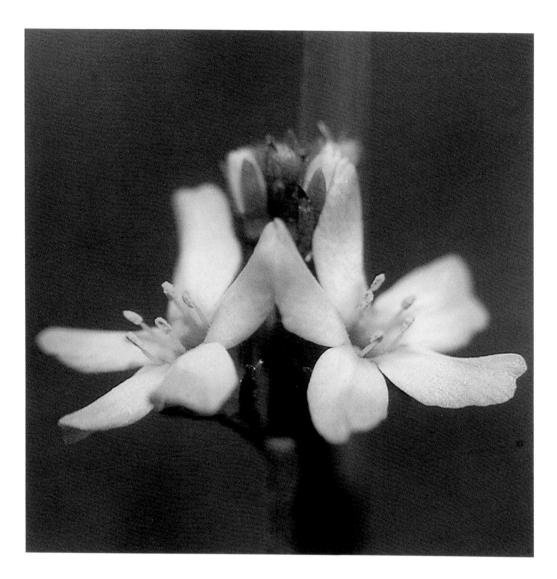

34. Water Violet: The Communication Flower
From Isolation to Togetherness

For those who in health or illness like to be alone. Very quiet people, who move about without noise, speak little, and then gently. Very independent, capable and self-reliant. Almost free of the opinions of others. They are aloof, leave people alone and go their own way. Often clever and talented. Their peace and calmness is a blessing to those around them.

Edward Bach

Water Violet relates to the potential to communicate and to the Soul qualities of humility and wisdom. In the negative Water Violet state you're prone to overly cultivating your "specialness," and withdrawing from the rest of the world in proud reserve.

The structure of the plant illustrates its essential energy: delicate but upright. What gives stability to the plant—the leaves—stays below the surface of the water.

People with strong Water Violet traits are usually well in control of their personalities. They present an image of unobtrusive superiority and calm self-control. In the eyes of others they may therefore appear unapproachable and almost flawless. Water Violet types always appear to have the air of being somehow different or special. Like a well-bred Siamese cat, they move silently with dignified delicacy, choosing their own way, above the influence of others. Upon observing such a person, one would automatically think, "It would be nice to be like that!" Yet despite their high degree of individuality, Water Violet people in the negative state have particular problems of their own.

A much admired yoga teacher in your community, for example, has a "together," independent manner but despite his superior qualities sometimes feels lonely and isolated. He finds it challenging to step down from the pedestal on which his students have placed him and approach them with ease. Gushing emotions are not his style—his affection has more spiritual roots. He sometimes does not know how far he should go, and when in doubt tends to be reserved.

People generally find it difficult to break through a Water Violet type's personal barrier, while others constantly ask him for advice and even try to make him into an emotional wastebasket. At times the drain on his energy from the demands of others becomes too much. Quite suddenly Water Violet types will inwardly shake their heads and come to the conclusion that they really are something different. They fall into negative behavior patterns, giving in to their typical weaknesses of pride and aloofness and withdrawing into their own shell where they are not to be disturbed. Just as on principle they do not meddle in the affairs of others, so do they reject third-party interference in their affairs, even when they are ill. They prefer to deal with problems on their own, keeping a stiff upper lip and blocking energy, which, in the long run, can lead to tension and stiffness.

People with marked Water Violet traits are much appreciated as superiors, not only because they are conscientious in their work but particularly because they have the ability to be something of a calm rock in the roaring surf of workplace emotions. They are almost always on top of things, but prefer to work tactfully and calmly in the background. The only thing they find difficult is making harsh decisions; they're always aware of everyone's particular situation. Unlike Vine, a Water Violet boss will never force an employee to do something. But if his expectations are not met for a long time, he will inwardly withdraw from that person.

Individuals in the negative Water Violet state who remain for too long inside their shell are not doing themselves a favor; they are separating themselves from the vital exchange of energies without which not even the most self-contained among us is able to exist. As a result the personality desiccates and hardens, which further restricts its interactions with its environment and, maybe more important, with itself. The error is that it has turned away from its Higher Self and refuses to understand that its specialness, while a gift, comes wrapped with an obligation. Rather than shutting themselves off from others in their uniqueness, Water Violet personalities should pass on their values in conscious or unconscious energy exchanges with others, and allow themselves to become an inspiring example.

People who are exceptionally tall frequently deal with Water Violet problems. Among Water Violet men, many will be loners or play the role of the gifted eccentric. Children who select a Water Violet stock bottle while making a spontaneous choice often wish to retreat from a specific situation—for instance, from going to kindergarten. People with a high potential for Water Violet will never sit down in the first row of their own accord. Teachers and people working in the healing professions often find themselves in Water Violet situations. A therapist may encounter the temporary feeling of being unable to make contact with her patients or may suddenly feel the need to withdraw completely from her practice. These are circumstances where Water Violet is indicated. The Essence also helps a teacher who feels an urge to retreat to meet students with an open mind and heart. Those must attend social functions but don't know what to say in such situations are usually more comfortable and communicate more easily after treatment with Water Violet.

Water Violet Key Symptoms

You are withdrawn and aloof; you have feelings of superiority and an inner reserve.

Behavior Pattern in the Blocked State

❀ You want to withdraw from a certain situation or relationship

❀ You feel isolated and not part of the group

❀ You occasionally are condescending and proud

❀ You won't permit others to become involved in your personal affairs

❀ You sort things out independently and won't burden others with problems

❀ You are considered to be antisocial or emotionally cold

❀ Because of your distance, others consider you to be conceited, disdainful, or arrogant

❀ You sometimes find it difficult to approach others

- You want to get down from your inner pedestal but don't know how

- You have problems engaging in discussions or party conversations

- You unknowingly make it difficult for others to make genuine personal contact with you

- You avoid emotional disputes because you find them exhausting

- You find it difficult to totally relax

- You rarely cry, trying instead to keep a stiff upper lip

- You want to physically withdraw

Even if only one or two of these patterns precisely match your present situation, you need Water Violet.

Positive Potential

- You're perfectly happy with yourself and act according to the saying "Live and let live"

- You keep a tactful distance but still feel in unison with other people

- You like to keep to yourself but know how to contact others when necessary

- Your actions are dignified and conscientious but you still prefer to stay in the background

- You serve as a model of a balanced, understanding, and independent person

Empowering Statements

- "I do belong."

- "I take part."

- "I allow closeness."

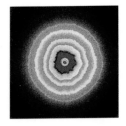

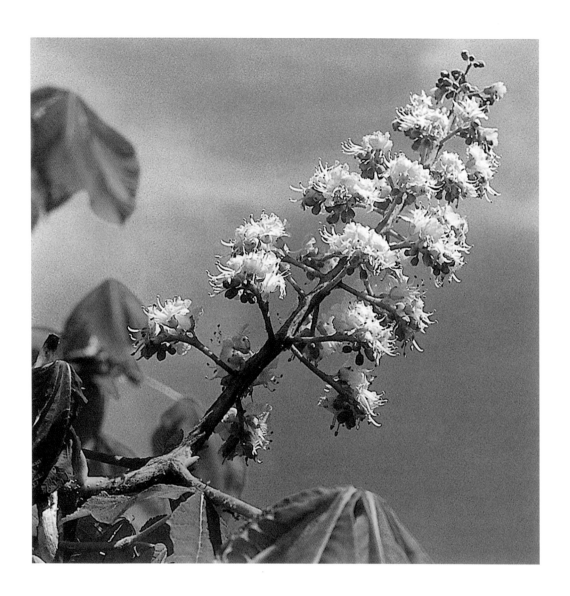

35. White Chestnut: The Thought Flower
From Mental Merry-go-round to Mental Quiet

For those who cannot prevent thoughts, ideas, arguments which they do not desire from entering their minds. Usually at such times when the interest of the moment is not strong enough to keep the mind full.

Thoughts which worry and will remain, or if for a time thrown out, will return. They seem to circle round and round and cause mental torture.

The presence of such unpleasant thoughts
drives out peace and interferes with being able
to think only of the work or pleasure of the day.

Edward Bach

White Chestnut relates to the Soul qualities of tranquillity and discernment. In the negative White Chestnut state you're the victim of unclear, disorganized thoughts. Here, for instance, is a familiar situation: You have experienced some disagreement at work. After two hours of hot debate everything seems to be settled satisfactorily. That night you're sitting in the bathtub, hoping to relax, but the dispute you had at work still rages on in your mind. You are now remembering everything you should have said. Over and over again you defend yourself to an imaginary work committee. Again and again you hear the derogatory remark made by a business partner—and yet you had held her in high regard. "Surely it can't be that she's proving such a disappointment to me. Should I sever my connection to her? And what about the big order that just came in? Forget about it," you tell yourself, "Consider it all dispassionately tomorrow morning—now it's time for bed and a good night's sleep." But sleep is out of the question. The swirling of your thoughts continues as you lie in bed, with the same arguments and counterarguments repeating themselves over and over. "Oh, if only I could turn off these thoughts!"

People showing strong White Chestnut traits do not go through this just once in a while, but frequently. Many are so used to these dialogues in their mind that they take them more or less for granted. In the negative White Chestnut state people are victim to an overbearing mental process that has gained the upper hand over all other aspects of the personality. During meditation some people in need of White Chestnut see their heads standing apart from the rest of their bodies. "In my thoughts I'm like a hamster in his wheel, not getting a single step ahead," said one man in the negative White Chestnut state. "My thoughts are like catchy tunes. They simply won't disappear from my mind and they completely control me." Others have said, "The other day I was so busy with mental arguments I almost ran into a streetlight." And, "My head is so full of mental chatter that I can't formulate a single clear thought when I'm in the office." These, too, are typical statements for the negative White Chestnut state. In his *Handbook of the Bach Flower Remedies*, Dr. Philip Chancellor wrote: "The Clematis person uses his thoughts to escape from the world, while the White Chestnut type would give anything to escape from his thoughts into the world."

Quite a few of these people suffer from chronic frontal headaches, particularly just above the eyes. Many have problems going to sleep, or their thoughts will wake them at four in the morning, refusing to go away. Often their faces will betray great mental tension. People in the negative White Chestnut state, similar to those in the negative Vervain state, tend to unconsciously grind their teeth.

There are differing hypotheses as to the origin of this negative state. Bach himself said that it occurs if the interest of the person in the present situation is not strong enough to occupy the mind completely. In such moments, insufficiently cleared thoughts seem to push up into the mind, hoping to be finally integrated.

In the negative White Chestnut state it appears that a process of selection at the mental level is not functioning as well as it should. The personality has not developed a constructive way to discriminate between thoughts and ideas that should be accepted and those that should be rejected. It greedily takes in everything that presents itself, and then finds itself confronted with a bundle of impulses, unable to integrate anything.

The ideas flutter about like papers in disarray on a crowded desk, the unimportant pieces concealing the important documents and generally causing consternation for the owner of the desk, who is overwhelmed and unable to tidy up and sort the important and urgent items from the rest.

In the negative White Chestnut state the personality has turned its back on guidance from its Higher Self and is consequently in the state of egotistical mental greed. Without its Inner Guidance to direct it toward the higher purpose of its Life Plan, the personality entertains too many thoughts, which circle, undigested, weighing down the mind. As soon as it once again accepts the guidance of its Higher Self, all mental impulses will automatically be selected and organized to serve the Life Plan. Thoughts that don't fit can be dropped and once again constructive thought processes will become feasible.

In the positive White Chestnut state the personality is able to let destructive thought impulses rush past like a nonstop train it has no desire to board. Calm and peace are the keynotes of its mental state. From the clear lake of its consciousness, the answers and solutions that are desired emerge of their own accord. People who are in the positive White Chestnut state are able to make constructive use of their powerful mental abilities.

Those who had little or no opportunity to talk to anyone when they were young have a propensity for White Chestnut; they had to come up with a conversation partner in their imagination. In diagnostic interviews, therefore, it is beneficial for White Chestnut types to have the opportunity to thoroughly talk things through. The treatment of speech problems, particularly stuttering, is often well supported with a combination of Vervain and White Chestnut. Other circumstances for which the use of White Chestnut should be fully explored are those times when thoughts seem to fly off in all directions just when it's necessary that the right thoughts materialize, such as those times when you have something important that you need to write or something important to express to a friend or partner.

White Chestnut Key Symptoms

Unwanted thoughts and inner dialogues persist and you're unable to get rid of them.

Behavior Pattern in the Blocked State

- Unwanted thoughts constantly come to mind and cannot be turned off

- A worry or event persistently gnaws at your mind

- Again and again you think about what you might have said or should have said

- Your mind sounds like a broken record

- You're mentally running in place, like a hamster in its wheel

- You experience incessant inner chatter, compulsive thought processes, or an echo in your brain

- You go over the same problems time and time again without coming to a solution

- Your mental hyperactivity prevents you from concentrating in everyday life—for instance, you don't hear when spoken to

- You're not thinking yourself—the thinking is running on its own

- You can't sleep because of the thoughts going around in your head, particularly in the early hours of the morning

- Mental tension causes teeth grinding and tightness around your eyes and forehead

Even if only one or two of these patterns precisely match your present situation, you need White Chestnut.

Positive Potential

- You have impressive mental capacities and use them clearly and constructively

- You concentrate well, working constructively with your mental powers

- Because you align yourself with your Inner Guidance, your thought impulses clarify and organize themselves

- Out of your inner quiet, solutions for every problem come up on their own

Empowering Statements

- "I feel the quiet."

- "I feel clear."

- "I guide my thoughts."

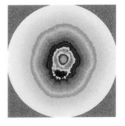

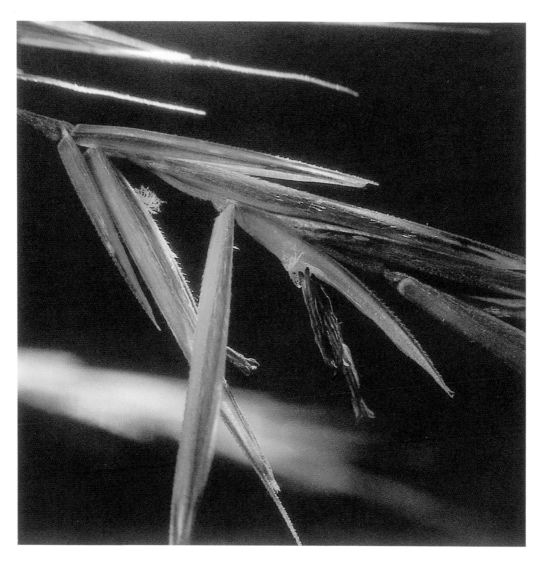

36. Wild Oat: The Vocational Calling Flower
From Seeking to Finding

Those who have ambitions to do something of prominence in life, who wish to have much experience, and to enjoy all that which is possible for them, to take life to the full.

Their difficulty is to determine what occupation to follow; as although their ambitions are strong, they have no calling which appeals to them above all others.

This may cause delay and dissatisfaction.

Edward Bach

Wild Oat relates to the Soul's potential for knowing one's inner purpose. If you're in the negative Wild Oat state, you don't know your true vocation, and are therefore unfulfilled and dissatisfied deep inside.

Imagine yourself being three years old and entering a toy store together with your mother for the first time. Bounty and color beckon everywhere. You are so overwhelmed that you don't know which way to turn. This is the basic feeling in the negative Wild Oat state. Typical Wild Oat people will already show this trait in their youth. They rarely belong to a firm group of friends, instead dipping in here or there but never getting fully involved. They usually have many talents and need to make no special effort to achieve anything—many things simply fall into their laps. Despite this, they are ambitious and want to achieve something special. On the other hand, they have only a vague notion as to what this may be.

Psychologically, the negative Wild Oat state may be traced back to parents who never recognized and acknowledged their child's special uniqueness. This missing affirmation is searched for in the activities of adulthood. Wild Oat types want to enjoy life, generally in rather unconventional ways. They don't want to go with the current, but want to steer their own craft. Unfortunately, they don't know the name of the port they want to head for. Because of this, they find it difficult to fit into society. They don't like to commit themselves, and sometimes this lack of definition causes them to end up in circumstances that aren't at their intellectual or spiritual level, resulting in further frustration.

Life is forever offering new opportunities to Wild Oat types. They will start many things, often pursuing a number of professions to great success, but will always lack that real inner certainty that permits a final, definite decision about their course. After a while, the work that was enjoyable for a time begins to pall, and the colleagues among whom they felt so much at home suddenly seem rather boring. Following a negative behavior pattern, they themselves tear down what they've built in order to move on to the next opportunity in the hope that it will bring them greater satisfaction.

Someone who has had no experience with such a state might well imagine that this creative unrest can be most stimulating, but in the long run the opposite is the case. People in the negative Wild Oat state feel that life is passing them by, despite all their talents and activities. They feel regret over their inability to wholly affirm anything, and are never able to really enjoy the fruits of their labor. They're always on the lookout for the right mate but never seem to find whom they want. Their condition may be understood as a continual state of mental puberty. The head is full of odd ideas, notions as to all the things they'd like to and ought to do. They seem still to be sowing their wild oats, squandering their energies in all directions rather than finally accepting the guidance of the Higher Self and working toward a single goal.

The error in the negative Wild Oat state is personality's excessive self-centeredness. In blind enthusiasm it's looking for goals and direction in the world outside, instead of realizing it merely needs to follow its Inner Guidance to discover that the decision, long since made, lies within.

If you're in the negative Wild Oat state, practice going for depth rather than breadth. You needn't fear that life will grow more boring. On the contrary, it will offer unimaginable new experiences. With every decision you make, ask yourself what your real inner motivation is. You need to realize that it is not a question of doing something special, but of doing the right thing in a given situation, and doing it as thoroughly and as well as possible. Know that your rich talents are needed within the context of the greater whole because everything we do is an essential part of a greater, meaningful process.

If you're taking Wild Oat, you'll experience a gradually increasing calm, clarity, and certainty in heart and mind. Little by little you'll gain a clearer picture of what it is you really want, and you will come to act intuitively rather than impulsively. At this point you can firmly align your many different talents to serve a higher goal, and even the most enticing new opportunities that may beckon will not make you let go of this. Life will continue to offer plenty of variety, but you'll be happier and more fulfilled.

In Bach Flower Therapy, Wild Oat can be used when you are looking for a vision for a new professional direction. In a "midlife crisis" Wild Oat helps to overcome inappropriate behavior patterns and assist in a renewed orientation in life.

Wild Oat Key Symptoms

You experience uncertainty about your ambitions; you're easily bored and are always looking for something new; you're dissatisfied because you don't know your purpose in life.

Behavior Pattern in the Blocked State

❀ You have only a vague sense of your goals; you can't find your direction in life, which leads to dissatisfaction, frustration, and boredom

❀ You're ambitious; you want to do something special but you don't know what it is

❀ You always feel driven toward exciting new projects

❀ You try many things without gaining real satisfaction at any of them

❀ You have many possibilities but don't feel called to any particular profession; hanging in the air in this way disheartens you

❀ You're frustrated because things are not as clear-cut for yourself as they seem to be for others

❀ You tend to become involved in too many things and spread yourself too thin

- Inwardly you don't want to commit and therefore you unconsciously end up in the same unsatisfactory situations

- Your professional or private life does not quite fit your type or abilities and you wind up wasting your talents

- You jump from one activity or subject to another, be it in your profession, in work, or during a conversation

Even if only one or two of these patterns precisely match your present situation, you need Wild Oat.

Positive Potential

- You recognize your own uniqueness

- You find your vision and come up with appropriate ways to live it

- You do many things well and find a way to simultaneously do several jobs successfully within your overall vision

- You know your inner calling and follow it

Empowering Statements

- "I know what to do."

- "I follow my vision."

- "I am fulfilled."

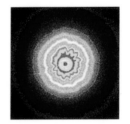

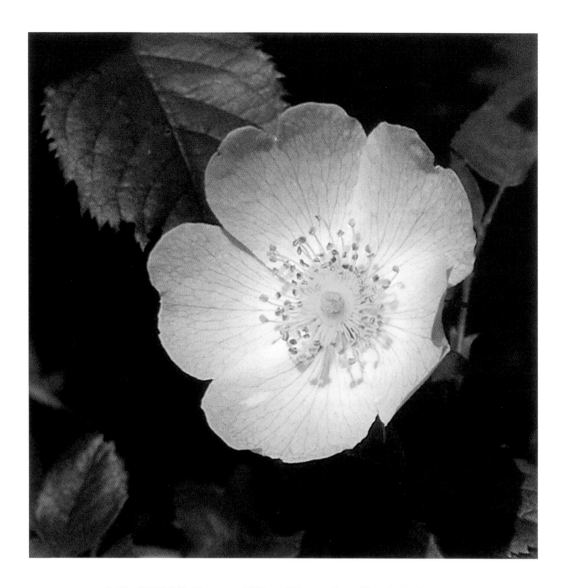

37. Wild Rose: The Zest for Life Flower
From Resignation to Devotion

Those who without apparently sufficient reason become resigned to all that happens, and just glide through life, take it as it is, without any effort to improve things and find some joy. They have surrendered to the struggle of life without complaint.

Edward Bach

Wild Rose relates to the Soul's potential for devotion to life and to joy in life. In the negative Wild Rose state, the principle of devotion is misunderstood and is applied at the wrong level. Instead of happily devoting yourself to your Life Plan, you have given in to fixed, negative expectations. This misunderstanding often arises during the first days of life—for instance, if your birth took a very long time or if, as a premature baby, you had to spend days or weeks in an incubator. Your little mind or spirit may have wondered whether its decision for life was an error and whether your life, in fact, might already be over. As a result, you abandon personal initiative and feel an apathetic resignation about life.

A Wild Rose patient cured of headaches due to chronic low blood pressure reported that she was born during the last days of World War II in Dresden during a night when bombs destroyed almost the entire city and tens of thousands of people lost their lives.

A baby who has been crying for her mother for hours will at some point give up hope of her mother ever coming to hold her. Feeling utterly deserted, in complete emptiness she resigns herself to her fate. Interest in life disappears and she becomes a being without energy, one who is merely vegetating, merely existing.

People in need of Wild Rose frequently seem half dead already, like dried plants that are barely hanging on. They have gone far beyond depression. They have capitulated, as people with a life sentence in prison might, with a dull acceptance of their fate. They believe the adverse circumstances in their lives—perhaps a chronic illness, a hopelessly inflexible marriage, or an unsatisfactory job—are beyond change. It no longer occurs to them that things could be different. In a voice empty of expression they say things such as, "It's in the family. I just have to live with it" or "As far as I'm concerned, it's all over anyway." To others they are often a puzzle, because their external circumstances do not always warrant such a negative approach. Because of this, those in the negative Wild Rose state are perceived as boring and make for tiresome company. Their apathetic lack of interest depresses the whole atmosphere. It's not surprising that the negative Wild Rose state has also been called "mental anemia" due to the fact that many inhibiting mental patterns make it impossible for the individual to call on the cosmic life energies and transform them for personal use.

The negative Wild Rose state is not always as apparent or clear-cut as in the examples above. At times it is very subtle and may combine with a Vervain state to result in a form of frantic compensatory activity, occasionally observed in successful people who work as managers or department heads. Identifying the negative Wild Rose state in your own personality tends to be very difficult. More prominent, compensating behavior patterns—Vervain, Rock Water, Vine—are able to push into the foreground and obscure the Wild Rose state because it is one of the Flower states with the least energy.

Once you take Wild Rose you'll gradually feel your spirits revive and begin to live again. Relieved, you'll will be able to become involved in life more and more as the days go on. The flow of vital energy eventually grows into an abundant stream and fills you with joyful expectancy and lively interest.

If children select Wild Rose in a spontaneous choice, it should be given to them even if you don't understand why it was chosen. Wild Rose is mostly used long term, though it has also proved helpful to relieve a temporary lack of energy during chemotherapy or low vitality after you've burned the candle at both ends sexually.

Wild Rose Key Symptoms

You experience apathy, a lack of interest and ambition, resignation, and inner capitulation.

Behavior Pattern in the Blocked State

- ✪ You give in to fate

- ✪ You no longer take yourself seriously

- ✪ You're resigned inside although circumstances don't seem all that hopeless or negative from the outside

- ✪ You feel absolutely no joy in life and have no inner motivation

- ✪ You've given up all efforts to make any changes in your life

- ✪ You accept your fate, unhappy home life, unsatisfactory job, chronic illness, and so forth

- ✪ You believe you've been burdened by bad genes

- ✪ Others sense an underlying sadness in you

- ✪ You experience chronic boredom, indifference, and empty feelings

- ✪ You no longer complain of your condition, believing it to be normal

- ✪ You always feel "wilted," with no energy at all; you are apathetic

- ✪ You speak monotonously and quietly

Even if only one or two of these patterns precisely match your present situation, you need Wild Rose.

Positive Potential

- ✪ You embrace life

- ✪ You develop initiative

- ✪ You find life exciting and interesting

- ✪ You feel an inner freedom and vitality

- ✪ You give yourself enthusiastically to life

Empowering Statements

- ✪ "I want to live."

- ✪ "I demand life."

- ✪ "I seize my chance."

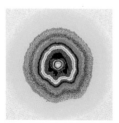

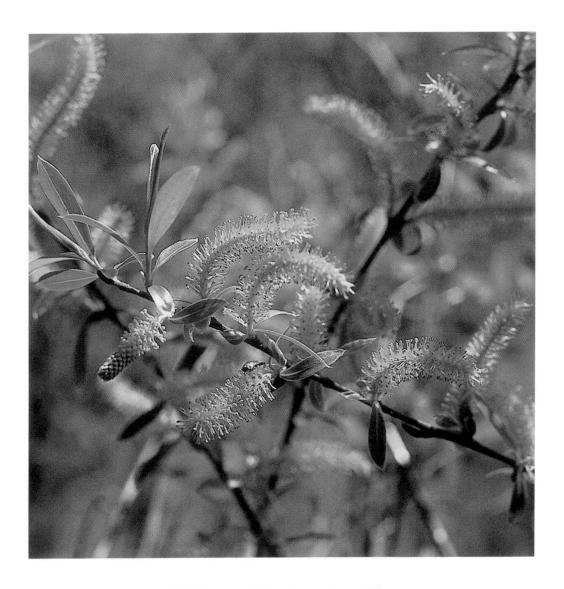

38. Willow: The Destiny Flower
From Resenting Fate to Taking Personal Responsibility

For those who have suffered adversity or misfortune and find these difficult to accept, without complaint or resentment, as they judge life much by the success which it brings.

They feel that they have not deserved so great a trial, that it was unjust, and they become embittered.

They often take less interest and are less active in those things of life which they had previously enjoyed.

Edward Bach

Willow relates to the Soul's potential to take full responsibility for yourself. If you're in the negative Willow state, you'll blame everyone and everything but yourself and have a negative attitude most of the time. On negative Willow days you rail at your fate, resenting the treatment you receive. You are unable to understand how others can be so cheerful and carefree. You begrudge them their good fortune and feel tempted to spoil their good mood. All of us have days like this, when we don't feel at all comfortable with ourselves. These are representative of the temporary negative Willow state.

Unfortunately, this state can develop into a chronic pattern, in which case it has a destructive effect on you and your entire surroundings. Just as one bad apple will sooner or later cause all the others in the basket to rot, so a person in the chronic negative Willow state tends to infect others by being a wet blanket and spoilsport. In the negative Willow state you feel that you're the hapless victim of a cruel fate that seeks you out again and again—"I don't deserve this. Life can be so unfair!" you'll complain, never considering how cause and effect may function in your life.

This is a state in which disappointments and resentment are strongly projected onto the outside world. It is often found among people who have passed the midpoint of life and unconsciously notice that few of their ideals and hopes have been realized. The head of a department who is getting on in age is passed over and a former colleague is promoted to manager instead. Subsequently he feels that the colleague is looking down on him. "Well, now that he's advanced he can afford to be like that," he'll say, his face careworn and the corners of the mouth turned down. "Had my parents not spent all their money on vacations and instead let me go to college, my career would have taken a better turn!" People in the chronic negative Willow state always grumble, surrounded by an invisible wall of negativity.

Such people may carry a grudge about a situation or against another person for years, never putting their cards on the table or trying to resolve it. For instance, the relationship between a woman and her daughter-in-law remains formal and polite for years and carries a constant tension that stems from the older woman's anger when her daughter-in-law and son moved to a new home of their own. For years she's never really been friendly and open toward her daughter-in-law, and when talking to her son will subtly criticize his wife. Her unspoken revenge has affected her physically in the form of repeated bouts with rheumatism. Her acrid anger never explodes, but instead quietly smolders. Though the daughter-in-law does the shopping for her rheumatic mother-in-law and washes the curtains for her, this is taken for granted, and receives neither mention nor praise from the older woman.

Willow types know well how to make demands but are not prepared to give in return. In the long run, this alienates all who initially feel friendly and helpful toward them until such positive and open people gradually cease their efforts and leave them alone. As a result, the chronic Willow type gradually grows more isolated and embittered, withdrawing more and more from life. Perhaps he liked to go to the bowling alley in the past but now goes less often, "because the new manager has been most unpleasant." Formerly a theater buff, she now stays at home, "because those new plays are either too superficial or too negative." Whichever way you look at it, in the negative Willow state only the negative side of life presents itself. A Willow patient recovering from an illness might say: "I'm feeling better, but not half as much as I may seem to be." It appears as though he wants to keep himself from letting any positive feelings or thoughts arise in heart or mind.

If you're in the negative Willow state you're a "victim," and this provides the perfect excuse for not accepting responsibility for your own destiny. You'll firmly continue to point to the outside world as the cause, absolutely refusing to acknowledge or even consider any connection between events and your own thoughts and actions.

What is the misunderstanding or error in the negative Willow state? Again it is due to a refusal on the part of the personality to accept the guidance of the Higher Self. In the Willow state you'll find it difficult to appreciate such guidance. You judge success in life not by inner experience but mainly according to material criteria. If he hasn't been able to keep his youthful physique, she hasn't received that honorary doctorate, or he hasn't managed to acquire that house in the country, there seems to be reason enough to rail against the Higher Self and fate. Unfortunately, such rumbles of disappointment aren't all there is to it. The personality also tries to block all further attempts at guidance from the Higher Self by negative stonewalling. Rather than work with the Higher Self, it will put up passive resistance. Thus it not only harms itself but also poisons the whole environment.

If you are caught up in a persistent negative Willow state, first of all you will have to learn to recognize and accept your own bitterness, your own negativity. Second, you must realize that every grumbling thought adds another brick to your growing wall of negativity, so that your personal sun is more and more blotted out. Everything we experience on the outside is the outcome of our own thoughts being projected outward, and all of us live in a world we imagined and created at some point or other. Anyone who feels like a victim will inevitably end up a victim.

The psychological roots of the Willow state date back to a time when a child experiences himself as one with his environment and cannot differentiate between cause and effect. If he's warned about a hot stove, he touches it anyway, gets burned, and the stove gets the blame: "You bad stove!"

It's easy to fall into a negative Willow state in the course of spiritual development. This often happens when you've become aware of too much negativity in yourself but your personality is not yet strong enough to integrate it all. Your anger is then projected onto the outside world; you often become very judgmental and make no attempt to cooperate.

For patients who visit one doctor after another or one naturopath after another in search of the treatment that will work (not recognizing that they, too, have a part in their healing), you will frequently find Willow is needed in combination with Vine.

Where the shadows are strong, however, there is also much light. In order to get out of the negative Willow state you have to train yourself to deliberately concentrate on the positive side of events. Because its cut branches are always replaced by new shoots, the Willow tree is a symbol not only of mourning but also of infinite knowledge and a wisdom that never fails.

People in the positive Willow state come to realize that they are not the victims but the architects of their destiny, and that the human mind has unlimited faculties that can help build a positive future. People who have overcome their negative Willow state therefore radiate faith, calm, and optimism. They know that all of us have the capacity to be masters of our own destinies.

When practicing the positive Willow state, it is recommended that you consciously study the laws of cause and effect. Additionally, it has been found beneficial to join a neighborhood initiative involved in resolving a common need, perhaps building a playground, establishing a walking team, or creating a neighborhood watch program.

Willow Key Symptoms

You feel self-pity, resentment, and bitterness; you feel you are a victim of fate.

Behavior Pattern in the Blocked State

❀ You feel that you are being held back or that there is no hope of being delivered from a situation

❀ You experience yourself as powerless

❀ You have an embittered attitude, resenting fate and feeling that you've been treated unjustly in life

❀ You don't feel responsible for your own situation, and are always blaming circumstances or others

❀ You don't think fate recognizes your efforts and input in life

❀ You believe life has failed to provide the things that you rightfully deserve

❀ You make demands on fate, but are not prepared to do anything for them

❀ You accept help from others and take it for granted

- You react defensively and with accusations, often appearing as a killjoy or a spoilsport

- You unconsciously try to put a damper on the cheerful mood and optimism of others

- You wear a sad, pouting face as you feel offended and withdraw more and more from life

- Your thoughts are spiteful and grudging due to the bitterness you feel in your heart

- Unspoken, smoldering anger rages inside but will not explode

- You're unable to accept your extreme negativity so nothing can change

- You are reluctant to admit that you're getting better when you are recovering from an illness, even if it's clear that you are

Even if only one or two of these patterns precisely match your present situation, you need Willow.

Positive Potential

- You actively take your life into your own hands

- You think constructively and know how to exert a positive influence on situations

- You take responsibility for your own fate

- You understand the principle "as within, so without," which means that you can attract positive or negative events, and you make conscious use of this principle

Empowering Statements

- "I have power."

- "I'm in control."

- "I take responsibility."

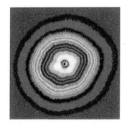

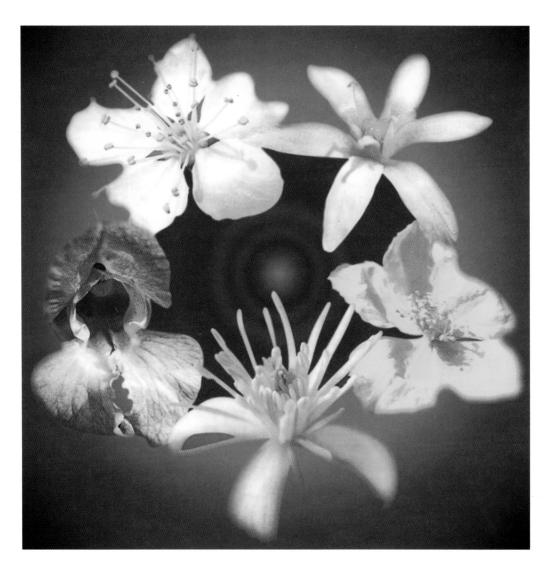

39. Rescue Remedy:
The First Aid or Emergency Remedy

In 1930 Edward Bach saved a fisherman's life with Rescue Remedy, the only combination formula in the Bach system. Since then it has provided the means to immediately restore calm and confidence in stressful situations—indirectly it has even been a lifesaver—for countless people all over the world.

Rescue Remedy works for everyone. This Flower combination has a universal effect because it addresses a transcending archetypal reaction pattern of mankind. This pattern is triggered through the synergistic interaction of five common negative behavior patterns that arise in response to stressful situations. When a certain level of feelings of being overwhelmed or threatened is reached and this pattern is activated, our whole personality becomes distorted and is stretched to its limits. Again, Bach was ahead of his time in describing what we have since discovered from stress research. The interacting patterns he recognized are:

- A reflex to play dead—for example, losing consciousness (Star of Bethlehem)

- Overreacting nerves, which lead, for example, to panic (Rock Rose)

- An exaggerated need to act immediately (Impatiens)

- Fear of losing control, as evidenced in tension or trembling (Cherry Plum)

- An impulse to deny reality as evidenced in, for example, the desire to lose yourself in dreams (Clematis)

Within a minute of taking Rescue Remedy, the body's self-healing mechanisms are reactivated. Rescue Remedy causes an emotional and psychophysical relaxation, which in turn is the best preparation for any necessary medical treatment. However, it cannot take the place of emergency medical treatment!

In the context of Bach Flowers the terms *emergency* and *shock* are defined more broadly than in conventional medicine: a shocking incident is anything that shakes up your energetic system. Some people are shocked when a door is slammed or by reading an unfriendly letter, while for others it takes a fall down the stairs or a serious accident to shock them.

Rescue Remedy also comes in a cream. Small shocks to the physical system such as burns, sprains, cuts, and sudden rashes can be treated with Rescue Cream. It can also be used in many other situations where there is a new or old shock present. Good results have been reported in the treatment of scars and bedsores, for instance. Rescue Cream contains Crab Apple in addition to the five Flower Essences in Rescue Remedy.

Typical Situations That Can Be Helped by Rescue Remedy

- When you're extremely disturbed—for instance, after a fight in the family

- If you have to face a difficult situation—for instance, a job interview or a public speech.

- When you've been frightened—for instance, because of an insect bite or a heart attack.

- If you work in a stressful environment—for instance, at a customer complaint counter.

Important Information on the Use of Rescue Remedy

- Rescue Remedy does not replace regular Bach Flower Therapy. At best it can be seen as a preliminary step to it. People who find themselves taking Rescue Remedy repeatedly are well advised to study the concepts of the five individual Flowers in this formula. They will most likely find that two or three of these are personal basic Flowers (see appendix A, Type-specific Remedies or Basic Flowers), in which case these Essences could be used as part of a personal combination.

- From time to time when necessary, Rescue Remedy can be taken in addition to regular Bach Flower Therapy.

- Rescue Remedy should be taken only on occasion and not on a regular basis. Some people will need it more often than others: While some may think of a visit to the dentist as a merely bothersome exercise, others are downright terrified—a situation that calls for the use of Rescue Remedy.

- Rescue Remedy can be used externally on bandages, compresses, and the like.

- Preparation and dosage of Rescue Remedy are described in chapter 8.

- Rescue Remedy is effective in plants and animals (see chapter 8, page 247).

- Rescue Remedy can alleviate a strong healing crisis (see chapter 8, page 233).

- A tip from a practitioner: Patients who are so unsettled when they come into the office that they can't speak about their feelings or are unable to fill out a questionnaire are best sent home to take only Rescue Remedy for two days before coming back for a new appointment on the third day.

Rescue Remedy can be effective in preventing menstrual cramps, gallbladder problems, colic, boils, epileptic seizures, migraine, and similar problems if it's taken early in the preliminary psychological phase of the condition, coincident with the first recognizable symptoms before the actual onset of illness. Later, once the phase of physical symptoms has begun, Rescue Remedy can do nothing to stop the progression of the illness or difficulty. The only way it can be of use at this point is to help the individual endure the process of the illness with more psychological or philosophical distance.

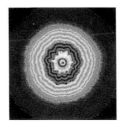

The Personal Emergency Mixture

Putting together a personal emergency mixture has often been a good first step before beginning regular Bach Flower Therapy. However, it makes sense to do so only when a personal behavior pattern frequently produces a situation that would respond to Rescue Remedy or when a situation that would benefit from Rescue Remedy always strongly triggers the same personal behavior pattern. For instance: You repeatedly experience jealousy (Holly) and overreact to it, which causes you to break down (Rescue Remedy). Your personal emergency mixture would therefore be Holly and Rescue Remedy. Or, every situation for which you could take Rescue Remedy triggers overwhelming guilt feelings (Pine). In this scenario your personal emergency formula would be Pine and Rescue. Or, if stressful situations always make you feel like a loser, your personal emergency mixture could be Larch, Willow, and Rescue.

Frequently Asked Questions

For further information, please match the *italicized terms* in the following questions with those from the alphabetized list of issues found in appendix A.

Is it possible to treat *plants* with Rescue Remedy?

Is it possible to combine *Rescue Remedy and painkillers?*

Is it possible to take Rescue Remedy as a *preventive measure?*

Is it possible to use *Rescue Remedy as part of a combination?*

How do I apply *Rescue Cream?*

What are the most common *Rescue Remedy applications?*

6

Finding the Right Bach Flowers

"No science, no knowledge is necessary, apart from the simple methods described herein; and they who will obtain the greatest benefit from this Godsent gift will be those who keep it pure as it is; free from science, free from theories, for everything in nature is simple."

Edward Bach

When first reading the descriptions of the Bach Flowers, most people feel that they need almost every one of them, or they immediately connect certain flowers with a specific friend, relative, or pet. This, of course, demonstrates excellent perceptive skills. But what causes this phenomenon?

Bach defined his thirty-eight Soul states as "character weaknesses of human nature." Today we speak of negative archetypal behavior patterns—such as hating, glossing over things, resisting, and giving in easily. As part of the collective subconscious, these patterns make up the repertoire of negative human behavior, independent of race, time, and culture. Because they reflect our basic human experiences, they are found over and over again in the myths, fairy tales, and proverbs of all cultures. Throughout history, great artists dramatized these behavior patterns in positive form as virtues and in negative form as vices. Since we are already using this array of behavior patterns on a daily basis, often without being aware of it, it is quite natural that when we read about them, they are immediately familiar to us.

Depending on the age we live in and its cultural, moral, and intellectual climate, these behavior patterns will appear in ever-changing shades and facets.* The Mimulus state seen in the fear of the plague in the Middle Ages appears today as the fear of AIDS. The intentional

---

* Some people misinterpret various shades of behavior patterns and argue that new discoveries and descriptions of flowers relate to new traits in human nature.

suppression of natural impulses in the extreme Rock Water state that was seen in the prudishness of many during Bach's lifetime appears today in the overly disciplined self-denial found in some fitness and health crazes.

It is the necessary yet exciting task of anyone who sets out to choose an appropriate flower combination to carefully study the endlessly varying manifestations of human nature and the very simple principles from which they arise.

Bach said that the correct diagnosis is reached after an interview by using intuition, observation, and the ability to empathize with another person. A deep knowledge of all thirty-eight behavior patterns is also indispensable and cannot be replaced by any kind of measurement, card reading, muscle tests, and so forth. (See *additional methods of diagnosis* in the alphabetized list of issues in appendix A.)

To learn how to apply Bach Flower Therapy the way Bach himself envisioned it, it is useful to begin with the following steps:

- ❀ Familiarize yourself with the description of each Flower

- ❀ Observe yourself to recognize your own typical behavior patterns

- ❀ Study human nature in all aspects of life

- ❀ Gather your own experiences by taking the Flowers

Familiarize Yourself with the Description of Each Flower

Everyone will have an individual approach to picking up this primary knowledge. Some people will start by systematically memorizing the attributes of the thirty-eight Flowers, beginning with, perhaps, Agrimony—the Honesty Flower.

More often, others simply start with those Flowers that are most appealing to them as they flip through the pages of this book. Probably these will be your own basic Flowers (see appendix A) that show your deeply rooted behavior patterns.* At first, work with these Flowers; the more you study them, the more other Flowers will spark your interest.

Observe Yourself to Recognize Your Own Typical Behavior Patterns

Look back on your life and identify the states that predominated at different stages. For instance, what were you like as a school-aged child? Were you an Agrimony type—cheerful on the outside, not wanting anyone to know what was going on inside? Or were you a Clematis type, always somewhere else with your thoughts?

Recall past crises and how you responded to

---

* Deeper analysis of each Flower state in respect to your own personality is available in my *Keys to the Soul* (Saffron Walden, Essex, England: C. W. Daniel Company, 1998).

them. Perhaps you received the shock of nearly drowning when you were a small child (Star of Bethlehem) and since then have felt anxiety about going in the water (Mimulus). The shock you experienced years ago may still be present in your energetic system. Now at last it can be released.

Observe your reactions when you are very tired, are in crisis, or have a difficult decision to make. In these moments, you experience your true personality with all its weaknesses and challenges at the times when they are not simply glossed over, intellectually justified, or hidden behind illusions.

Pay attention to the way others react in your presence, and to how your environment mirrors your own actions. Do others complain repeatedly about the same shortcomings in your personality? Do they say you are too critical, too good-natured, or too impatient?

If you are completely certain that one of the flowers definitely does not apply to you, it's likely that you may have a blind spot—this flower might be of great importance to you.

Finally, ask yourself which characteristics you most admire or despise in others. These might be traits you have yet to discover in yourself.

Study Human Nature in All Aspects of Life

Human nature shows itself everywhere in our daily environment at work, with family, or with friends, as well as in art and in literature. Study the nature of those around you—for example, what kind of behavior pattern does your daughter use when she needs to tell you something uncomfortable? Does she play the victim and accuse you of something (Willow), or does she try to play down the situation (Agrimony)?

Be playful when learning about Bach Flowers. Imagine the natures of your favorite movie and TV characters, or even characters in familiar fairy tales. Which Bach Flower would benefit each of them? Cinderella, for example, is a Centaury type, put upon by all the family and too weak-willed to stand up to them. She never feels herself to be a victim and therefore would not need Willow. The stepmother is clearly a Chicory type; she manipulates her daughters to fulfill her own ambitions. When Cinderella finally marries her prince, her stepsisters can no doubt do with a few drops of Holly to overcome their hatred and envy.

The classics also provide rich examples for diagnostic practice. What remedy would you prescribe to Hamlet? Most important of all would be Scleranthus for his indecision ("To be or not to be?"), then Mustard for his deep melancholia, and Cherry Plum for obsessive, suicidal thoughts. And what of Faust? If he could have a clear goal and a vision of his Life Plan, he might never sell his soul to Mephisto. He makes a clear case for Wild Oat due to his dissatisfaction and search for meaning.

It takes a more sensitive mind to spot

archetypal Soul states in the visual arts. For example, *The Scream*, the famous work by Edvard Munch, would be indicative of the Rock Rose state. Fascinating but even trickier to see are the states that can be read into the faces of famous portraits or the states that can be heard in a piece of music.

Gather Your Own Experiences by Taking Bach Flowers

Many people have their first experience with Bach Flowers when they are given to them by a doctor, therapist, or practitioner. Others may have received them from a friend or relative who was helping them to deal with a crisis situation.

In reading through this book, it is a common beginner's mistake to feel that you must immediately take the Flowers that most attract you. While these are very likely some of your personal basic Flowers, it is useful to take them only when they address a problem that is bothering you at a specific moment. You may tend to be generally indecisive but the Flower would be appropriate to take only when you are having trouble making a specific decision, such as which of two job offers to accept by the end of the week (Scleranthus). A well-chosen combination of Flowers will be effective within a few days or even hours during an acute crisis. The speed and clarity of this kind of success will then motivate you to take further steps in using Bach Flower Therapy.

In gathering personal experience with the Flowers, it is important to know that there are different levels of difficulty that they can address.

Level A: Acute crisis. A crisis situation might be fear before going to a class reunion, problems with a colleague at work, or a misunderstanding with your child's teacher at school.

This is the most frequent and most important level of self-treatment and a beginner is advised to start at this level. Since the symptoms in an acute condition are easier to see, it is easier to successfully choose the right Flowers to take without engaging in an interview or requiring help from others.

Working at this level, you will find it helpful to use the situation questionnaire in chapter 11. Additional hints can be found in the information regarding choosing combinations (chapter 11) or possibly under *spontaneous choice* in the alphabetized list of issues in appendix A.

For your final decision, read up on the Flowers you selected in chapter 5 and keep in mind that **even if only one or two of these patterns precisely match your present situation, you need the Flower.**

In cases where you find it difficult to decide between two Flowers, start with the reference table in chapter 9, and look up the comparisons in that chapter.

Level B: Character weakness. Time and again chronic, deeply ingrained negative behavior patterns become stumbling blocks to our personal development and spiritual growth. They might include chronic lack of self-confidence, constant indecisiveness, extreme shyness, and all kinds of excessive behavior, such as working, eating, drinking, or smoking far too much. It is recommended that you attempt this kind of self-exploration in collaboration with a practitioner or therapist, or with a friend well versed in Bach Flowers.

A chronic problem is best approached at times when it becomes acute. For example, if you have a difficult relationship with your father, the problem will usually become acute shortly before an impending family reunion and treatment would be most effectively started at that time. For Flower selection, refer to the entire double questionnaire in chapter 10.

Level C: Supportive treatment for cases of acute or chronic physical illness. To support the psychological aspects of an acute physical problem—a broken leg, for example—follow the same strategy as for Level A. Ask yourself, "What are my present psychological reactions to this problem?" Are you impatient? Anxious? Skeptical?

In cases of a chronic illness such as psoriasis or asthma, you are well advised to inform other medical or psychological professionals whom you are working with of your supportive treatment with Bach Flowers. For your Flower selection, refer to the entire double questionnaire in chapter 10.

Scope and Limits of Self-Treatment

The Five Golden Rules for Self-Therapy

1. **Take Flowers only when you feel a *definite need* for support in a current crisis.** The Flowers' energies are nature's gift—do not misuse them for frivolous experimentation or "Soul cosmetics."

2. **Determine the Flowers you need according to acutely present and *consciously recognizable* negative states.** For this, you do not need deep psychological analysis or esoteric rituals. The problems you are able to tackle here are clear and tangible. Then, over time, by continuing to take Bach Flowers on a regular basis, conditions that are hidden deeper within you will be uncovered and brought to your consciousness. They will reveal themselves to you in a natural order, as though you are peeling the layers of an onion. Each will manifest at precisely the time when you are ready to confront it and are able to work it out.

3. **Take *personal responsibility* for your final choice.** No matter what method you use to arrive at your selection of Flowers, whether self-observation and study of the Flower concepts or use of

nonverbal means—a pendulum, kinesiology, spontaneous choice, or electronic measurement—in the end, you need to consciously evaluate your decision within yourself. Reading the material here can help you do this, as can discussion with a partner. Always ask yourself, "Do these Flowers really represent the problem I am dealing with right now?" Any Flowers that are not pertinent *at this time* should be held back for reconsideration in the future.

People who do not focus on the present condition, and instead experiment with any number of Flowers at the same time, will touch upon different kinds of problematic issues without getting a proper hold on any of them. Experience has shown that a mixture of this kind does not provide a lasting effect and will not support further developmental steps.

4. **Try to understand how the Flowers in your *combination* interact to address the various aspects of a *recurring behavioral pattern*.** In time this will facilitate your understanding of the psychological connections between the particular Flower states. A well-selected combination will have a harmonizing effect not only on the specific situation it was chosen for, but also on the behavior pattern you might exhibit in another

similar set of circumstances. For example, a woman needs Red Chestnut, Centaury, and Olive. She cares for her mother in an exaggerated manner (Red Chestnut), she is unable to refuse any of her mother's wishes (Centaury) and thus has becomes exhausted (Olive). Through taking the Flowers and working with their principles, she recognizes that she is repeating the same behavioral pattern with friends and colleagues time and again. Eventually, this pattern is resolved both with her mother and in the other situations.

5. **Learn to recognize *when to talk to an experienced Bach Flower practitioner or a therapist*.** It has often been seen that after people successfully take one or two Flower combinations of their own choosing, they find that they have come to a standstill. This is understandable because although acute negative Soul states have been harmonized, to achieve further development you have to get down to the nitty-gritty—and self-perception in this respect is naturally somewhat cloudy. Almost certainly you have come to a blind spot. Talking to an outside expert at this point will provide you with new perspectives and valuable points of view. It has been proved beneficial to alternate between talking to an expert and self-treating a time or two with your own Flower combination.

At this point it must be stressed once again that Bach Flower Therapy cannot take the place of professional psychotherapeutic or medical treatment!

Additional Advice Generated from Many Years of Experience

❀ Don't expect overnight miracles or an experience exactly like that of a friend. No two people are the same and every problem is unique.

❀ In any situation where you are so overwhelmed that you have lost contact with your Inner Guidance and can make no choice for yourself, Rescue Remedy will help.

❀ Keep a *reaction record* with daily observations of changes in your feelings and mental states (see appendix A). Positive changes from taking Bach Flowers are sometimes so subtle that they may escape notice at first; with harmony restored you might take your new self for granted or recognize it as the norm. This is logical because each correct combination of Flowers brings you closer to your true personality. Dreams can be frequent while taking Flowers, as can new ideas and insights. These should be recorded. It may also happen that the next deeper or older layer of a problem reveals itself, which then can be treated with a subsequent mixture. Having notes helps you track the course of your development more consciously, helps you use the Flower impulses optimally, and works to establish reference points for determining future combinations.

Frequently Asked Questions

For further information, please match the *italicized terms* in the following questions with those from the alphabetized list of issues found in appendix A.

Is it possible to take *all thirty-eight Flowers* in just one combination?

Is it possible to take specific Flowers as a *preventive measure?*

How many Flowers should be combined into a single mixture?

Is it possible to choose Bach Flowers according to their *positive potential?*

What are *type-specific remedies* or *basic Flowers?*

What is the compatibility of each Bach Flower with the others?

What can I expect from a *spontaneous choice?*

Is *taking single Flower Essences* more effective than taking combinations?

Are there *standard combinations* for specific problems or situations?

What happens if I take the *wrong choice of Bach Flowers?*

How do I set up *reaction records?*

Is it advisable to give a dose of Flowers without a person's *awareness of the administration?*

What are the advantages and disadvantages of *additional methods of diagnosis?*

Is there such a thing as a *correct* or incorrect *combination?*

Is there a *general mixture for everyone starting treatment?*

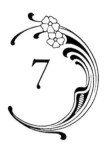

How to Help Others through Bach Flowers

After you have experienced the positive effects of Bach Flowers on yourself for a year or so, you will likely be able to begin using them to help others. Bach called it "serving you neighbors," meaning all those who are your relatives, friends, and colleagues—in other words, the people you know well.*

Be careful not to push your services on others. Instead, talk with them about Bach Flowers and the possibilities the therapy holds. Then wait and see if the person you talk with is really interested in going further. You may find it very difficult to let the other person make his or her own decision, particularly when you have a distinct feeling of how much a combination of Bach Flowers would help your friend or colleague; he or she may be involved in a serious crisis at the moment, such as the death of a spouse or an escalating problem at work. Do bide your time. When the initiative comes from the Inner Guidance of your friend's Higher Self, the combination will be more effective (Heal Thyself principle).†

Frequently the combination you give will be enough to help your friend tackle a crisis alone, but at other times it will be the first indication that there is an existing problem in definite need of professional medical or psychotherapeutic help. Either way, your friend will have benefited from your help. In addition, some friends will learn to apply the Bach Flowers to help themselves—a benefit for you and them in your future use and study of Bach Flowers.

To make sure that you're really ready and able

---

* The professional treatment of others is subject to varying laws, depending on the country in which you live.

† This does not apply to the use of Rescue Remedy or to the personal Bach Flower combinations given to children.

to help another person and that your care isn't just compensating for needs of your own, remember to take a quiet moment to explore your personal motives. "Why is it that I want to help others? Do I truly wish to serve them, or do I have an additional reason such as a desire to gain influence, recognition, companionship, or remuneration?"

The more these and other limiting personal motives stand out—they are, of course, always present to some degree—the poorer the results will be in the long run because your actions are not guided by your Higher Self and will not be in tune fully with spiritual laws.

Another interesting question may be why the other person has chosen you for a partner. Did she come on her own? Did somebody else send her to you? Does she really want to make a change in her life, or does she merely want to have a good cry? Does she take seriously Bach Flower Therapy, or is it simply an activity that allows some social interaction?

The more clearly you understand your neighbor's motives, the easier it is to decide whether to offer him assistance, politely decline to help, or recommend that he talk to a trained professional.

Work on your personal unfolding and development must continue to take priority. To paraphrase Bach: The greatest gift we can give to another is to be happy and full of hope ourselves, for in that way we shall pull him up from his depression. In other words, if your own vibra-tions are in harmony, they will aid other people to harmonize their own vibrations—even without taking any Bach Flowers.

The following are the most important principles of diagnosis in Bach Flower Therapy:

⊛ It is your partner's *emotional and mental states that* need to be studied in detail; the physical* state needs neither observation nor interpretation.

⊛ To make your choice of Flowers, it is important to have an *interview* and to *put yourself into your partner's shoes.*

⊛ Bach stressed that in an interview, you must trust your *intuition*, the communication from your Higher Self. It is often experienced as sudden flashes of awareness that occur when the mind and emotions are synchronized.

Inner Preparation

Before each interview, keep in mind that your purpose is more than merely "turning off" a negative feeling.

---

* An interpretation based on the correspondence of psychological states to body parts might suggest, for instance, Holly as a Remedy for heart problems. This, however, is not the appropriate approach for a Bach Flower diagnosis. In an appropriate approach for a Bach Flower diagnosis, the important question to ask the patient is: What are your mental and emotional reactions to your problem? For example, is the patient without hope, full of despair, or very impatient?

- We are all consciously or unconsciously on a journey to fulfill our Life Plan and to find our true Self, with the support of our Inner Guidance.

- Our times of crisis occur when we are cut off from our Inner Guidance and have come to a dead end.

- The deeper reason we have become cut off is the misunderstanding or misuse of spiritual laws.

- The negative behavior patterns defined by Bach provide information about where our misunderstandings come from. They help us recognize where and how we have acted against either the law of Unity or the law of Inner Guidance.

- However, these same behavior patterns are also indicative of our positive qualities and the spiritual potential lying dormant within us, abilities we are unable to use in the moment because our misunderstandings have blocked them.

- As an interviewer I am a traveling companion on a joint search for a way out of the dead end.

- Foremost in any Bach Flower interview is to help the other person understand and accept responsibility that it is his and only his doing that got him where he is and it is only his doing that will turn his life in a new direction.

- Your interview partner needs to gain absolute confidence that now, with the energetic support of the Flowers, this step is a real possibility.

- The more deeply you yourself understand these principles and become a living example of them in your daily life, the more effectively you will be able to communicate them to your partner. Furthermore, the subconscious of your partner receives and responds to your vibration directly and this even has a positive energetic effect on the Flower mixture that is used.

- If before every interview you attempt to connect with your own Higher Self, it will be possible to avoid the typical mistakes that arise from our personality such as moral judgments, intellectual interpretations, missionary ambitions, projection of our own ideas, and internal righteousness.

- Don't be discouraged if this endeavor sometimes turns out to be less successful than you hoped. Trust that any heartfelt conversation is a step in the right direction for both you and your interview partner, and is a valuable human experience.

The First Impression

When a person you are interviewing comes into the room, you will get a first impression that includes messages for an intuitive choice of Flowers. Take note of this impression and find out during the session if some of those Flowers are indeed appropriate.

Please note that the following general association clues are not the specific building blocks shown in chapter 11.

What is the impression I get from my interview partner? How do I perceive him? How does she strike me?

Shy, sensitive, timid	Mimulus, Aspen, Centaury, Crab Apple
Muted, restrained	Honeysuckle, Gorse, Wild Rose
Lacking concentration	Clematis, Chestnut Bud
Is difficult to grasp	Centaury, Clematis, Cherry Plum, Agrimony
Unapproachable, far away	Star of Bethlehem, Mustard, Cherry Plum, Clematis
Apathetic, without initiative	Star of Bethlehem, Mustard, Wild Rose, Olive
Weak	Wild Rose, Centaury, Olive
Discouraged, resigned	Elm, Gentian, Mustard, Gorse, Wild Rose
Depressed	Gentian, Mustard, Gorse
Tense	Vine, Rock Water, Agrimony, Impatiens, Vervain, Star of Bethlehem
Inhibited	Water Violet, Larch, Cherry Plum, Star of Bethlehem, Mimulus
Stressed, nervous	Rock Rose, Agrimony, Impatiens, Scleranthus, Crab Apple, Cherry Plum
Impatient, driven	Impatiens, Vervain, Chestnut Bud
Aggressive, agitated	Holly, Impatiens, Vine
Overtaxed, overwhelmed	Elm, Olive, Centaury, Star of Bethlehem
Feels under pressure	Cherry Plum, Impatiens, White Chestnut
Self-centered	Heather, Rock Water, Water Violet
Imposing, possesses a strong personality	Chicory, Holly, Vine
Proud, arrogant	Water Violet, Vine
Demanding, goal-oriented	Vine, Vervain, Chicory
Pushy	Vervain, Heather
Rigid, frozen	Rock Water, Star of Bethlehem

Structuring a Bach Flower Interview

Because a talk with a person you know will most likely be of an informal nature, more so than one in a professional's office,* it is important to have a structure and keep it in mind so that you don't overlook important elements of the interview.

An effective Bach Flower interview should include the following five elements:

1. Clarifying the conditions of the interview.

2. Discovering what led up to the present crisis and what currently accompanies it.

3. Assessing the problem and making a preliminary choice of Bach Flowers.

4. Finalizing your choice for a Flower combination.

5. Motivating and encouraging your interview partner to take action.

Clarifying the Conditions of the Interview

Before the interview takes place, it's a wise idea to clarify a few things, even if over the phone. Questions such as "What do you know about Bach Flowers in general?" and "What do you expect from me or from Bach Flower Remedies?" would be a good place to start. You must also try to determine whether the person is really seeking support in making a change or just looking for a way to let off steam. In the latter case, a Bach Flower interview will not be needed.

It is also important to establish how much time should be set aside for the interview (a length of approximately an hour is suggested; open-ended interviews tend to lose their focus) and what fee or trade is expected, if any.

Discovering What Led Up to the Present Crisis and What Currently Accompanies It

Find out first what event occurred just before the crisis started (an accident, quarrel, or bad news, for example). Then check for additional pertinent circumstances: Is anyone else directly involved? Is the person you are interviewing currently under medical or psychological care or has he been previously institutionalized? (Even among friends, these facts are frequently kept secret.) In many cases, it would be important for the professionals in other fields to know that their patient is taking Bach Flowers.

You might find yourself in a situation where the other person is in a serious and acute physical or psychological crisis (your interview partner is no longer able to control his physical or psychological reactions) and is refusing appropriate professional help. In such a case it is your responsibility to insist that he get professional help. If he continue to resist, you should inform his family and can only recommend Rescue Remedy.

---

* See also my *Original Bach-Blütentherapie: Lehrbuch für die Arzt und Naturheilpraxis* (Neckarsulm, 1996).

Assessing the Problem and Making a Preliminary Choice of Bach Flowers

Start with your first intuitive impressions (see box on page 220). What do you sense in the other person? Is he muted, under pressure, depressed? Make a note of these first impressions. Then observe more precisely.

What are the person's emotional and mental reactions to her problem? This is the most important point to observe (remember to observe and not analyze!). What patterns become apparent? Make a note of the Flowers that immediately come to your mind.

Use all of your senses in your observations. How does your interview partner speak? Does he speak with conviction (Vervain) or authority (Vine)? Does she report in a timid, fearful voice (Mimulus)? Does he say, "I have given up hope" (Gorse) or "I am very impatient about . . ." (Impatiens)?

Body language will also provide you with clues. What is his posture—loose or tense (Rock Water)? Does she shift around in her seat (Impatiens)? Is her smile a true reflection of her feeling, or is it worn to convince the world (Agrimony)? Does he have tense wrinkles on his forehead (White Chestnut)?

According to experience, people start talking about the issue that bothers them the most during the first five or six sentences of the interview. With more practice, during this phase you will be able to determine three or four of the Flowers needed.

However, be aware that some people will reach the main issue only at the very end of an interview or even after it has finished.

If your impression is that you haven't understood completely, keep asking questions until you are absolutely sure about the person's state. This strategy is most appropriate in cases where your interview partner regularly uses conditional forms of speech ("I guess I should . . ."), speaks in generalizations ("One should . . ."), or answers in the form of a presumption ("I suppose my husband . . ."). To ask further questions is not an indiscretion. Rather, it helps your partner to recognize the problem more clearly and be more focused about finding a solution. When you ask a question, make sure that your partner has ample time for a reply—if there's a quiet moment, respect it and wait before continuing with the next question.

Try to take notes without interrupting the flow of the conversation or hindering your ability to listen.

Ask for further background information only if the description of the present situation is inconclusive. In the end, most crisis situations have a basis in unresolved conflicts with parents or other significant people, undigested experiences, strokes of fate, or problematic belief systems. Because all of us have had previous personal experiences in these areas that may underlie crises, be careful not to let your own experiences influence you.

Further, don't abandon your role as an observer by judging what you hear and responding with phrases such as "I don't like that" or by interpreting what you've been told and remarking, "I am sure that happened because of . . ." Instead, ask questions such as: "Have you had a similar crisis before?"; "How did you resolve the crisis at that time? Was it by giving in?" (Centaury); "Did you demand your own way?" (Vine); "Did the crisis simply end on its own, with you being left behind as the victim ?" (Willow).

This line of questioning automatically takes you deeper into your interview partner's life history. Continue by exploring which issues, psychological or physical, she hasn't completely come to terms with and that may still be playing a part in this crisis. For example, has there been some disappointment in love or a professional setback? Are there upcoming events that she is more apprehensive about than she'd like to admit or is even aware of, such as a new job, a divorce, an operation, a move?

Keep coming back to the present situation. Try to relate the behavior pattern of a previous crisis to the current situation: "It appears that you are acquiescing now in the same way that you did in your last marriage" (Centaury). If it turns out that an old situation is still having particularly debilitating effects today, your interview partner should be seeking professional help.

At this point, recheck the pertinent Flower patterns by asking direct questions: "Are you afraid to start the new project?" (Mimulus), or "Do you get suspicious when you see people talking together and looking at you?" (Holly). You can also ask more than one question about the same topic in order to further clarify the pattern: "Do you feel fearful when you have to work as part of a team?" (Mimulus); "Do you prefer to work in the background?" (Water Violet); "Are the others working too slowly for you?" (Impatiens); "Are you trying to control the team?" (Vine); or "Are you diplomatic with people so that they will do more of what you want?" (Chicory).

Resist any temptation to find a solution for your partner's problems. This is not your job. Remember: "Heal thyself." Give him help only for self-help. Allow the other person to realize her own mistakes and find her own solution.

At this point in the interview you probably have determined a number of appropriate Bach Flowers. If you feel that it is still necessary, this would be the right time to use a nonverbal diagnostic method to round out your picture. For instance, your interview partner's quick spontaneous choice (see appendix A) may illuminate an aspect you have overlooked if the chosen Flower is one you haven't considered yet. This would then require further investigation. If, for instance, your partner picks White Chestnut, your question might be, "Does this situation worry you so that you wake up during the night thinking about it?" This would allow you to determine whether the choice of White Chestnut is genuinely indicative of the problem or relates to a momentary situation such as worry over an expiring parking meter outside. White Chestnut would be included only if its choice reflects the larger problem.

Finalizing Your Choice for a Flower Combination

At this point take all the Flowers you have considered and discuss them with your partner. The goal here is to determine which Flowers represent the most acute aspects of the situation and therefore should be included. If necessary, refer to chapter 5 under "Behavior Pattern in the Blocked State" for each Flower.

If you have difficulty deciding between two Flowers, refer to chapter 9 for precise comparisons.

Don't push your partner to take a Flower he resists, even if you're absolutely sure that it's needed. This is your partner's combination, and his process. Make note of this Flower, though, for future sessions.

Now the time has come for the last—perhaps most important—part of the meeting.

Motivating and Encouraging Your Partner to take Action

On many occasions your interview partner will not be able to identify with a particular Flower

concept. The reason might be that you didn't find the right words* when you explained the concept or that the entire interview has taken on a destructive tone. In cases where your interview partner responds with a statement such as "I didn't know that I was that bad," it's obvious that your meeting got off on the wrong foot. At the conclusion of an interview that proceeded positively, your partner will feel a sense of "Aha!" or "I see!" and will be looking forward to developing her positive potential with the help of the selected Bach Flowers.

Go through the selected Flower combination once again and explain to your partner how each Flower can support the constructive resolution of the current crisis. For example, Beech, the Tolerance Flower, will support you in developing tolerance toward your colleagues so that you no longer need to be overly critical of them. Larch, the Self-Confidence Flower, helps you build your self-confidence so that you begin to trust more in your abilities and no longer compare yourself with others.

Encourage your partner to start working immediately with the impulses from each of the Flowers. If his particular crisis involves a colleague at work, he should pay attention to his reaction when a similar situation arises after taking the Flowers. It's possible that he will quickly

---

* Behavioral states do not always appear exactly as they are described in books. They can manifest differently depending on how they combine with other states (see the introduction to chapter 5).

begin seeing the situation more objectively and responding to it with greater calm.

Ask your interview partner to keep a reaction record (see appendix A) both for his own benefit and for use in possible future interviews.

Following the First Interview

While taking the Bach Flowers, your partner should have the opportunity to talk with you. There may be a misunderstanding of some sort, or a new question may arise for her. In any case, you should plan a follow-up meeting for three weeks after the first interview to discuss your partner's experiences with the present mixture. Of course, it's possible that the combination will elicit the desired effect in this time, allowing your partner to resolve the crisis on his own. Celebrate the success together.

Alternatively, your partner will ask for further assistance. In this case, go over the changes that have taken place in the three weeks and determine which states have been resolved and which need further attention. Have other Flower patterns become more acute at this point, possibly those you considered during the first interview? Or have new negative states developed in the meantime? Discuss in detail with your partner any modification of the mixture you decide upon at this time.

Sometimes during a second or third interview both partners realize that the problem is much deeper than they originally thought it would be. At this point it is your responsibility to support him in seeking proper professional help.

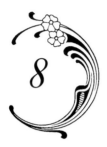

8

Original Bach Flower Therapy in Practice

Preparation, Dosage, and Administration

Once you have decided on the Flowers either you or your interview partner will take, you can then pick the appropriate method of preparation, dosage, and administration to use.

Two Classic Methods of Preparation

Water Glass Method. This method is particularly recommended

❀ During the beginning phase of Bach Therapy

❀ In acute or extreme states

❀ At times when you're planning to take the Flowers for only a few days

Every morning fill a large glass with water and add two drops of each Flower from the stock bottles (four drops of Rescue Remedy, if this is part of your combination). Take the liquid in small sips throughout the day until the glass is empty. This gradual dosage is more intense because each sip provides a fresh impulse of energy. In cases of very acute problems it's possible that you may need to take more than one glass a day before the state requiring harmonization has subsided.

People who travel a great deal may choose to use a small water bottle in place of a glass for dosage.

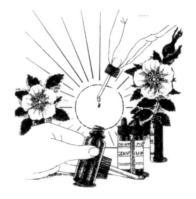

Mixing Bottle Method. This method is recommended for the treatment of chronic negative behavior patterns or those continuing for a longer duration.

Fill a dispenser bottle (with a dropper)* with three parts water to one part drinking alcohol (see below for suggested types of alcohol). To this add one drop of each Bach Flower Essence you have chosen for each ten milliliters of liquid in your bottle. (Add two drops, if using Rescue Remedy.) For dosage, see below.

You can find out where to purchase bottles at most places where Bach Flowers are sold. The most useful size for adults is thirty milliliters and for children, ten to twenty milliliters. Those who work away from home will find it practical to prepare two bottles, one to keep at home and the other to keep at work. If only you will be using your bottle for future Bach Flower applications, you may simply rinse it in hot water when you have finished your treatment. If your bottle will be used by others, however, it's recommended that you boil or sterilize it first.

Types of Water and Alcohol

Which kind of water to use. Bach recommended the use of springwater, meaning "healthy water from natural sources." Today's equivalent would be high-quality tap water, water from your own well, filtered water, or commercial mineral water without carbonation.

Water from mineral springs that have a reputation for healing certain ailments is not recommended, since these waters have a strong vibration of their own and are not neutral enough. Also not appropriate are distilled or demineralized water because they lack "impregnability." The use of techniques that change the vibration of water has not been proved to have a long-term, positive effect on Bach Flower mixtures.

Taking the undiluted essence straight from the stock bottle has a strong, immediate effect, but experience tells that it does not as last as long. It seems that water is a necessary medium to store the energetic impulses of the Flowers and to make them more long lasting.

The role of alcohol. Alcohol merely serves to preserve the water. Either cognac or grape alcohol (which is already part of the stock-bottle mixture) is fine, but any other clear spirit with less than 46 percent alcohol content (92 proof) is acceptable. Children and those who must avoid alcohol may use mixtures made without it to the same effect. (See the end of this chapter and "*Alcoholic*" in appendix A for further information.)

Raspberry vinegar or glycerin may be used as an alternative preservative.

---

* The sizes of bottles vary between ten and fifty milliliters. For bottles that measure in fluid ounces only, note that one ounce equals almost thirty milliliters. In some books and leaflets you will find two drops recommended for a thirty-milliliter bottle. Dr. Bach often spoke of "a few" drops and I have found the above suggestions to be both practical and effective.

Additional Methods of Application

When physical ailments are present during treatment with Bach Flowers, people may have the impulse to use the drops directly on the afflicted area of their body as well—for instance, on rashes, swollen glands, or around the ears after a sudden loss of hearing. This seems to work when the Flowers are also being taken internally.

Compresses with Rescue Remedy

Add no less than six drops from the stock bottle to a container with two cups of water. Use as a soaking medium for a compress.

Baths. An evening bath with Bach Flowers has been shown to be beneficial in relieving exhaustion and promoting relaxation or when you feel like you are coming down with the flu or similar illness. While recommendations for dosage may vary, it's best to use no more than five drops of each chosen Essence—ten in the case of Rescue Remedy—to one full bathtub.

Storage of Bach Flower Essences

Sets of Bach Essences and single stock bottles can be stored at room temperature inside a cupboard and away from sunlight, just like homeopathic remedies. Bach Flower Essences are more energetically stable than high potency homeopathic remedies, however, so things such as computers, refrigerators, and automobiles do not affect them.

Perishability

The contents of stock bottles will keep indefinitely despite the fact that, for legal reasons, dates are printed on the packages. Rescue Cream, just as other medical or cosmetic salves, will keep for many months, and the contents of mixing bottles will last at least three to four weeks. If you wish to keep the contents of a mixing bottle longer—Rescue Remedy is one you might want to have available—it's recommended that you increase the alcohol content to 50 percent or more.

Old mixtures are still energetically effective, even in cases where the water has turned milky. Rather than simply being discarded, they should be used in a bath, or should be returned to nature by adding them when watering your plants.

If the combination you are taking has been prepared without alcohol, it will last as long as the water will keep. Therefore, in summer it is advisable to keep these mixtures in the refrigerator.

Dosage and Administration

There is no danger in varying the dosage* of Bach Flower Remedies for individual needs, as there would be with homeopathic remedies. The standard dosage for the Water Glass Method is two drops daily from the stock bottle into a glass of

---

* With respect to dosages, experience has varied widely. Some recent recommendations have been found to be substantially higher or lower than Bach's original guidelines. In any case, it's recommended that you start with Bach's original guidelines and then find out for yourself which dosage works best for you.

water. For the Mixing Bottle Method, it is four drops directly on the tongue, four times a day.

Higher dosage. When first beginning Bach Flower Therapy, many people feel the need to take a mixture more frequently. They like to prepare several glasses of water with the remedy or, if using the Mixing Bottle Method, administer drops up to fourteen times a day. It's advisable to answer this need because it often brings the breakthrough that leads to a successful treatment. Most people shift to the standard dosage after about a week.

Lower dosage. A few people intuitively feel the need to reduce the dosage. Those who have already found that they do better with smaller amounts of homeopathic or other natural remedies are advised to start with one drop, once a day, and increase the amount gradually to up to four drops, four times a day.

Dosage for children. Observation indicates that children will usually express very clearly how much more or less they want to take in relation to the standard dosage. Parents are advised to carefully follow these requests.

Dosage of Rescue Remedy. Fill a small glass with water or another beverage (such as juice or tea). Add four drops of Rescue Remedy and drink all of the liquid within fifteen minutes by taking small sips. If you fail to achieve the results you anticipated within this time frame, prepare another glass of liquid.

There may be situations in which no fluids are available or the person in need of treatment is unable to drink. Rescue Remedy can then be administered by placing drops from the stock bottle directly onto the lips, gums, temples, inner wrists, elbows, area around the heart, or the thyroid.

Recommended times of day for dosage of drops. In order to achieve the fullest effect, take the drops about ten minutes before a meal or at least thirty minutes after. Before swallowing, keep the fluid in your mouth for a few seconds. You might take the drops:

- ❀ A few minutes after brushing your teeth in the morning

- ❀ Between noon and one o'clock in the afternoon

- ❀ In the afternoon between four and six o'clock

- ❀ At night before going to bed

Duration of dosage for a combination. In cases of acute crisis, it's best to take Essences on a short-term basis in a glass of water. Drink one glass each day for one to four days. During this time the combination of Flowers should be modified according to any changes in your state.

- ❀ Most typical crisis situations will require one or two mixtures that will be taken for eighteen to twenty-eight days each.

- For the treatment of chronic behavior patterns, take the mixture for eighteen to twenty-eight days, reevaluate and adjust the mixture accordingly, and take this new mixture for the next eighteen to twenty-eight days. Continue reevaluating and adjusting the mixture every eighteen to twenty-eight days as long as is necessary.

- In long-term treatment or for older people, use the same mixtures for five to eight weeks.

- For further information on the *duration of Bach Flower Therapy*, see appendix A.

Duration of dosage for Rescue Remedy.

- During an acute crisis it can be taken several times a day.

- During critical long-term stress—if your workload doubles, for example, because a colleague is ill or on vacation—Rescue Remedy can be taken daily when needed, even for more than a few days.

- For older people, refer to the end of this chapter

Combining Bach Flowers with Other Forms of Therapy

Because Bach Flower Therapy is effective on a different energy level than any other form of medication, combining it with other drugs or therapies is possible. The Flowers bring you closer to yourself and help you to feel motivated, which usually increases the effect of other medications. Indeed, it often happens that those taking Bach Flowers are finally able to open up to or benefit from forms of therapy or treatment they had previously resisted or found to be ineffective. Psychotherapy, surgery, or a much needed retreat, for instance—may suddenly seem like a helpful treatment option.

The first two of the following combined therapies have proved to be the most effective.

Bach Flower Therapy and psychotherapy. Psychologists experienced in using Bach Flowers agree that for those clients taking Flowers, much time is saved in psychotherapy because Bach Essences help them to get off to a better start with better focus and decreased resistance. An added benefit is that those who have taken Bach Flowers have an additional tool to use once psychotherapy has come to an end.

Bach Flower Therapy and natural or physical methods of cleansing and detoxification. These forms of therapy or treatment and Bach Flower Therapy complement one another well because what one achieves on a physical level the other addresses on emotional and mental levels.

Examples of these physical forms of therapy include fasting, colon cleansing, water treatment, shiatsu, and acupressure massage.

Bach Flower Therapy and conventional medicine. Conventional forms of medicine have proved to be more effective when taken together with Bach Flowers. When used with the agreement of the treating doctor, dosages of pharmaceuticals such as cortisone, beta-blockers, antibiotics, and the use of antidepressants can often be reduced or stopped altogether. However, in combination with such drugs Bach Flowers will sometimes have slower and more subdued effects. **Please note:** It is not advisable to alter the dosage of your medication without the knowledge of your doctor.

If you aren't certain whether you should use Bach Flower Therapy in conjunction with your medication, you might consider a trial with Rescue Remedy. If Rescue Remedy has an effect, even a modest one, it's certain that other Essences will do their job.

Bach Flowers and other forms of subtle therapy. Other forms of therapy that influence finer levels of energy—acupuncture, homeopathy, chakra massage, prenatal therapy, and so on—may have increased effectiveness if used in conjunction with Bach Flower Therapy. It's recommended, however, that you have one practitioner prescribe both methods, or at least have the two prescribing practitioners in close contact concerning your case. Using Bach Flowers jointly with these kinds of treatments may result in overstimulation (which can usually be alleviated by using Rescue Remedy). High-potency homeopathic remedies and Bach Flower Remedies should be used alternately for best results.

Frequently Asked Questions

For further information, please match the *italicized terms* in the following questions with the terms in the list of alphabetized issues in appendix A.

Is it possible to use Bach Flowers in *spray form?*

Are Bach Flowers in *globuli (pellet) form* useful?

Is it useful to *carry Bach Flower Remedies close to the body* all day?

Is it useful to put Bach Flowers at your *bedside or under your pillow* at night?

Are Bach Flowers even more effective in *homeopathic potentization?*

Do *coffee, alcohol, and nicotine* have adverse effects on Bach Flowers?

Is it possible to *overdose* with Bach Flowers?

Courses of Development and Typical Reactions

"What will happen after I take my first Bach Flower combination? What can I expect? What do I need to be prepared for?" Questions of this kind have no general answers because each of us reacts to Bach Flowers according to our own character structure; some of us react slowly and hesitantly, others quickly and decisively.

Other differences are determined by the situation we wish to harmonize—it may be an acute crisis (level A; see chapter 6) or a chronic state (level B; see chapter 6). The more acute the situation, the faster we will become aware of the Bach Flower effect; the more open we are and the less we predetermine the outcome, the more freedom our Inner Guidance has to give new impulses that initiate changes.

The intention and focus of a Bach Flower interviewer strongly catalyze the effectiveness of each mixture. This explains why combinations chosen experimentally or "for fun" are less effective: at the time the Flowers were chosen, there was no clear mental goal or true, deep wish that stood behind the choice.

A well-chosen combination often will "fire" the first time it is taken—as though an energetic link spontaneously forms to reestablish a connection that has been missing. People who are very sensitive often experience this reconnecting immediately:

"I felt as though a switch was being flipped."

"I had to take a very deep breath."

"Suddenly everything inside of me became brighter."

"There was a pleasant tingling sensation that went through me."

"Following the very first sip I felt a sensation around the scar of an old injury on my calf. It felt as if it got a fresh supply of blood."

Two Classic Courses of Development

Bach Flowers set harmonizing impulses that may be "digested" or taken into your system in different ways. The following is one possible response scenario: An acute crisis that has come about recently (for instance, a serious fight with your grown-up son) is softened; your jumble of feelings dissolves; and with a clear mind, you suddenly have confidence to tackle the problem from a different angle. A crisis with strong chronic components, however (for instance, losing a job causes your chronically low self-esteem to sink even lower), will generally follow one of two possible types of response patterns to the Flower Remedies:

Beginning with an upward trend. The first Flower combination is experienced positively. You see the light again, possibly you are able to sleep through the night for the first time in years—you may even feel surprisingly confident. Experiencing all of this gives you a glimpse of how you really are and what your Life Plan really holds in store for you. It puts you back in touch with your Inner Guidance and encourages you to trust the process and the possibilities for change, which you are finally able to do because you've experienced how things could be, or how your Life Plan has meant things to be.

Close to three weeks later, though, around the time when you've finished the first combination, your condition worsens. This phase is characterized by strong physical and psychological changes—and now your deeper, inner work begins. You truly begin to deal with your negative behavior patterns in a way that becomes more and more conscious. Finally, with the ups

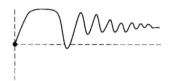

Beginning with an upward trend

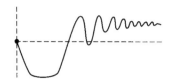

Beginning with a downward trend

and downs slowly leveling, you come to terms with these tendencies. Usually, two or three combinations after your condition begins to worsen, the positive potential becomes stabilized.

Beginning with a downward trend. The second typical reaction pattern is seen more often in people who have physical problems that accompany those that are psychological or emotional. Shortly after taking the first dosage, you have a feeling that everything is becoming worse; the negative feelings and physical symptoms intensify. These reactions, however, are not side effects; instead they are the first indications of the healing process, comparable to the term *aggravation* in homeopathy.

Just as a numb or paralyzed limb that is suddenly reenlivened or a painful, long-repressed thought that resurfaces in your consciousness can create pain or hurt, these shifts can cause you to experience discomfort. Just as there are waste products to be expelled by the physical body during a healing crisis, so too is there psychological waste that you must become aware of and release before it can, as Bach put it, "melt like snow in the sun."

Your Inner Guidance will not, however, allow more to surface in your consciousness than you are able to handle at any given time. Under the influence of the Flower impulses, it reveals exactly those problems that, according to your Life Plan, can be understood and solved at the time. One blockage after another is "peeled away"—much like the layers of an onion—as you go back into the past, often touching upon traumatic situations from childhood.

It is very important to understand this phase of perceived worsening as a positive step in the healing process. Usually this state lasts for only a few days before changing—sometimes abruptly, sometimes gradually—for the better. After this initial change, wavelike changes can be expected until the positive potential becomes stabilized.

How to Deal With a Healing Crisis

If a healing crisis overwhelms you, there are two possible ways to deal with it:

❀ Gradually reduce the frequency and/or dosage—if necessary, all the way down to one drop, once a day. In addition, you might take Rescue Remedy in a glass of water.

⚘ If you feel it's right to do so, gradually increase the frequency and/or dosage up to fourteen times a day, four drops each time, depending on your need. This will most likely shorten the difficult phase.

Terminating Bach Flower treatment in order to wait for a better time has not been found to be helpful at all. The same inner conditions will still be present and will become active whenever you decide to start up again.

Commonly Occurring Reactions

As a general rule you should accept any reaction, try to take in the experience as consciously as possible, and go along with whatever need arises. Indeed, it's the purpose of this reaction to help restore the energetic equilibrium.

During the first three days you may experience:

⚘ Feelings of being set free, of happiness, lightness, or being uplifted, which are expressions of the new connection with your Inner Guidance

⚘ Increased everyday activity; you begin a project that has long been delayed

⚘ Increased interest in exercising or getting out into nature

⚘ Inner unrest, irritability, or dizziness as expressions of your inner struggles

⚘ Increased need for rest and sleep, particularly if you normally need little sleep—the inner work you're doing takes up a great deal of extra energy that is no longer available to your physical body

⚘ A desire for cleansing: taking showers, fasting, and so forth

⚘ Bodily cleansing in the form of sneezing, diarrhea, frequent urination, swelling of lymph nodes, or sudden rashes (your body is responding on a number of levels to the shifts initiated by the Flower Essences)

⚘ Reduced desire for stimulants such as coffee, nicotine, and alcohol

Stronger reactions are to be expected with simultaneous fasting or use of therapies that work with subtle energies. In these cases it is recommended that you take fewer drops less frequently during the day.

During the first few months you may experience:

⚘ Changes in your facial expression, a softened, soulful look in your eyes

⚘ More vitality and a positive outlook

⚘ Increased sensitivity, stronger reactions to changes in the weather, and increased awareness of your moods

⚘ Extreme eating and drinking habits beginning to return to normal

- Others noticing positive changes in your behavior before you yourself notice them: "My wife said that I'm not as easily irritated as before"

- Relationships becoming more relaxed

Insights That Come through Dreams

Of all reactions in Bach Flower Therapy, the content of dreams might be the most interesting to observe because it shows most clearly the working of Inner Guidance. It has been noted that people who take a well-chosen combination will react with a symbolic dream during one of the first two nights of treatment. Analysis of hundreds of such dreams show three man recurring patterns:

- A basic personal conflict is presented symbolically—for instance, you're trying to find the central bus station but can't locate it

- An inner cleansing process is expressed metaphorically—for instance, you dream of a large number of washing machines doing your laundry in the basement

- A blocked personal potential is revealed—for instance, you dream that you discover a new room in your house that you've never seen before

Observing these symbolic expressions in dreams makes it possible to recognize developmental and consciousness-building processes at an early stage. Not only do dreams show your current state, but they also suggest the direction in which you should look for your next step.

It's known that all humans dream at night, though we don't all remember our dreams in the morning. The failure to recollect dreams is not a sign that a Flower combination has not been chosen well.

When You Are Not Aware of Any Reaction

There are various reasons for a Bach Flower Therapy to be blocked. The most likely possibility would be that the combination of Flowers is the wrong one, or that it has not been taken frequently enough.

Another possibility is that the negative psychological state stems from a level different from what can be reached by the Flowers. For instance, during menopause hormonal changes trigger mood swings that cannot be fully harmonized by Bach Flowers alone.

It's often the case that a therapy is blocked because you have expectations far beyond what Bach Flowers can achieve over a short period of time, or that you expect you will become an altogether different person. It's important to remember that treatment—particularly of chronic behavior patterns—takes a great deal of patience.

Another cause may stem from the fact that some people believe "more is better" and try several different therapies at the same time without going deeply into any of them. This rarely leads to any satisfactory results.

It's possible that you're unable to connect with Bach Flowers because someone else talked you into trying them. In this case it would make sense to stop the treatment and start again only when you really want to do it for yourself.

A standstill can frequently occur when you've reached a critical point—you've come too close to a problem that you unconsciously aren't ready to let go of. Perhaps a transformation would lead to painful changes that you aren't quite ready to accept, such as the separation from a partner or a career change. In this case it's advisable to stop therapy until you've accumulated enough inner strength to take your next step.

Finally, phases of stagnation can occur when you've reached a turning point in self-treatment. What can you do? In this case, try not to work against your resistance, but instead work with it. Examine the states you are experiencing now. Are you impatient (Impatiens)? Are you discouraged and in doubt about whether the flowers are really working (Gentian)? Do you wonder which direction to take (Wild Oat)? These are a few examples to give you ideas and a starting point for a new combination. If you aren't able to sort out the situation for yourself, talk with someone you trust.

Frequently Asked Questions

For further information on this subject, please match the *italicized terms* in the following questions with those from the alphabetized list of issues in appendix A.

How long does it take to see the *first effects* from taking a combination?

What should the total *duration of Bach Flower Therapy* be for a given situation or behavior pattern?

How will I know *when I can stop taking a specific combination?*

Must I *consciously study the Flowers in my combination* in order for them to work?

Should I always expect a *healing crisis as a first reaction?*

Are *healing crises common for children* during Bach Flower Therapy?

Is it possible to *combine drugs or other medicines with Bach Flowers?*

Can a person with *allergies* take Bach Flowers?

Is it possible for Bach Flowers to become *habit-forming?*

How strong is the *placebo effect* with Bach Flowers?

Do some people show *no reaction* to Bach Flowers?

Is it necessary to finish a *personal combination that is no longer needed?*

Do baggage *scanners at airports* affect Bach Flowers?

Applying Bach Flower Therapy

While the successful application of Bach Flower Therapy in other areas awaits official acknowledgment and acceptance by the experts, two of the first areas to embrace the use of Bach Flowers—with well-documented positive results—were the treatment of children and the treatment of pets.

A few projects focusing on the use of Bach Flowers to treat preschool children with behavioral problems and school-age children with learning disabilities suggest it would be extremely valuable for the Flowers to be used as part of an official psychological preventive health care program in schools. These projects were successful in part because the people who initiated them were well trained and experienced both in their own field of expertise and in the use of Bach Flower Therapy.

Bach Flowers would also be of great help in many areas of rehabilitation, such as following cancer treatments and in recovery from heart attacks. Interest in the use of Bach Flowers in treatment of the mentally ill and in drug rehabilitation is also slowly growing. The future holds much promise in these areas.

Additionally, both social workers and their clients have found Bach Flowers to be very beneficial during their work together. A few very successful applications within the prison population have also been reported.

Supportive Treatment in Physical Illnesses

It is recommended that Bach Flowers be used as a supportive measure in cases of physical illness including everything from recurring colds, eczema, asthma, pollen allergies, migraine, acne, psoriasis, other allergies, and blood pressure problems to gastrointestinal problems, multiple sclerosis, Alzheimer's, cancer, and AIDS. Most of the time it is possible to improve the psychological states such as resignation, hopelessness, and impatience that often accompany illness. In an ideal case the Flowers enable you to understand the mental error at the root of the illness (see chapter 2, page 20) , which can lead the way to real healing. You may discover, for instance, why it is that you suffered a fracture on your right hand the same day you planned to move to a new apartment, or what message your repeated attacks of migraine or psoriasis may be sending you.

However, it's important to note that while books associating the body's organs, systems, and parts with our attitudes or behavior have become rather popular, with regard to Bach Flower Therapy no general connection has been made between particular physical symptoms and specific Flowers. Not every heart patient needs Holly, and not every kidney problem calls for Mimulus. The only connections to be drawn in this respect are those involving the "primary diseases of mankind" presented by Bach in the third chapter of his book *Heal Thyself* (see also chapter 2 of this book).

To determine the right combination to accompany the healing process in physical illness, the first question to ask is: "How am I reacting to my current illness right now?" Do your heart problems cause you to feel guilty (Pine)? Are you afraid it may become a chronic problem (Mimulus)? Are you reminded that your mother died from her heart problems (Honeysuckle)?

The second question to ask is: "What benefits do I get or what can I avoid by having this illness?" Do your heart problems cause your family to take care of you all the time (Heather)? Do you avoid moving to another location because, as a heart patient, you're unable to take the stress associated with a move (Mimulus, Walnut)?

It is usually best if an experienced therapist helps you make associations of this kind. It's frequently the case that these behavior patterns were adopted in early childhood and may therefore call for psychotherapeutic treatment.

Bach Flowers and acute illnesses. In the beginning phases of an acute illness—for instance, when you feel as though you're coming down with the flu—it's helpful to take Rescue Remedy in a hot beverage or bath before going to bed. This allows reharmonization to take place during the night so that the immune system has enough energy to deal with the virus.

It often doesn't pay to use a mixing bottle for a personal combination of Flowers during an acute illness. If you are at home, you have the opportunity to respond to each feeling that comes up with the appropriate Flower Essences in a glass of water. Initially you may have feelings of needing protection and wanting to be spoiled a little (Heather, Willow). The next day you might experience vague fears that something more serious is causing the illness (Aspen, Mimulus). When things are getting better, you'll likely grow impatient (Impatiens).

Bach Flowers and chronic illnesses. When used as a supportive treatment with patience and care, Bach Flowers can at times lead to miraculous results. This does not mean, however, that all physical symptoms will disappear.

To avoid triggering a healing crisis, it is important to take small steps. Only clearly observed, negative states should be treated. For example, people who have been taking many drugs for a long time often complain of being tired (Olive), feeling dazed (Clematis), feeling resigned (Gorse), or feeling like a victim of fate (Willow). These flowers would then be used in the first treatment combination.

Once the initial states have been reharmonized, usually after two or three Flower combinations, enough motivation and strength are restored to work on the deeper causes of the illness. It may be that it is caused by a misdirected guilt that drives the person to "pay off a debt" (Pine). Another issue may be the person's unconscious uncertainty over whether or not to accept the challenge of life (Scleranthus).

In this phase of treatment, the combination will change little, if at all, for the next six to eight weeks. Small relapses are to be expected, but over time they will be less severe and less frequent. Medication that had been necessary up to now can often be reduced gradually—only after consultation with your doctor.

In cases of chronic illness, Bach Flower Therapy has accomplished its goal if the patient can say: "I've become a different person now"; "I'm planted more firmly in my life now"; "I've learned how to cope with my chronic illness and I experience less pain"; "Now I really understand the reason for my illness." At this point, appropriate forms of therapy can more readily resolve or ease the remaining symptoms of a chronic illness.

Bach Flowers and rehabilitation. When faced with a serious operation or a life-threatening problem, most of us will gain important new insights or find a new resolve to make changes in our life. During rehabilitation, after the immediate threat has been addressed, the support of Bach Flower Therapy can be an invaluable help. The proper combination can aid you in clarifying what is really true for you, and can assist you in holding to it and manifesting it. Your chance for starting a new life can grow tremendously.

Bach Flowers for those with incurable diseases or those near death. Bach Flowers have provided many a blessed moment for those with incurable diseases and those who are dying. Be-

cause the ill or dying person is depleted in strength, deep-rooted negative behavior patterns are often strongly displayed, making it easy to identify the appropriate Flowers for treatment. If a person declines to take the Flowers, it's important to respect this decision. It often makes more sense for the caregiver simply to give Rescue Remedy, if the patient is willing, and to take the chosen Flower combination him- or herself—this will help because the caregiver is attuned to the same circumstances as the patient. The relationship between the patient and anyone who is particularly close to him or her is very intense at this time, and the harmonizing effect from a mixture that a caregiver has taken will be transmitted directly to the patient.

Many relatives will think about giving Honeysuckle (let go of the past), Red Chestnut (let go of others), and Walnut (making the transition). While this is done with the best of intentions, it is often the case that these Flowers are not needed and that others, or Rescue Remedy alone, would be more appropriate to the particular situation. If you, as a caregiver, think of giving these Flowers, honestly ask yourself the following questions: "Am I presuming that the person is definitely dying?"; "Is it somehow my wish for it all to be over?"; "Am I the one having trouble with this process?"; "Whose feelings do I really have in mind here?"; "Do these Flowers belong to the sick person or am I the one who is unable to let go in this situation?"

There is no debate, however, concerning the

use of Rescue Remedy to accompany the dying. Even when a patient is in intensive care and is unable to take it internally, Rescue Remedy can be applied to the forehead, the wrist, or the soles of the feet.

It is never too late to use Bach Flowers, especially Rescue Remedy. People have related again and again that when dying friends or relatives took Rescue Remedy they experienced their last few days in a more humane and harmonious way and most passed away peacefully in their sleep.

Bach Flowers for Children

In chapter 5 of *Heal Thyself*, Bach describes the "true relation" between parents and children.

> *If properly understood, there is probably no greater opportunity offered to mankind than this, to be the agent of the physical birth of a soul and to have the care of the young personality during the first few years of its existence on earth. The whole attitude of parents should be to give the little newcomer all the spiritual, mental and physical guidance to the utmost of their ability, ever remembering that the wee one is an individual soul come down to gain his own experience and knowledge in his own way according to the dictates of his Higher Self, and every possible freedom should be given for unhampered development.*

Most psychological problems that show up later in life have their roots in life's first seven years.

Therefore it stands to reason that many physical and psychological problems later in life might be avoided through using Bach Flowers during these early years. According to leading pediatricians, approximately 80 percent of a child's symptoms such as stomachaches and headaches are psychosomatic responses. Unfortunately, today even these problems are treated more often than one might imagine with heavy weapons such as psychopharmacological drugs. Knowing this, parents who have seen the results that are possible with Bach Flowers would certainly not want to be without them.

Although many people think that it's difficult to treat children, it's really very simple. Generally, you may follow the same guidelines as for adults. Included here are a few additions and some of the experiences that have been reported.

Bach Flowers for babies and toddlers. Rescue Remedy and Walnut or Star of Bethlehem and Walnut are combinations that help both mother and child to overcome the strain of the birth. They can help both to feel at home in their new state of being when added to the first bath after the birth. This use has been successful in thousands of cases.

Because a nursing baby has a symbiotic tie to the mother, both mother and child naturally have need for the same Flowers; a breast-feeding baby will receive the Flower impulses with the mother's milk.

Apart from Rescue Remedy, which can be

given whenever there's too much excitement, babies normally do not need their own Bach Flower combinations. On the other hand, it would be valuable to the child for everyone else who influences the climate in the household to take Bach Flowers—not only the nervous mother or the father suffering from stress, but also the overly enthusiastic grandparents, aunts, and older siblings who take part in the child's upbringing.

When toddlers show their first individual character traits, Bach Flower combinations may be given to address acute problems for short periods of time. Spontaneous choice is a helpful tool in these cases. A pediatrician gave this account: "I spread the little bottles on a blanket, let the baby crawl around on it, and observe which ones the baby plays with. The other day a baby grabbed the Impatiens bottle and didn't want to let go of it. The surprised mom recalled that she had been waiting for weeks for her daughter to finally start walking."

For toddlers, ten to twenty milliliters prepared without alcohol is sufficient. This dosage is recommended as a starting point, but you need to pay attention to how much and how often the child likes to take the drops and adjust the dosage accordingly. There should be no danger of aggravation as long as acute problems are the only ones treated. When a negative state in a baby does keep recurring despite a well-chosen combination, it indicates that the situation is being triggered by another member of the fam-

ily system. If this person is treated with the appropriate Flowers, the problem should resolve.

Bach Flowers from childhood to emerging puberty. As is the case for adults, children can benefit from Bach Flowers in three different kinds of situations.

1. **Preventive health care.** One day little Katy, who usually is agile and doesn't miss a beat, comes home from school very tired, very quiet, and seemingly dazed. Grandma says, "I wonder what she's coming down with?" At this point if Katy is given Clematis she'll likely bounce back from being "not quite present" to being her spirited self again. Using Bach Flowers may prevent a physical illness from taking hold or, if it doesn't prevent it, will at least cause the symptoms to be much lighter than they would be otherwise.

2. **Overcoming an acute crisis.** Jealousy over a new sibling, panic about scary images in a movie, fear of the first day of school, and resistance to homework are all situations that can respond dramatically within twenty-four hours of taking ten to twenty milliliters of the appropriate Bach Flower combination.

3. **Parallel treatment of chronic problems.** Long-lasting effects in the treatment of problems like asthma, bedwetting, and chronic eczema can be

achieved only when both the child and at least one other family member (usually one or both parents) are simultaneously treated. When the child alone takes the Bach Flowers, he or she will show some improvement for a while but will relapse the moment the climate at home turns unfavorable.

If you take your child to a Bach Flower specialist, it's best to report on the presenting problems without the child's presence in the room. Next, the specialist and the child need time to themselves to talk and determine the right Flower combination.

Conditions for Which Pediatricians Recommend Bach Flowers

Sleeping disorders

Bed-wetting

Fears

Difficult teething

Eating or digestion problems

Aggression

Headaches and migraine

Difficulties at school

Prone to infections

Dyslexia

Eczema

Stuttering

Allergies

Asthma

Neurodermatitis

Hyperkinetic syndrome

General recommendations. The younger a child is, the more useful is *spontaneous choice* (see appendix A) in helping to select the correct Bach Flower combination.

As far as is possible, talk with your child in his own language about the Flowers that have been chosen. It's very important that he doesn't see Bach Flowers as a kind of bandage for little problems but rather as an ally that can help him to develop and grow stronger.

As evidence of their growing autonomy, many children have given their mixtures a name like "my courage drops" or "my patience drops." As part of this developing independence, children will need to decide for themselves whether or not to take the drops.

It's important to note that because children are much closer to their Higher Self than adults, who have built up years of resistance, they will react quickly and with extreme precision to the Essences. Actual experiences seem to bear this out. For example, a four-year-old comes in from playing outside to remind his mother that it's time to take his drops. Two days later, however, the same child refuses to take any more—he has registered unconsciously that his equilibrium has been restored. Another account tells of a mother who is about to give some drops to her little daughter but confuses bottles and offers the child drops from her son's combination instead. The little girl screams until the mother notices her mistake, after which the daughter takes the drops without further ado.

It's worth noting that it's not a good idea to try to convince a child to take drops simply because everyone else in the family is taking them. Nor is it a good idea to insist that a child finish a combination if it is being resisted.

Bach Flowers and puberty. During this phase of development, Bach Flowers can help alleviate the strong mood swings that are so typical at this age. Most of the time parents are no longer accepted as the people to decide upon the combination. Indeed, they aren't best suited to do so; because parents usually play a part in the psychological turbulence of the adolescent, they cannot judge objectively. If it appears that a psychological problem is a serious one, the young person should be encouraged to meet with a neutral Bach Flower specialist who also has psychological training.

The family combination. Observations of spontaneous choices made by young children have indicated that the Flowers chosen were not only important for the children themselves but also addressed key difficulties within the family as a whole. A family can be described as a system in which everyone reacts to everyone else. Therefore it often makes sense to treat several members or the entire family at the same time. Family combinations came into being because some family system practitioners did not have enough time to research and prepare individual mixtures for each family member and, understanding the nature of reactions within the fam-

ily structure, developed instead one combination that could be used to treat all members. Such combinations have proved successful in various acute crises. During the interview, states are isolated that apply to everyone in the group. This combination is then made into a mixture that each person takes. Family wellness organizations have found this approach very beneficial despite the fact that it doesn't exactly follow the classic method of Bach Flower Therapy.

Frequently Asked Questions

For further information on this subject, please match the *italicized terms* in the following questions with those from the alphabetized list of issues in appendix A.

Is it possible to *manipulate* children with the help of Bach Flowers?

Is it a good idea to suggest a *continuous intake of Bach Flowers* for children so their life will be better later?

Does the *alcohol content* in the stock bottles have a negative effect on babies?

Bach Flowers during the Female Life Cycle, Pregnancy, and Birth

Recommending Bach Flowers to women is like carrying coals to Newcastle. In Bach Flower workshops at least 75 percent of the participants are women, and mothers are usually the driving force behind introducing Bach Flowers to the family. Dr. Heide Göttner-Abendroth, noted for her research into the historical epoch of matriarchal societies, postulates that Bach received his inspiration from sources that have their origin in these times, when all forms of healing were the responsibility of women. It's interesting that midwives were among the first groups of people to embrace Bach Flower Therapy. The Flowers' natural therapeutic approach based on observation and self-regulation fit closely with feminine thought and feelings. These advantages are slowly being discovered in specialized fields of conventional medicine that deal with women's health. In many hospitals, even university hospital gynecology departments, Rescue Remedy is being used regularly to assist the birthing process.

Various specialists in different medical areas have found Bach Flowers valuable in the following situations:

- **Parallel treatment of PMS** (premenstrual syndrome)—important Flower Essences are Rock Water and Pine

- **Libido dysfunction** among women and men—Wild Oat as part of a personal combination has been recommended along with psychotherapy

- **Childlessness,** after physical causes have been ruled out—usually Walnut is involved in the combination

- **Tendency to miscarry**—if at a psychological level there is an unconscious indecision on the question of truly wanting the pregnancy, Scleranthus and Water Violet are Flowers of choice in this context

- **After an abortion or a miscarriage**—Star of Bethlehem, Red Chestnut, Pine, and Mustard have proved helpful as part of the individual combination

- **During pregnancy,** to stabilize mother and fetus—finding just the right Flowers for this time isn't easy because the mother's feelings change a great deal, and the state of the unborn child is already playing a role; it's recommended that the mother treat herself by using spontaneous choice and that she take the Essences in a glass of water instead of preparing combinations for long-term use

- **To prepare for and accompany birth,** it's best to prepare a "personal Rescue combination" for emergencies (see chapter 5); when contractions stop, for example, this can be applied directly to the belly

- **During the postnatal phase,** Olive and Mustard are added to the personal combination

- **When nursing ends,** Red Chestnut and Walnut are helpful when added to the personal combination

- **During menopause,** mood swings respond well to Honeysuckle, Scleranthus, and Mustard; the deeper aspect of this process is the mental reorientation to the coming phase of the individual Life Plan—deeply rooted negative behavior patterns become very apparent at this time and present an excellent opportunity for successful Bach Flower Therapy in conjunction with psychotherapy (which has also proved valuable during midlife crises in men)

❀ **After surgery for cancer** it is necessary to attempt a complete psychological reorientation; during this difficult time Centaury, Agrimony, Walnut, and Holly are only a few of the Flowers that can help "open the gates to a new life"

Treating the Elderly

Older people often say that their nerves have become much more sensitive, and that they are much less resistant to stress. The subtle effects of Bach Flowers are thus ideal for them.

When older people are open, it's surprising how quickly they respond to Bach Flowers. Long-standing family quarrels or inheritance disputes may be suddenly resolved and brought to a happy ending or an older person can be helped in her ability to cope with illnesses or handicaps with more composure and peace of mind.

At the same time there are understandable situations in which a senior citizen may have become rather embittered and closed-minded through strokes of fate or many difficult years of serious chronic illness and will only hesitantly show any reaction to Bach Flowers.

Some older people will strictly refuse to use personal combinations of Flowers, while at the same time demanding to be given Rescue Remedy or their personal emergency mixture (see chapter 5). It's important to respect these wishes because they may reflect a lack of spiritual reserves for dealing with conflicts of the past. Some elderly people simply wish to make it through the day.

You will be of much greater help to an elderly family member if you yourself take the Flowers you would like to give her (see page 239, Bach Flowers for Those Who Are Dying).

As long as older people who are very ill still wish to take Bach Flowers, certainly allow them to, even if you're unable to perceive any effects. They wouldn't ask for them if they hadn't experienced a distinct reaction.

In senior citizen housing and nursing homes, Bach Flowers are widely used with positive results and have been instrumental in reducing the use of psychopharmacological drugs and sleeping pills.

Bach Flower Therapy for Addicts, the Mentally Challenged, and Psychiatric Patients

In the hands of well-trained specialists in all three fields, Bach Flower Therapy has produced wonderful results.* The positive experiences during the last ten years strongly suggest that additional Bach Flower training would be beneficial for people involved in psychiatry, addiction rehabilitation, and the care of those who are mentally or physically challenged.

The deciding factor for success in these complex and difficult areas is the simultaneous treatment of people who are intimately involved with the patient. Children and adolescents in particular have at times been saved from institutions when the parents were included in the treatment.

In treating addicts, involving those who are codependent is extremely important. A drug addict once wrote in a memorable letter: "Since the day my parents started taking Bach Flowers it has been a lot easier for me to cope with my illness." If you're a member of a support group, becoming acquainted with Bach's message and using the Flowers yourself will give you a better understanding of dependencies, which in turn will help you to take advantage of opportunities for positive changes.

Addictions. There is often no immediate effect of Bach Flowers on people who are seriously addicted to drugs or alcohol† and tremendous skill and patience is required on the part of the therapist. Early in treatment, more help can usually be offered to the relatives. Bach Flower

Therapy will assist them to break the up-and-down pattern of exaggerated support alternating with resignation or rejection as well as any tendency to lay blame. The turning point for the addict comes when he is ready to question his self-destructive behavior and makes a conscious decision to change. This is the moment when Bach Flowers will provide the all-important impulses to support the new motivation.

Mental retardation. Many case studies have shown that giving Bach Flowers to patients and their parents at the same time for more than one year can result in very positive developments. In one case a patient who was unable to leave her bed for twenty years became able to use the bathroom by herself and could be fed at the table. Choosing the combinations for patients takes a lot of empathy and intuition, since they're often unable to deal with even a spontaneous choice. After interviewing the personnel in charge and observing the patient, only nonverbal diagnostic methods are available.

Psychiatric patients. People who suffer from depression, anxieties, eating disorders, and borderline personality disorder can profit from Bach Flower Therapy if they are interested. In the hands of experienced specialists, the use of Bach

---

* For additional information and the description of cases refer to my book *Original Bach-Blütentherapie,* (Krone & Fischer, 1999), a textbook for conventional medical doctors and natural healers.

† For alcoholics, it is necessary to prepare Flower mixtures without alcohol. Placing the drops in boiling water, hot tea, and so forth will allow most of the alcohol to evaporate and will not affect the potency of the remedies. Additionally, the drops may be massaged into the temples or the inside of the elbow.

Flowers is most important when setting an overall course of treatment, at crisis points in treatment, and during rehabilitation because they help the patient to access and express his deepest human needs. It's very important to strike a good balance among chemical, psychiatric, and the more subtle Bach Flower treatments.

However, while it is possible to take Bach Flowers in combination with any kind of psychopharmacological drugs, please do not experiment on your own.

Bach Flower Therapy for Pets

It has been said that animals are soulful beings subject to their emotions in a more direct way than we humans are. Therefore, when our pets are sick or in pain, Bach Flowers may be an even greater gift for them than they are for us.

Animals very much like taking drops. A veterinarian who administered Holly to a bull visited the animal four weeks later only to witness the bull immediately approaching to greet him and wait for another dose. In another case, a parrot who had been pulling out his feathers spontaneous chose Impatiens out of the many bottles that were held up to its cage and subsequently improved quickly with the treatment.

The daily experience of many veterinarians confirms that there is a close relationship in animals between psychological disharmonies and organic problems. Thus it's possible to transcribe Bach's general recommendation "Do not treat the disease—treat the person" to the realm of animals: "Do not treat the illness—treat the animal!"

It has been shown that animals react surprisingly quickly to the positive impulses from Bach Flowers, resulting in harmonization within a short period of time. An animal who is very shy and scared, for instance, will overcome this with the help of Mimulus, growing more at ease within a few days. In general, you will find that the duration of the therapy is much shorter than in humans.

In contrast to humans, an animal doesn't have the opportunity to take part in consciously overcoming negative psychological states. Character problems that are due to breeding are influenced only while the drops are being given, but such behavioral problems often come back when the Flowers treatment is stopped. There are also cases where the behavior traits are so deeply ingrained genetically that the Flowers have no effect.

If you wish to use Bach Flowers with your pets, it is important to first make sure that the behavior problem does not have a physical cause. Bach Flower Therapy cannot and does not attempt to take the place of a veterinarian's treatment.

People who keep and treat animals speak about successful treatment with Bach Flowers in cases that deal with acute emotional problems such as fears and aggression, or with behavioral problems such as uncleanness and difficulty adapting. Other important fields of successful application are emergencies of all kinds, like vet visits and births. Supportive treatment when there are chronic physical problems such as long-term diarrhea, eczema, and hair loss has shown only mixed results.

When an animal does not respond to a Flower combination and you have no idea why, it is often helpful to look to the people and conditions in its surroundings. Pets usually are subject to many different relationships with the people and other animals in the household or yard. Often it is the pet that most clearly reflects a conflict taking place among other members of its world—perhaps a hidden fight between partners or somebody's sorrow. You may misinterpret the animal's behavior, not realizing that he is simply crying for help without knowing how to express it. Such problems are easily reversed when the condition among the others is resolved.

Experienced practitioners know to study the surroundings and in particular to analyze the animal's relationship with its main companion. Much as in the relationship between mother and child, animal and companion share an energetic bond that is very sensitive to any kind of change. Chronic problems in pets therefore respond more favorably when treatment with Bach Flowers is given to both human and pet.

Typical cases at the veterinarian's office reveal that many people are not aware of their responsibilities to the animals they keep. Tasks that ought to be obvious, and that are suited to the animals particular needs, are frequently omitted due to lack of knowledge, laziness, or misdirected love for the animal. Everyone who plans to adopt a pet needs to provide the necessary natural environment (sufficient space, nourishing food, and so on). If you're inexperienced with animals, you should seek professional advice. Damage caused by the inadequate care of an animal cannot be repaired with the help of Bach Flower Therapy.

Responsible animal companions take good care not to demand too much of their pets in terms of work or sporting activities. By helping to keep these areas balanced, the activities will not lead to the development of physical problems later on. Bach Flowers should not be given out of exaggerated ambition to improve the performance and endurance of an animal. The main purpose of Flowers is to improve and harmonize the animal's quality of life.

Determining the appropriate Flowers for your pet. Just as for humans, start with the negative emotional state of the moment. Of course you won't be able to ask your cat, "How do you feel right now?" Next to characteristics of type and breed, however, every animal displays individual character traits that are easy to see. Exceptions from the norm then become readily apparent. How does the animal react? Is she scared or unusually wild? Does she keep to herself? Is she aggressive, timid, or nervous?

People who have treated animals say that a combination of two to four Flowers is usually sufficient. Remember to give the Flowers only at times when your animal shows these negative behavioral or emotional symptoms.

If your animal doesn't react favorably to the treatment, it has been beneficial to choose a combination that reflects your own emotional state instead. Thus check the momentary feelings that dominate your—and therefore your pet's—daily life. In this manner you will not only help your pet but perhaps find out something new about yourself as well.

Preparation, dosage, and administration. For normal use, dilute Bach Flower Essences from the stock bottles just as you would for human consumption.

There is no standard dosage for animals. The essences are applied according to individual needs. Experienced practitioners, however, have suggested a few guidelines for general use:

1. **Small animals** (dogs, cats, birds, and so forth) receive four drops, four times a day, from the mixing bottle when they are full grown. Newborns and very young animals are given a dosage of one or two drops, and older ones two or three drops, four times a day.

2. **Large animals** (cows, horses, and so forth) receive ten drops, four times a day, from the mixing bottle. When they are newborns the dosage is four or five drops, and for those more than a few weeks old, give five or six drops, four times a day.

When giving Bach Flowers to an animal, it is important not to force him or cause him any stress. There exist no set rules for how to administer them, but the following are some suggestions.

If you have a small animal, you can place the drops directly on the tongue from the mixing bottle dropper while holding the animal on your lap, petting it, and talking to it lovingly. Another method is to mix the drops in with the food or water. Cats tend to be very finicky, though, and may refuse to eat this mixture. Some people put the drops on the animal's nose or paws, which causes the pet to lick itself clean.

Large animals will take the drops directly from a spoon onto the tongue or gums. Or you can put the drops on bread or fruit, which the animal will usually eat without a problem.

There may be a rare case in which an animal refuses all methods of application. As a last resort you can put a few drops, several times a day, on the fur in the area of the forehead, massaging them in while talking in a sweet voice. After a few days of this regimen, most animals will take to one of the methods above.

Giving Rescue Remedy directly from the stock bottle. Depending on the size of the animal, two to ten drops of Rescue Remedy can be added directly to your pet's water or food.

Table for Use When Choosing Between Two Flowers (page 252)

Flower Name	Agrimony	Aspen	Beech	Centaury	Cerato	Cherry Plum	Chestnut Bud	Chicory	Clematis	Crab Apple	Elm	Gentian	Gorse	Heather	Holly	Honeysuckle	Hornbeam
Agrimony	–		11	1	2	3								4			
Aspen		–				25			7								
Beech	11		–	12													
Centaury	1		12	–	16				17			18					
Cerato	2			16	–	29											
Cherry Plum	3	25				–										26	
Chestnut Bud				29			–		30			31					
Chicory								–						58	61		
Clematis		7		17			30		–							40	
Crab Apple										–							
Elm											–	46	52				47
Gentian				18			31				46	–	53				
Gorse											52	53	–			65	69
Heather	4							58						–			
Holly						26		61							–		
Honeysuckle									40				65			–	
Hornbeam											47		69				–
Impatiens						27	32								62		
Larch				19	22						48	50	75				70
Mimulus	5	8		78		79								59			
Mustard									41			51	54			66	
Oak											86						
Olive				20							49		90				71
Pine										44							
Red Chestnut		9		98				36								99	
Rock Rose		10				101											
Rock Water		13				104			45					105			
Scleranthus					23		33										
Star of Bethlehem	6								42							67	
Sweet Chestnut						28					111	112	55				
Vervain				14				37						60			
Vine				15				38							63		
Walnut		115		21	116												
Water Violet																	
White Chestnut						122			123								
Wild Oat				126	24		34					125					
Wild Rose						35			43				56			68	72
Willow								39					57		64		

Impatiens	Larch	Mimulus	Mustard	Oak	Olive	Pine	Red Chestnut	Rock Rose	Rock Water	Scleranthus	Star of Bethlehem	Sweet Chestnut	Vervain	Vine	Walnut	Water Violet	White Chestnut	Wild Oat	Wild Rose	Willow
		5									6									
		8					9	10							115					
									13				14	15						
	19	78			20		98								21				126	
	22									23					116			24		
27		79						101	104			28					122			
32										33								34	35	
							36						37	38						39
			41									42							43	
						44			45								123			
	48			86	49							111								
	50		51									112						125		
	75		54		90							55							56	57
		59							105				60							
62													63							64
			66				99					67							68	
	70				71														72	
–								73					74			118	124			
	–	76				94										119			77	
	76	–				95	80	81				82				120				
			–		91							83	84			121			85	
				–	92	96			87				88	89						
			91	92	–														93	
	94	95	96			–			97											
		80					–	100								117				
73	81						100	–			102	103								
			87			97			–				106	107						
										–								108		
		82	83				102				–	110							127	109
		84					103				110	–								
74			88						106				–	113						
			89						107				113	–		114				
							117								–					
118	119	120	121										114			–				
124																	–			
										108								–		
	77		85		93							127							–	
												109								–

Differences and Similarities among the Bach Flowers

The following list, to be used in conjunction with the reference table on the previous two pages, will help you when you find it difficult to make a choice between two Flowers that have a common aspect. With each pair, listed numerically from 1 to 127, is the description of a particular state shared by both Flowers along with the different way this state is expressed by each of the two. These descriptions are based on over twenty-five years of practical observations from my teaching and consulting practice. They seek to clarify key psychological differences at work behind a pattern and can also be used to help formulate questions in an interview.

How to Use the Reference Table When Choosing Between Two Flowers

Find the two Flowers you wish to compare by locating one on the horizontal row at the top and the other in the vertical column at the left. The intersecting field tells you which number to look up. For example, if you're comparing Agrimony and Centaury, you'll go to number 1 in the list of pairs below.

From the information there you can create a question from each side to ask your interview partner (or yourself). For example: "At times when you put up with a situation, do you give in because you want to avoid disturbing the peace? (Agrimony). Or is the situation such that you don't even recognize that you have gone along with a request because you are so good-natured that you can't refuse?" (Centaury).

If your partner answers yes to both questions, and both apply to the situation at hand, then both Flower Essences are to be included in the mixture. You will find this to be the case fairly often.

1. Agrimony or Centaury? Both tend to give in to others because—

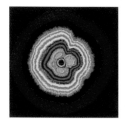 **Agrimony:** You'd like to act differently, but you give in to a situation in order to avoid disharmony.

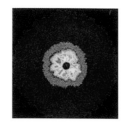 **Centaury:** You give in to situations without noticing that you're giving in—because of your good nature you're unable to refuse a request.

2. Agrimony or Cerato? Both like to follow established rules or do what's "in"—

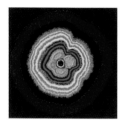 **Agrimony:** You use this behavior to mask your true feelings.

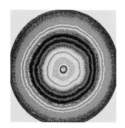 **Cerato:** You are looking for a type of insurance because you're not sure of your own ideas or may not have an opinion.

3. Agrimony or Cherry Plum? Neither wants to show feelings because—

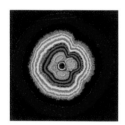 **Agrimony:** You want to avoid quarrels or a negative atmosphere. You appear nervous.

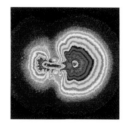 **Cherry Plum:** You're afraid to face your own feelings, which you've pushed aside because they might burst beyond your control. Your body may appear blocked.

4. Agrimony or Heather? Both can talk excessively because—

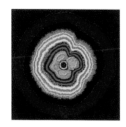 **Agrimony:** You try to play things down, push them under the rug, or distract from a subject at hand.

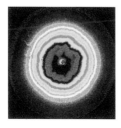 **Heather:** By constantly talking about your problems, you may get attention and help (which, in turn, you're unable to accept).

5. Agrimony or Mimulus? Both will at times be shy and hesitant because—

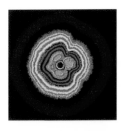

Agrimony: You're determined to avoid causing any conflict or dispute.

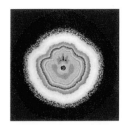

Mimulus: You're naturally sensitive and cautious, so you'll act only when it's absolutely necessary.

6. Agrimony or Star of Bethlehem? Neither will show real feelings because—

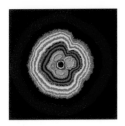

Agrimony: You don't want to.

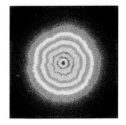

Star of Bethlehem: You're still in shock from something.

7. Aspen or Clematis? Both may appear as though they aren't really paying attention or are thinking about something else because—

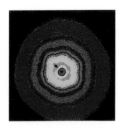

Aspen: Your antennae are seeking to locate imagined dangers, such as strange vibrations or ghosts.

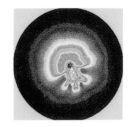

Clematis: Mentally you're involved some-where else—thinking of a vacation spot or solving a new problem.

8. Aspen or Mimulus? Both are fearful—

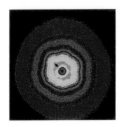

Aspen: You don't know the reason for your fear; it's a "something is lurking in the dark" kind of feeling.

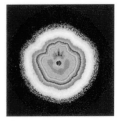

Mimulus: You're well aware of the reason for your fear: a dog, the dentist, an exam, or the like.

9. Aspen or Red Chestnut? Neither is able to keep clear boundaries because—

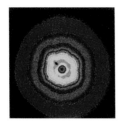

Aspen: You're too open to outside influences and impulses and take them in unconsciously, absorbing, for instance, the stressful atmosphere in a mall.

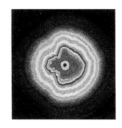

Red Chestnut: You become aware of your own needs only through projecting them onto others, whom you are tied to psychologically.

10. Aspen or Rock Rose? Both are afraid—

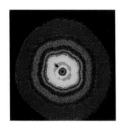

Aspen: The fear sneaks up on you and is not clearly defined—for instance, the fear felt in a dark cellar.

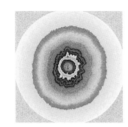

Rock Rose: The fear is acute, is thought to be life-threatening, and is felt in every part of your body—for instance, the panic felt during a thunderstorm. In children, especially, a Rock Rose state can grow out of an Aspen state.

11. Beech or Agrimony? Both suppress their needs and feelings because—

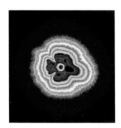

Beech: You can't accept your own flaws and instead criticize others for the same things. A stingy person, for instance, will criticize a partner for saving money.

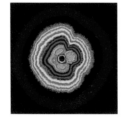

Agrimony: You distract yourself and others from problems by putting the difficulties into a humorous context: "Penny wise, pound foolish."

12. Beech or Centaury? Frequently neither will voice an opinion because—

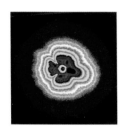

Beech: You try to veil your own criticism with exaggerated tolerance. You may stop nagging altogether and say, "Everything is great" (the compensating Beech state).

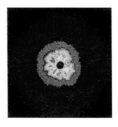

Centaury: In the presence of stronger personalities (such as Vine), your own opinion is smothered; you lose touch with it and it doesn't get expressed.

13. Beech or Rock Water? Both have strong ideas about the way things ought to be—

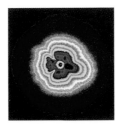 **Beech:** You criticize freely what you don't like: "They shouldn't put so many preservatives in the food!"

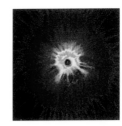 **Rock Water:** Locked in your own belief system, your only care is for yourself and doing things perfectly: "As long as I eat only raw foods, I'll be healthy."

14. Beech or Vervain? Both tend to have problems with being tolerant because—

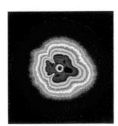 **Beech:** You're unable to accept another's faults or nature. The criticism is often an attempt to keep from facing these qualities in yourself.

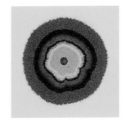 **Vervain:** You're unable to tolerate it when a "good" or "helpful" idea is rejected; you then try even harder to convince others of how right it is. These battles to convince others also serve the purpose of assuring yourself.

15. Beech or Vine? Neither is concerned about the feelings of others because—

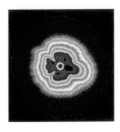 **Beech:** You tend to find your own feelings and those of others irritating, so you don't want to be involved with them and instead proceed rationally.

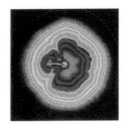 **Vine:** The feelings of other people take second place to your need for dominance. The fulfillment of your own personal needs and plans is of sole importance.

16. Centaury or Cerato? Both have problems defining themselves and standing up for themselves because—

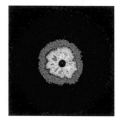

Centaury: In order to be acknowledged and due to your inborn helpfulness, you get pulled in to work for other people's interests while neglecting your own Life Plan. You have a soft heart.

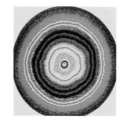

Cerato: In childhood your intuitive development was suppressed and subsequently shriveled. Therefore you don't trust your own intuitive impulses and seek outside assurance. You're easily thrown, at times acting like a child who is unable to say anything. (Both states are often found together.)

17. Centaury or Clematis? It can be difficult to fully understand or get hold of either because—

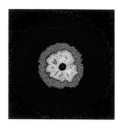

Centaury: Your will is weakly developed so your needs are not clearly expressed.

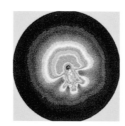

Clematis: You find it difficult to confront reality so you mentally escape to another world.

18. Centaury or Gentian? Both tend to give up easily because—

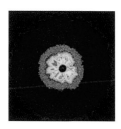

Centaury: Your will is not strong enough to hang in there and persevere.

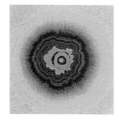

Gentian: You lack basic trust in a positive outcome; you get thrown off easily—any little setback casts doubt on your decision.

19. Centaury or Larch? Both may react in an overly modest and compliant way because—

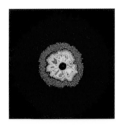 **Centaury:** You lack self-determination.

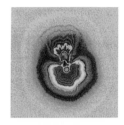 **Larch:** You lack self-confidence.

20. Centaury or Olive? Both may complain about weakness and loss of energy because—

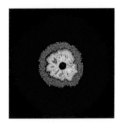 **Centaury:** In wishing to be helpful, you tend to unconsciously overextend yourself.

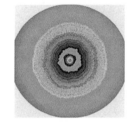 **Olive:** After constant physical and/or psychological strain, your reserves are empty and you shy away from any further activity.

21. Centaury or Walnut? Both have difficulty actualizing themselves because—

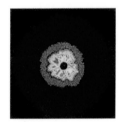 **Centaury:** You're unable to say no, thus allowing others to determine your next step. It's important for you to improve your personal willpower.

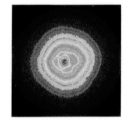 **Walnut:** During phases of orientation you tend to give up on decisions you've already made due to the influence of others. You have to learn to stick to your guns.

22. Cerato or Larch? Both can delay getting things started because—

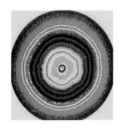 **Cerato:** You lack confidence in your own judgment; you're afraid to make a mistake.

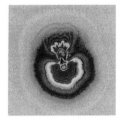 **Larch:** You're afraid you aren't able to do it.

23. Cerato or Scleranthus? Both have difficulty sticking to decisions because—

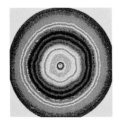 **Cerato:** You'll keep on consulting further sources that will naturally come up with contradictions.

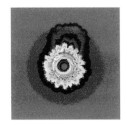 **Scleranthus:** You keep alternating between two poles. Trying to solve the problem alone, you don't ask others for advice.

24. Cerato or Wild Oat? Both have problems with inner direction because—

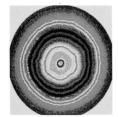 **Cerato:** You doubt your inner voice and repeatedly discount the first thing that comes to mind.

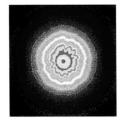 **Wild Oat:** You want to do something special but you don't know what it is, so you try many things without any real satisfaction.

25. Cherry Plum or Aspen? In extreme (pathological) states both appear to be compulsively influenced because—

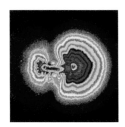 **Cherry Plum:** You have long controlled or suppressed your feelings and they are threatening to break loose.

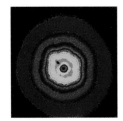 **Aspen:** You're so wide open to your surroundings that you are flooded by them. You can't deal with it all and passively go along with the strongest impulse you feel.

26. Cherry Plum or Holly? Both can be under extreme emotional pressure—

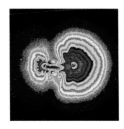 **Cherry Plum:** While fighting for composure inside, you appear unnaturally calm only to explode at the wrong time over a minor incident.

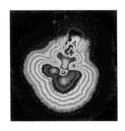 **Holly:** You spontaneously express your feelings and let off steam aggressively as rage, anger, or tantrums. Or, you may react harshly and retreat distrustfully.

27. Cherry Plum or Impatiens? Both appear to be under pressure because—

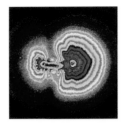

Cherry Plum: You struggle for self-control, suppressing your feelings; you feel like a time bomb that's ticking.

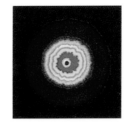

Impatiens: You feel pressured by time and always feel pushed to be on the go (this is part of your constitution); you feel like a sprinter just before the race starts. (Both are part of the Rescue Remedy formula.)

28. Cherry Plum or Sweet Chestnut? Both states are similar—your reaction, whatever it is, is extreme (e.g., extreme fear, extreme despair). At times they even appear one after the other—

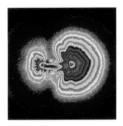

Cherry Plum: You're afraid that you are being taken over by long suppressed feelings, sometimes fearing that you may go mad.

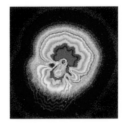

Sweet Chestnut: You feel that you have reached the utmost limit of your endurance and are afraid you can't go on. You feel extreme despair, as if this is the dark night of your soul.

29. Chestnut Bud or Cerato? Both will appear naive or foolish to others because—

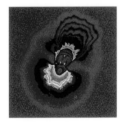

Chestnut Bud: You tend to repeat the same mistakes because you're unable to fully integrate your experiences. Possibly you may have a constitutional learning disability or one based on your upbringing.

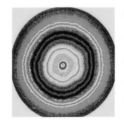

Cerato: You'll ask the same questions again and again of different people and—without success— believe you must solve problems on a mental level alone.

30. Chestnut Bud or Clematis? Both will complain frequently about their lack of concentration because—

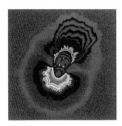

Chestnut Bud: Your thoughts are racing ahead so you're unable to focus on the problem at hand.

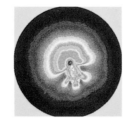

Clematis: Much of your attention is tied to other planes, and little energy remains to deal with present tasks.

31. Chestnut Bud or Gentian? Both have a "sputtering," stop-and-start pattern because:

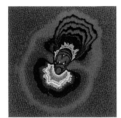

Chestnut Bud: You keep making the same mistake, which forces you to start over again and again.

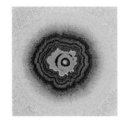

Gentian: Unexpected difficulties or disappointments are often so dispiriting that you tend to give up, and then have to remotivate yourself to start anew.

32. Chestnut Bud or Impatiens? Both will complain about feeling driven inside because—

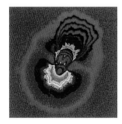

Chestnut Bud: You jump ahead of yourself in your mind and don't give enough attention to taking grounded steps.

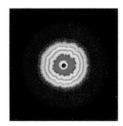

Impatiens: You race through life because you're determined not to lose any time.

33. Chestnut Bud or Scleranthus? Both show specific, repeating energetic patterns—

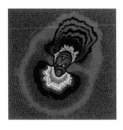

Chestnut Bud: You follow a stop-and-go pattern, alternating between phases of learning and stagnation.

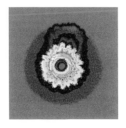

Scleranthus: You display an up-and-down or yes/no pattern of polarized thinking and behavior.

34. Chestnut Bud or Wild Oat? Both will complain about not really getting on with their lives because—

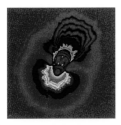

Chestnut Bud: You don't work deeply with your experiences and so must repeat them often.

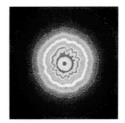

Wild Oat: Despite having made many promising attempts, you still haven't found your calling, and waste energy in secondary pursuits.

35. Chestnut Bud or Wild Rose? Wild Rose can be taken in all cases where Chestnut Bud is indicated but has not resulted in a positive outcome—

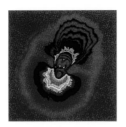

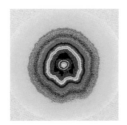

Wild Rose: This may revive a zest for life; a lack of it may have caused the learning disabilities. In this case, take it for several weeks.

36. Chicory or Red Chestnut? Both care too much about others and their fate—

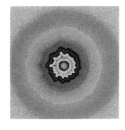

Chicory: You try to be indispensable, often due to fear of losing someone or something. You give a great deal in order to receive, and wind up interfering with others' lives.

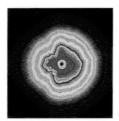

Red Chestnut: You tend to merge with another person, sense his or her feelings and needs more strongly than your own, and get involved with them as if they were your own.

37. Chicory or Vervain? Both are sure they know what is good for another person, and try to convince another to do something because—

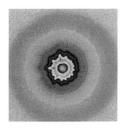

Chicory: You unconsciously expect to be paid back for such "good" deeds.

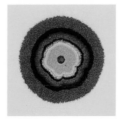

Vervain: You have missionary intentions— the desire to fight for a good cause; personal recognition is of lesser importance.

38. Chicory or Vine? Both try to influence others and to get others to do what they want—

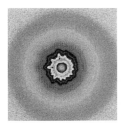

Chicory: You try to obligate another person diplomatically—for instance, by giving a present and later asking for a favor.

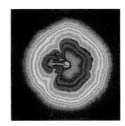

Vine: You express personal wishes directly and expect them to be granted.

39. Chicory or Willow? At times, both tend to feel cheated, betrayed, or deceived because—

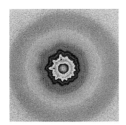

Chicory: You feel you've been inadequately repaid for all the help you've provided (often because its volume was unwanted); your investment didn't pay off.

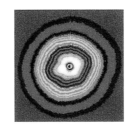

Willow: You expect fate to bring you only good things and are disappointed when you don't get them. You are unwilling or unable to see your personal involvement in a situation and don't accept responsibility.

40. Clematis or Honeysuckle? Neither can generate enough energy to tackle problems at hand because—

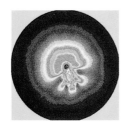

Clematis: You are uninterested in reality and escape to a speculative vision of the future or invented dream world.

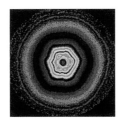

Honeysuckle: You are nostalgic, comparing your present mood of dissatisfaction to past happier days and holding on to them.

41. Clematis or Mustard? Both appear unapproachable at times because—

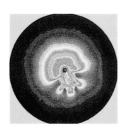

Clematis: Living in a world of your own, you don't wish to be disturbed.

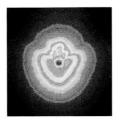

Mustard: You've sunk into a melancholic pit where you cannot be reached.

42. Clematis or Star of Bethlehem? Neither is mentally available at times because—

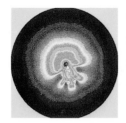

Clematis: You're actively involved in another realm, such as a day-dream.

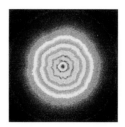

Star of Bethlehem: You've had a shocking experience; you're still numb and unable to react.

43. Clematis or Wild Rose? Both have little interest in actively changing their present life situation because—

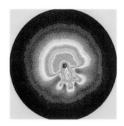

Clematis: You are not clearly conscious of reality and you prefer to dwell on things that might be instead of facing those that are.

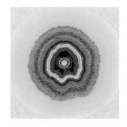

Wild Rose: You have little zest for life and therefore don't care what happens.

44. Crab Apple or Pine? Both feel physically or psychologically dirty or impure from actions, beliefs, or other involvements of their own because—

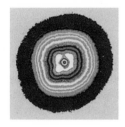

Crab Apple: You simply feel dirty and want to be clean again as soon as possible.

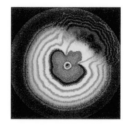

Pine: You judge yourself for moral lapses and blame and diminish yourself.

45. Crab Apple or Rock Water? Both can be compulsively focused on the physical body—

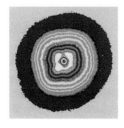

Crab Apple: You're easily disgusted with your body—with your sweat, for instance—and so take showers many times a day.

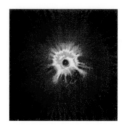

Rock Water: You try to master disturbing physical drives through stringent self-discipline.

46. Elm or Gentian? Both can be despondent, depressed, and willing to give up because—

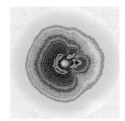

Elm: You've exhausted your energy during a passing episode of high performance that over-taxed you.

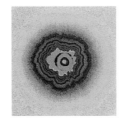

Gentian: Unexpected resistance or disappoint-ment quickly takes away your courage, confirming your latent negative expectations.

47. Elm or Hornbeam? Both are convinced they won't be able to master a certain task at hand—

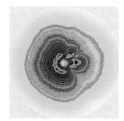

Elm: This is a passing state. You believe you are not able to bear the responsibility despite the fact that you've mastered similar jobs with ease in the past. Here, the task is made too important.

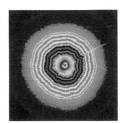

Hornbeam: Particularly in the morning, you believe you lack energy to deal with the day's usual routine work. In the evening it turns out you were able to do it all but the next morning the feeling is back. The task here is disliked and diminished; it's a bother-some duty.

48. Elm or Larch? Both are afraid to fail because—

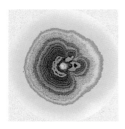

Elm: During times of overwork, you worry against your better judgment, even though you've done similar jobs successfully in the past.

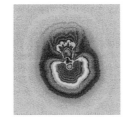

Larch: You basically believe you're less capable than others. You feel inferior because you're constantly measuring yourself against those who are more successful.

49. Elm or Olive? Both have overdone things because—

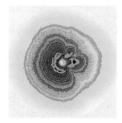

Elm: You overidentifiy with the tasks at hand and feel too responsible. You don't delegate enough work to others.

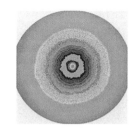

Olive: You simply don't stop until you have reached "the end of the line" and are physically and psychologically exhausted. Further obligations are out of the question; you need rest.

50. Gentian or Larch? Both give up too early because—

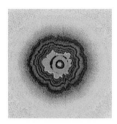

Gentian: Due to your pessimistic attitude, you easily exhaust your emotional reserves.

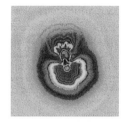

Larch: You believe yourself incapable and therefore give up before you've even begun.

51. Gentian or Mustard? Both may get depressed—

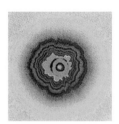

Gentian: You're aware of the specific cause of the depressed state, perhaps a disappointment or even fate. In a mild case you may feel pessimistic and skeptical.

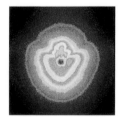

Mustard: You're unable to determine a concrete cause; you go in and out of the depressed state. In mild cases you may have an inexplicable inner heaviness and lack of motivation.

52. Gorse or Elm? Both can appear resigned in an acute situation—

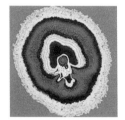

Gorse: You've really given up on possible improvements or positive changes.

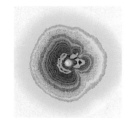

Elm: You experience short periods of resignation until your perspective clears again. During a crisis you may feel old and used, but you'll return to your former vitality after a little rest or vacation.

53. Gorse or Gentian? Both have negative expectations—

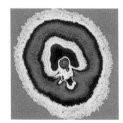

Gorse: You're unable to imagine a positive change—for instance, in the case of a chronic disease.

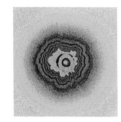

Gentian: In order to avoid disappointments, you prefer to expect a negative outcome.

54. Gorse or Mustard? Both are frequently a weight on others because—

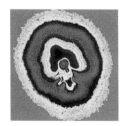

Gorse: You've resigned yourself to circumstances and given up hope.

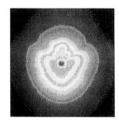

Mustard: You're under a "black cloud" and others must constantly pull you away from it.

55. Gorse or Sweet Chestnut? Both believe their state is hopeless because—

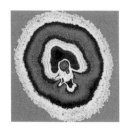

Gorse: You're resigned because you're unable to imagine any other possibility. The state threatens to become chronic.

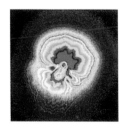

Sweet Chestnut: In an acute crisis, you feel hopelessness and deep despair because you cannot find a way out anymore.

56. Gorse or Wild Rose? Both are obviously resigned—

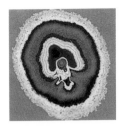

Gorse: You're aware of the reasons but can possibly, through some new approach, be motivated to try again.

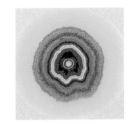

Wild Rose: On a very deep level, there is often an unconscious refusal to live that leads you to turn yourself off in certain areas of your life.

57. Gorse or Willow? Both frequently identify with the role of victim—

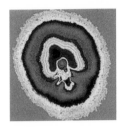

Gorse: You're convinced that you must put up with a negative situation and passively suffer.

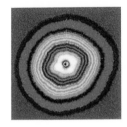

Willow: You rail at fate for being so unfair, try to find others who are at fault, and become embittered.

58. Heather or Chicory? Both have a strong psychological neediness—

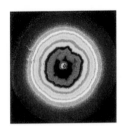

Heather: You need your surroundings as a kind of mirror and proof of existence. You are like the needy child—being self-centered, you cannot give, and consume the energy of anyone you talk to.

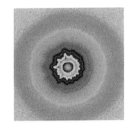

Chicory: You are like a puppeteer pulling the strings of those around you to fulfill your own personal needs. You are the needy mother—you give to others in order to get back what you want.

59. Heather or Mimulus? Both radiate self-directed worry—

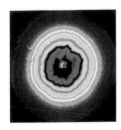

Heather: You'll describe your fears without hesitation when asked.

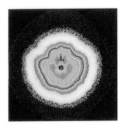

Mimulus: You'd rather not have to talk about your fears.

60. Heather or Vervain? Both may be very pushy—

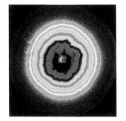

Heather: You talk incessantly about yourself and your personal affairs.

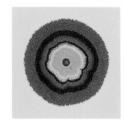

Vervain: You talk with great fervor about something "good" or "important" trying to win others to your cause.

61. Holly or Chicory? Both have disappointment and hurt feelings—

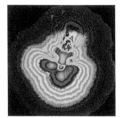

Holly: In the past, the way you expressed your feelings was misinterpreted or ignored. You took this personally and now react with distrust, irritation, or feelings of revenge.

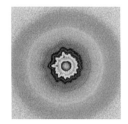

Chicory: Growing up, you received little loving care, so you now use your own loving care as an object of trade; you invest and give, in order to receive.

62. Holly or Impatiens? Both will overreact forcefully at times—

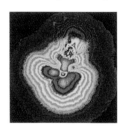

Holly: Due to your anger you may scream or even throw things. You will calm down again, but you don't forget.

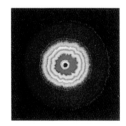

Impatiens: Due to your nature, you can "blow up" when others are too slow. The anger will subside as quickly as it surfaced. You don't carry a grudge.

63. Holly or Vine? Both may have very strong personalities—

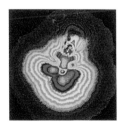

Holly: Feelings are predominant; you have a fiery disposition.

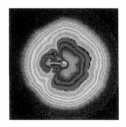

Vine: Willpower is the dominant trait; you have a cold disposition.

64. Holly or Willow? Both are easily offended because—

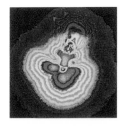 **Holly:** You're very sensitive emotionally and misinterpret or are easily hurt by what others say.

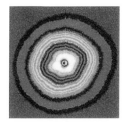 **Willow:** You were expecting something else and feel you weren't treated fairly.

65. Honeysuckle or Gorse? Both appear reserved or muted because—

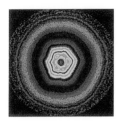 **Honeysuckle:** You've retreated mentally from the present and dwell in the past.

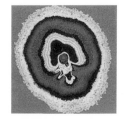 **Gorse:** You have fallen into a state of resignation.

66. Honeysuckle or Mustard? Both appear absent and difficult to reach because—

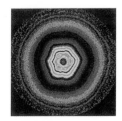 **Honeysuckle:** Your mental and psychological orientation is turned toward the past.

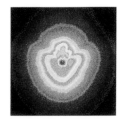 **Mustard:** You're under a black cloud, so you're isolated from the world around you.

67. Honeysuckle or Star of Bethlehem? Both are very helpful in coming to terms with undigested psychological experiences—

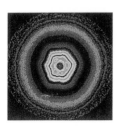 **Honeysuckle:** You still vividly remember all details of the experience.

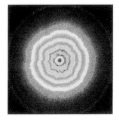 **Star of Bethlehem:** You don't want to look at the experience. You would rather avoid even touching upon it.

68. Honeysuckle or Wild Rose? When one or both of these are chosen spontaneously and cannot be confirmed in the interview, it may indicate—

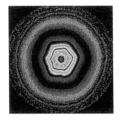

Honeysuckle: An unresolved deep experience that you had a long time ago.

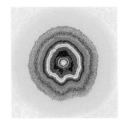

Wild Rose: You turned off some part of yourself a long time ago. In this case, take Honeysuckle or Wild Rose for several weeks.

69. Hornbeam or Gorse? Both can lack motivation because—

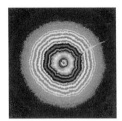

Hornbeam: You believe you lack the strength to accomplish the task at hand.

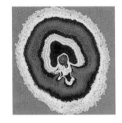

Gorse: It doesn't make sense to you to pursue the matter any further; "What's the use?"

70. Hornbeam or Larch? Both believe they can't deal with certain tasks because—

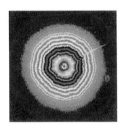

Hornbeam: You lack inner drive and seek support from stimulants such as coffee, tea, cigarettes, and telephone conversations.

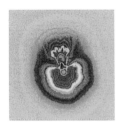

Larch: You're convinced you lack necessary skills.

71. Hornbeam or Olive? Both will complain about exhaustion and being asked to do too much because—

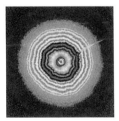

Hornbeam: Everyday activities are too routine, lacking any tension/relaxation stimulus, which leads to mental lethargy. Unexpected tasks, however, immediately summon new energy.

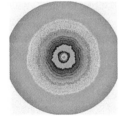

Olive: You have experienced great strain and now find further activity impossible. You're simply too exhausted and shy away from everything.

72. Hornbeam or Wild Rose? Both find it difficult to get going because—

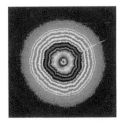 **Hornbeam:** Your inner drive has faded. You seek a jump-start from outside yourself, through stimulants or phone calls.

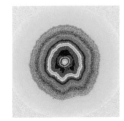 **Wild Rose:** On a deeper level your motivation to do something is gone, so you don't even consider change. You initiate nothing on your own.

73. Impatiens or Rock Rose? Both may appear hectic—

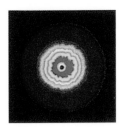 **Impatiens:** You're moving at top speed inside; you try to finish everything immediately and get upset with people who are slow.

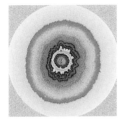 **Rock Rose:** Due to your inner panic, you lose perspective and run around like a chicken with its head cut off.

74. Impatiens or Vervain? Both feel a strong inner drive because—

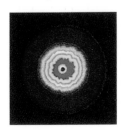 **Impatiens:** You wish to take care of all duties as quickly as possible.

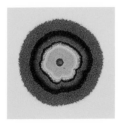 **Vervain:** You're possessed by a plan or an idea and push to realize it.

75. Larch or Gorse? Both believe they're unable to change a given situation because—

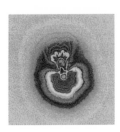 **Larch:** You believe you lack the necessary skills to do anything about it.

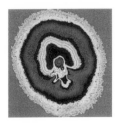 **Gorse:** You believe your situation is hopeless.

76. Larch or Mimulus? Neither is willing to get going with a task at hand because—

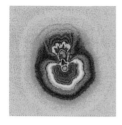 **Larch:** You're convinced you're not up to the task.

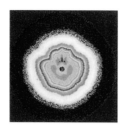 **Mimulus:** You become disheartened when you imagine the things that might go wrong.

77. Larch or Wild Rose? Both will frequently mention that they're putting up with a situation or have come to terms with it because—

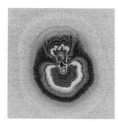 **Larch:** You lack the self-confidence to deal with it.

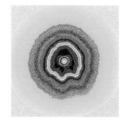 **Wild Rose:** You have a generally apathetic attitude toward life.

78. Mimulus or Centaury? Both may appear weak because—

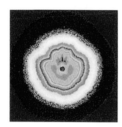 **Mimulus:** You have a natural tendency to be fearful.

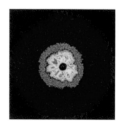 **Centaury:** You have a lack of will and self-determination.

79. Mimulus or Cherry Plum? Both have fears they don't want to talk about—

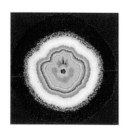 **Mimulus:** You know about your fears but must be asked to describe them.

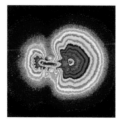 **Cherry Plum:** You find it difficult to describe the fears because you're afraid that they'll take over if you talk about them.

80. Mimulus or Red Chestnut? Both can describe their fears—

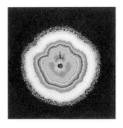

Mimulus: The fears are for yourself and your ability to cope with your own life.

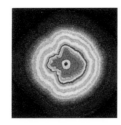

Red Chestnut: The fears are about others who are close to you and their abilities to cope.

81. Mimulus or Rock Rose? Both have fear—

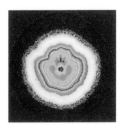

Mimulus: You have enough distance from your fears to describe them and possibly do something about them.

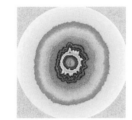

Rock Rose: You're totally overcome by your fears; you panic and react mindlessly. Among Bach Flowers that deal with fear, the Rock Rose state is the most acute. It's therefore an important part of Rescue Remedy.

82. Mimulus or Star of Bethlehem? If it is part of their basic character, both radiate a certain timidity and vulnerability—

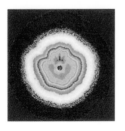

Mimulus: You try to avoid feared situations and procrastinate as long as possible.

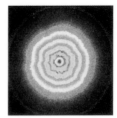

Star of Bethlehem: You don't want old, painful wounds to hurt again, so you quickly shut yourself off in advance when you feel they might be touched.

83. Mustard or Star of Bethlehem? Both can find it difficult to talk and may act as if they're numb because—

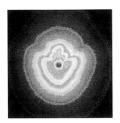

Mustard: A heavy, dark cloud is surrounding you and weighing you down.

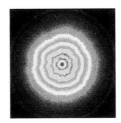

Star of Bethlehem: You are still frozen; you haven't yet recovered from a severe blow.

84. Mustard or Sweet Chestnut? Both feel trapped and don't know any way out because—

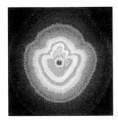

Mustard: You suffer passively, having no idea how or why you got into the situation.

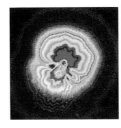

Sweet Chestnut: You're conscious of and still actively involved in the climax of a crisis, and thus fear breaking down.

85. Mustard or Wild Rose? Both can be indifferent or apathetic because—

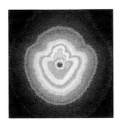

Mustard: You've fallen into a depression that keeps you from active participation in everyday life.

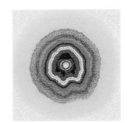

Wild Rose: You've closed down some part of yourself and can no longer motivate it.

86. Oak or Elm? Both tend to go beyond their limits because—

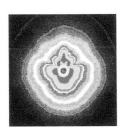

Oak: You feel obligated to complete a task you've started—at any price—or to keep a promise despite changed circumstances.

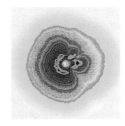

Elm: Due to a very strong sense of responsibility, you don't acknowledge your personal limits.

87. Oak or Rock Water? Both are often seen as stubborn by those around them because—

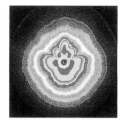

Oak: Once you've made a decision, you feel you must stay with it to the bitter end, even if changed circumstances have made the decision questionable.

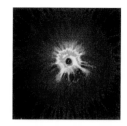

Rock Water: You'll stick to a self-determined set of principles with ironclad resolve, rigidly denying your personal needs.

88. Oak or Vervain? Both will at times strain the limit of their energy because—

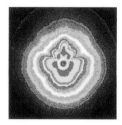

Oak: You feel obligated to persevere at all costs.

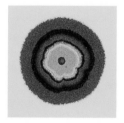

Vervain: Your enthusiasm drives you to give 150 percent.

89. Oak or Vine? Neither will give in easily because—

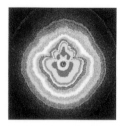

Oak: You won't allow yourself to ease up; you're determined to do your duty.

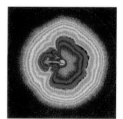

Vine: You won't give in to others; you're determined to realize your own interests.

90. Olive or Gorse? Both will say they can't rouse themselves to get going again because—

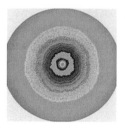

Olive: You're exhausted.

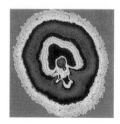

Gorse: You've resigned yourself to the situation.

91. Olive or Mustard? In the extreme state, both may be unable to take any action because—

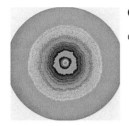

Olive: You've used up all energy reserves.

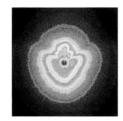

Mustard: You feel trapped under a big black cloud and are unable to get out from under it by yourself.

92. Olive or Oak? Both can look at work as a heavy load or an unloved duty because—

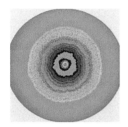

Olive: You're exhausted and need rest.

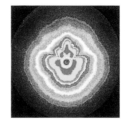

Oak: Due to a sense of duty, you've overdone it and now lack motivation. Frequently a long-standing Oak state will shift into an Olive state.

93. Olive or Wild Rose? Neither may show any initiative because—

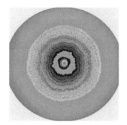

Olive: You're too exhausted.

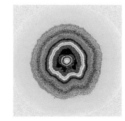

Wild Rose: You're unconsciously tired of life in general.

94. Pine or Larch? Both may frequently feel worthless because—

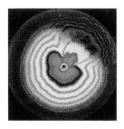

Pine: You believe you aren't living up to your own unrealistic moral values. You lack self-acceptance.

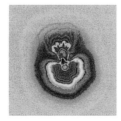

Larch: You believe you're less able than others. You lack self-esteem.

95. **Pine or Mimulus?** Both can be afraid of whatever is coming next because—

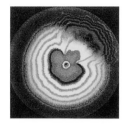 **Pine:** You're afraid you will do something you'll feel guilty about and that others will blame you.

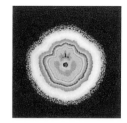 **Mimulus:** You're overly sensitive to many daily situations, so you constantly worry about what will happen.

96. **Pine or Oak?** Both are very demanding of themselves—

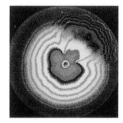 **Pine:** You try to live up to your overly idealized moral values.

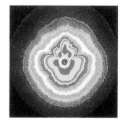 **Oak:** You try to live up to your extreme personal sense of duty.

97. **Pine or Rock Water?** Both suppress their needs and deny themselves many things because—

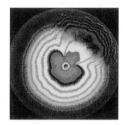 **Pine:** You believe you don't deserve to have your needs fulfilled.

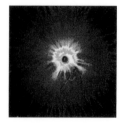 **Rock Water:** You try to become a better, more pure person by disciplining yourself.

98. **Red Chestnut or Centaury?** Both frequently do what others want them to do because—

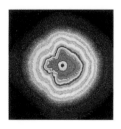 **Red Chestnut:** Your emotional ties to another person are too strong.

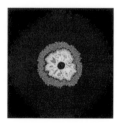 **Centaury:** You surrender without resistance to a stronger personality.

99. Red Chestnut or Honeysuckle? Both find it difficult to part from someone because—

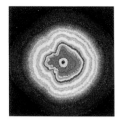 **Red Chestnut:** You're invisibly tied to the other person as if by an umbilical cord.

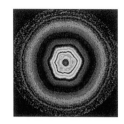 **Honeysuckle:** You're determined to hold on to the past situation and won't accept any change.

100. Red Chestnut or Rock Rose? Both may develop a panicky fear—

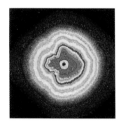 **Red Chestnut:** You feel fear for another person.

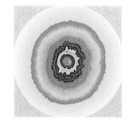 **Rock Rose:** You feel fear for yourself.

101. Rock Rose or Cherry Plum? Both may develop an extremely tense fear because—

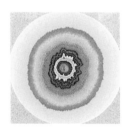 **Rock Rose:** You become extremely excited by an immediate threat.

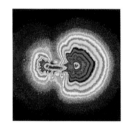 **Cherry Plum:** You're afraid you won't be able to control emerging emotional chaos. Both Flowers are part of Rescue Remedy.

102. Rock Rose or Star of Bethlehem? The two states are frequently mixed up because after a shock, one tends to shift to the other—

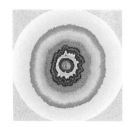 **Rock Rose:** A shock causes an active panic (a storm of activity). You may, for instance, react by screaming.

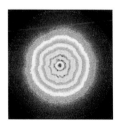 **Star of Bethlehem:** A shock results in a "death reflex," a passive state of numb rigidity. You're unable to react. Both Flowers are part of Rescue Remedy.

103. Rock Rose or Sweet Chestnut? Both have reached their emotional limits and see no way out—

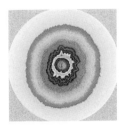

Rock Rose: You feel acute fear in a situation, are gripped by panic, and react mindlessly.

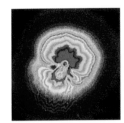

Sweet Chestnut: You've gotten yourself into an extreme crisis. You have no idea how to escape and fear that it may destroy you. In extreme situations it may be helpful to combine Rock Water and Sweet Chestnut.

104. Rock Water or Cherry Plum? Both have a tendency for self-repression because—

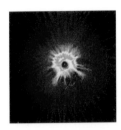

Rock Water: You wish to master your physical urges, instincts, and desires.

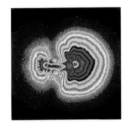

Cherry Plum: You're determined to control the emotional chaos within you.

105. Rock Water or Heather? Both can be very involved with themselves because—

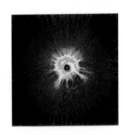

Rock Water: Your own tasks and disciplines have your complete attention.

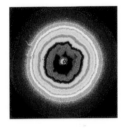

Heather: You lack sufficient emotional energy reserves and need whatever is left for yourself.

106. Rock Water or Vervain? Both are open to self-improvement techniques and progressive ideas because—

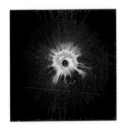

Rock Water: You're eager to employ these techniques yourself for your own path to perfection.

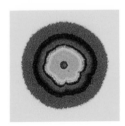

Vervain: You're totally enthusiastic and want to get everyone around you involved.

107. Rock Water or Vine? Both will demand and expect a lot because—

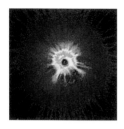

Rock Water: You demand a lot from yourself in terms of self-discipline.

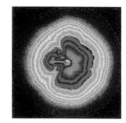

Vine: You expect others to work hard to realize your own ideas.

108. Scleranthus or Wild Oat? Both find it difficult to make decisions because—

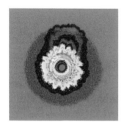

Scleranthus: At first one decision seems right and later the other does, so you're torn between the two.

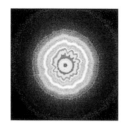

Wild Oat: You have no clear goal and are steadily searching for better solutions, so you avoid making decisions.

109. Star of Bethlehem or Willow? Both can feel powerless because—

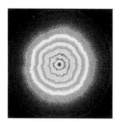

Star of Bethlehem: Deep shock prevents you from reacting right away.

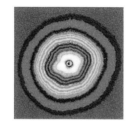

Willow: You feel that fate is treating you unfairly. You're unable to see that you have something to do with it.

110. Star of Bethlehem or Sweet Chestnut? Both appear temporarily unable to act because—

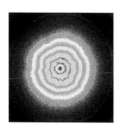

Star of Bethlehem: You haven't yet overcome a personal blow.

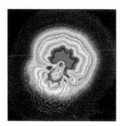

Sweet Chestnut: You're at your wit's end and have no idea what else you could do.

111. Sweet Chestnut or Elm? Both are fearful about breaking under the load they're carrying because—

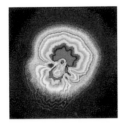

Sweet Chestnut: You're experiencing a deep life crisis, possibly requiring you to revise important life decisions.

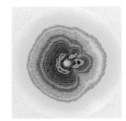

Elm: You're experiencing a temporary crisis in performance and most likely need to change the way you work.

112. Sweet Chestnut or Gentian? Both have a bleak outlook because—

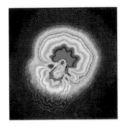

Sweet Chestnut: You're in the acute phase of a difficult life crisis.

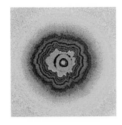

Gentian: You tend to be skeptical and have a negative outlook; this mood is frequent.

113. Vervain or Vine? Both have great willpower and are goal oriented—

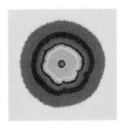

Vervain: Your goal is an altruistic one, and other people need to be convinced of its advantages.

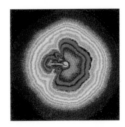

Vine: Your goal is an egotistical one, and others are used to accomplish it.

114. Vine or Water Violet? Both may appear proud and arrogant because—

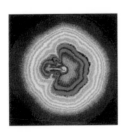

Vine: You know exactly what you want and usually succeed in getting it.

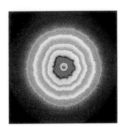

Water Violet: You're independent and prefer to stay in the background.

115. Walnut or Aspen? Both may have the feeling of being under some kind of influence or spell because—

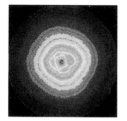 **Walnut:** You're still tied to someone who was an authority figure for you, or are tied to current academic theories, conventions, promises, oaths, and so on. It's important to break these "spells."

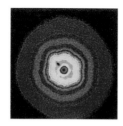 **Aspen:** You're under the influence of self-created, scary fantasies such as demonic powers or aliens. It's important to develop a more realistic view of things.

116. Walnut or Cerato? Both can be swayed to give up their opinion because—

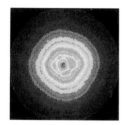 **Walnut:** You are in a process of change; a new beginning is taking place, and you lack personal experience to draw upon.

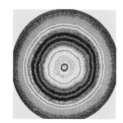 **Cerato:** You place more weight on other people's advice than on your own ideas.

117. Walnut or Red Chestnut? Both let themselves be influenced easily because—

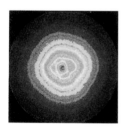 **Walnut:** You are in a new phase of development and are in a state too delicate to resist.

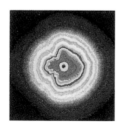 **Red Chestnut:** You're emotionally tied to another person.

118. Water Violet or Impatiens? Both enjoy working independently because—

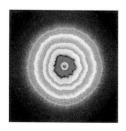 **Water Violet:** When alone you find it easier to follow your individual style of working.

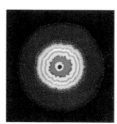 **Impatiens:** You work faster than others.

119. Water Violet or Larch? Both tend to be reserved because—

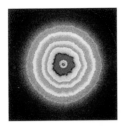 **Water Violet:** You need a certain inner distance from the people around you.

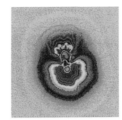 **Larch:** You feel you're of little importance or not very capable.

120. Water Violet or Mimulus? Both have difficulties dealing with "the masses" because—

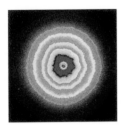 **Water Violet:** You feel like you don't belong.

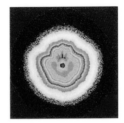 **Mimulus:** You find it strenuous and it takes too much energy to protect yourself.

121. Water Violet or Mustard? Both may appear unapproachable because—

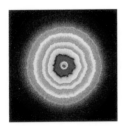 **Water Violet:** You withdraw inside yourself.

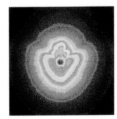 **Mustard:** You're lost in depression.

122. White Chestnut or Cherry Plum? Both appear to be under a lot of pressure—

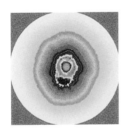 **White Chestnut:** The pressure comes from your thoughts, which you can't turn off.

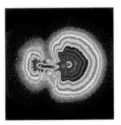 **Cherry Plum:** The pressure comes from your emotions, which you want to control.

123. White Chestnut or Crab Apple? Both become fixated on what irritates them—

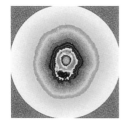 **White Chestnut:** Unwanted thoughts keep intruding and are dominating your thinking. You're unable to stop them.

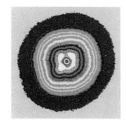 **Crab Apple:** You must compulsively restore the customary order in your personal environment before you are able to turn to anything else.

124. White Chestnut or Impatiens? Both are under pressure—

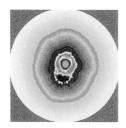 **White Chestnut:** You're pressured by your thoughts.

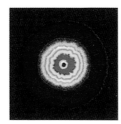 **Impatiens:** You're pressured by time.

125. Wild Oat or Gentian? Both are repeatedly frustrated because—

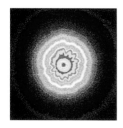 **Wild Oat:** Despite being successful, you have an inner uncertainty about your life's goal.

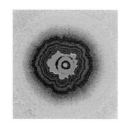 **Gentian:** You become frustrated about a project as soon as you experience any adversity.

126. Wild Rose or Centaury? Both tend to appear weak and lacking in vitality, but they don't complain about it because—

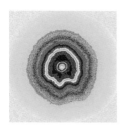 **Wild Rose:** You have little motivation for life in general.

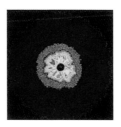 **Centaury:** You have little willpower to stand up for yourself.

127. Wild Rose or Star of Bethlehem? Both may be apathetic because—

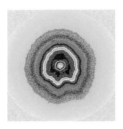

Wild Rose: You lack zest for life.

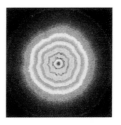

Star of Bethlehem: You are still in shock from any experience, no matter how big or seemingly small.

10

The Double Questionnaire and Final Choice Checklist: Tools to Assist Beginners

How to Use These Tools

The Questionnaires and Final Checklist are recommended for use until you are comfortable with the Building Blocks in chapter 11 or are so familiar with the Flowers that you don't need to use either. They can be used in two different ways:

1. For treating yourself during times of acute personal problems.

2. For interviews with others.

   The questionnaires build upon each other and should be used in the order presented. In particular, using the Final Choice Checklist alone is useless because you need to do the deeper work of recognizing and clarifying the problem first. Used by itself, this checklist would lead to a superficial choice of Flowers.

   After reading or hearing a question, your response should come from a spontaneous "gut feeling" and not a carefully thought through answer. Most important, mark only the questions that clearly reflect your current situation—that is, things that have been bothering you in the last few days. Do not mark other issues that have a generally fitting ring to them but aren't part of the problem now. If the Flowers that address these issues were also included, they would prevent you from getting a clear picture of the current pattern, and ultimately your mixture would not be as effective.

1. **Define the problem (e.g., conflict, stress, frustration) you wish to work on.** Write it down in no more than three to five sentences or help your interview partner to write it.

2. **Fill out the Present Situation Questionnaire on page 290.** The Situation Questionnaire assesses current negative states.

It is designed to answer the question "How am I reacting to the current problem?" or "How are you reacting to your current problem?" These negative patterns may have resulted from:

- A reaction to external circumstances—for example, panic about blocked streets after a snowstorm (Rock Rose).

- A reaction to a current accident or illness —perhaps being impatient after a skiing accident or an operation (Impatiens).

- A reaction to the behavior of others—for instance, being angry after a fight with your spouse (Holly).

The answers to these questions will indicate the Flowers needed in your present situation. However, since these Flowers address your current situation, not all of them need to fit your basic character.

If your circumstances are changing quickly, you can simply take these flowers using the Water Glass Method (see chapter 8).

Sometimes in a first interview a person will have so many current problems that you can't determine what the main difficulty is. At these times, it may be advisable to use only the Present Situation Questionnaire and the Final Choice Checklist.

3. **Define in writing the goal or desired change.** Simply put, what do you (or what does your interview partner) wish to change or accomplish? In setting your goals, it is important to make them realistic and to describe them in specific and precise terms. If possible, try to imagine how you'd feel after having reached your goal. By doing this, you will be able to see more clearly the negative patterns that hinder you from getting there.

4. **Fill out the Character Questionnaire on page 292.** What are the negative behavior patterns that keep you (or your interview partner) from implementing your goal? This question will take you to a deeper level of awareness. You will identify individual behavior patterns that are part of your character or have taken root very early in life. You have probably used these patterns again and again in similar situations.

From many years of experience I've learned that almost every effective combination of Bach Flowers will contain flowers that address issues from the Present Situation Questionnaire and those you identified with the help of the Character Questionnaire.

You will frequently wind up feeling that too many Flowers (more than eight) are needed. In such cases, proceed to the following step.

5. **Go through the Final Choice Checklist on page 295.** Use the Final Choice Checklist to answer the question "What is most bothersome right now?" Once again, in filling out the checklist it's very important to

concentrate on the present situation alone and to give your answers quickly and spontaneously.

6. **Fill out the Evaluation Sheet.** Make a copy of the Evaluation Sheet (page 298) prior to your assessment and write on it the suggested Flowers from all your lists. Referring to the descriptions in chapter 5, familiarize yourself with the Flowers that appear in all of the columns, and then read about the others you've listed.

Now from the information you have at hand, make a conscious decision about which Flowers you or your interview partner will take. If you still find it difficult to decide between two of the Flowers, you might also consult the Flower comparisons in chapter 9.

Here's an example of how these questionnaires might work:

1. **The problem.** I have to cancel a family get-together, a weekend trip, because I'm swamped both at work and at home—I need the weekend to catch up on things. I feel guilty disappointing my family, especially because the same thing has happened before.

2. **How am I reacting to the current problem?** (See the Present Situation Questionnaire.) My reactions now are:
   > I feel like an exhausted fighter—Oak
   > I am panic-stricken inside—Rock Rose
   > I feel guilty—Pine

3. **The goal—what do I wish to change or accomplish?** I'd like to be able to organize my tasks better and finish them. I want to be able to tell people about my decisions without feeling guilty.

4. **What are the negative behavior patterns that keep me from implementing my goal?** (See the Character Questionnaire.) What holds me back is:
   > I'm so enthusiastic that I overdo things—Vervain
   > I don't know if I really want to be doing this—Wild Oat
   > I'm too connected to other people's feelings. I always know how they will feel, which makes it difficult for me do things they won't like—Red Chestnut

5. **Final Choice Checklist—which reactions and negative behavior patterns are most bothersome right now?**
   > My guilt feelings—Pine
   > My panic—Rock Rose
   > My need to endure at any cost—Oak
   > My excessive zeal—Vervain
   > My strong connection to others' feelings—Red Chestnut

6. **Evaluation.** This (simplified) example would call for the combination of Pine, Rock Rose, Oak, Vervain, and Red Chestnut. Most likely, it will take more than one combination to solve this problem.

Present Situation Questionnaire

How am I reacting to my current problem?

(In an interview: How are you reacting to your current problem?)

Right now I'm feeling guilty. I am blaming myself.	Pine
Right now I'm feeling uncertain. I question my own judgment and follow the advice of others.	Cerato
Right now I'm feeling distrustful; emotionally hurt; hostile; angry; jealous; or vengeful.*	Holly
Right now I'm feeling as though I'm not quite here; my mind is preoccupied with other things.	Clematis
Right now I'm feeling irritated because things are too disorderly; I feel dirty, nauseated, or disgusted; I feel the need to clean up.*	Crab Apple
Right now I'm feeling abandoned; as though Fate has treated me unjustly; poor me!	Willow
Right now I'm feeling driven to impose my will, to succeed.	Vine
Right now I'm feeling tired; I don't have the energy and initiative to face the day's work.	Hornbeam
Right now I'm feeling unstable and too easily swayed; I wish I could be true to myself.*	Walnut
Right now I'm feeling melancholy, sad, and depressed, and I don't know why.	Mustard
Right now I'm feeling inferior; as though I'm a loser; less able than others; as though I'm a second-rate person.*	Larch
Right now I'm feeling like an exhausted fighter still on duty by myself; there's no way I will quit now.	Oak

_____

* Only one of the words or phrases must apply.

Right now I'm feeling afraid. I'm scared of [enter specific person or situation.]   Mimulus

Right now I'm feeling too soft and too nice; I can never say no.   Centaury

Right now I'm feeling nostalgic; I just can't let go of [enter relationship or situation].   Honeysuckle

Right now I'm feeling overwhelmed by my responsibilities; I can't go on any longer!   Elm

Right now I'm feeling indifferent; I've given in to the situation.   Wild Rose

Right now I'm feeling undecided, scattered, dissatisfied; uncertain whether this what I really want.*   Wild Oat

Right now I'm feeling impatient; everything is moving too slowly!   Impatiens

Right now I'm feeling needy; I need affection and sympathy.   Heather

Right now I'm feeling as though I have to grin and bear; I'm pretending that things are all right.   Agrimony

Right now I'm feeling reserved; I want to withdraw and be left alone.   Water Violet

Right now I'm feeling perplexed because I'm still making the same mistake.   Chestnut Bud

Right now I'm feeling bothered by unwanted thoughts and persistent inner dialogue; I just can't tune them out.   White Chestnut

Right now I'm feeling up against a wall; I'm desperate and I have no idea how to go on from here.   Sweet Chestnut

Right now I'm feeling very enthusiastic—150 percent committed!   Vervain

Right now I'm feeling as though I'm still in shock; I haven't digested it yet.   Star of Bethlehem

Right now I'm feeling torn between two things; I'm really out of balance.   Scleranthus

Right now I'm feeling drained, zapped, exhausted.   Olive

Right now I'm feeling like an athlete in training, mercilessly denying myself everything.   Rock Water

Right now I'm feeling defeated and without hope; I'm resigned.   Gorse

Right now I'm feeling vaguely threatened; I can't get a handle on my fears.   Aspen

Right now I'm feeling unloved; I feel hurt or disappointed because I expected   Chicory
more gratitude or appreciation for what I've done.*

Right now I'm feeling completely absorbed by my fears for someone else;   Red Chestnut
I don't even know what I feel myself.

Right now I'm feeling discouraged; skeptical; despondent.*   Gentian

Right now I'm feeling as if I'm sitting on a powder keg ready to explode;   Cherry Plum
I'm barely able to control myself.

Right now I'm feeling irritated—maybe I'm just too critical and intolerant;   Beech
maybe it would be better not to criticize at all.*

Right now I'm feeling panic-stricken; I've lost my mind and my nerves   Rock Rose
are on edge.

Character Questionnaire

What are the negative behavior patterns that keep me from implementing my goal?
(In an interview: What are the negative behavior patterns that keep you from implementing
your goal?)

I hold myself back because I'm timid and scared; I'm afraid it will involve   Mimulus
too much effort and stress.

I hold myself back with my low self-esteem; I don't believe I can do it.   Larch

I hold myself back with my strong need for harmony; I dislike ugly disputes   Agrimony
and arguments.

I hold myself back because I'm completely exhausted and everything takes   Olive
too much effort.

I hold myself back by being too sensitive; when I think about changing this, I'm taken over by strange feelings I can't quite describe.   Aspen

I hold myself back with my constant criticism of others and myself; there are many things that disturb me but it's impossible for me to turn a blind eye.   Beech

I hold myself back with my wish to please; I can't say no.   Centaury

I hold myself back with my tendency to live in the past; I just can't forget how it used to be.   Honeysuckle

I hold myself back with my lack of inner drive; I always feel like it's Monday morning and I just can't get going.   Hornbeam

I hold myself back by fearing that I'll lose control of myself; if I let go of my feelings, I don't know what I'll become.   Cherry Plum

I hold myself back by distrusting others and feeling jealous; I can easily become aggressive.   Holly

I hold myself back with my lack of inner direction; it's difficult for me to know what I really want.   Wild Oat

I hold myself back by blaming myself for everything; if I make this change I know I'll find things to feel guilty about.   Pine

I hold myself back because I'm very vulnerable; I'm afraid of being hurt again as I was before.   Star of Bethlehem

I hold myself back by not being able to stick to my decisions; first I prefer one solution, and the next moment I prefer another.   Scleranthus

I hold myself back with my extreme sense of duty; I feel as though I always have to keep struggling on.   Oak

I hold myself back by being so driven and enthusiastic; I always seem to overdo it and get on others' nerves.   Vervain

I hold myself back with my strong sense of fairness; I can't see an unjust situation without having to do something about it.   Vervain

I hold myself back by doubting my judgment. I always check with others, just to make sure.	Cerato
I hold myself back because I tend to panic easily; I feel totally helpless just thinking about it.	Rock Rose
I hold myself back by being overly disciplined. I'm always setting standards for myself that are too high.	Rock Water
I hold myself back by being overly ambitious; I always want to have things done my own way.	Vine
I hold myself back by being picky about details and cleanliness; when things aren't just right, I get nervous.	Crab Apple
I hold myself back with my feelings of hopelessness; it's no use anymore.	Gorse
I hold myself back by being so absorbed in myself; I don't pick up on other people's concerns.	Heather
I hold myself back with my dreaminess; I seem to lack any interest in reality.	Clematis
I hold myself back with my impatience; I'm unable to wait for things to happen.	Impatiens
I hold myself back by being too sympathetic; I know exactly what the other person will feel and become overly concerned for him or her.	Red Chestnut
I hold myself back with my melancholy disposition; at times it paralyzes me.	Mustard
I hold myself back with my apathy; deep inside, I don't care about improving the situation.	Wild Rose
I hold myself back with my tendency to be aloof; I find it difficult to jump in and mingle with others.	Water Violet
I hold myself back with the steady stream of chatter in my head; I'm unable to concentrate on what's important.	White Chestnut
I hold myself back because I'm too easily influenced; I always let others	Walnut

interfere with my plans instead of staying true to myself.

I hold myself back by not really paying attention; I tend to make the same mistakes over again.   Chestnut Bud

I hold myself back with my skepticism; I just don't expect things to end well.   Gentian

I hold myself back with my exaggerated sense of responsibility; it keeps me from putting on the brakes before I feel overwhelmed.   Elm

I hold myself back because I expect too much from others; I get involved and then expect recognition or gratitude in return.   Chicory

I hold myself back because I tend to let something go until there is no way I can do anything about it.   Sweet Chestnut

I hold myself back with my self-pity; I'm resentful and see myself as a victim of circumstance.   Willow

Final Choice Checklist

What is most bothersome right now?
If possible, please check no more than six responses.

My anxiety   Mimulus

My lack of self-esteem or feelings of inferiority   Larch

My need for harmony   Agrimony

My lack of energy and exhaustion   Olive

My vague fears   Aspen

My intolerance   Beech

My inability to say no   Centaury

My tendency to dwell on the past   Honeysuckle

My mental weariness	Hornbeam
My inner emotional pressure	Cherry Plum
My anger, envy, jealousy, etc.	Holly
My lack of clear inner direction	Wild Oat
My feelings of vulnerability, shock, and numbness	Star of Bethlehem
My tendency to blame myself for others' mistakes	Pine
My indecision	Scleranthus
My need to endure at any cost	Oak
My excessive zeal	Vervain
My inner uncertainty	Cerato
My panic	Rock Rose
My exaggerated self-discipline	Rose Water
My need to dominate	Vine
My tendency to be picky about details and cleanliness	Crab Apple
My hopelessness	Gorse
My tendency to be too self-absorbed	Heather
My dreamy and unrealistic nature	Clematis
My impatience	Impatiens
My tendency to be too tied to someone emotionally	Red Chestnut
My deep gloom	Mustard
My apathy	Wild Rose
My isolation or tendency to retreat	Water Violet

My never-ending thoughts   White Chestnut

My inability to be true to myself   Walnut

My tendency to repeat the same mistakes   Chestnut Bud

My negative expectations   Gentian

My tendency to be overly responsible   Elm

My possessiveness or need to manipulate   Chicory

My despair, desperation   Sweet Chestnut

My bitterness   Willow

Evaluation Sheet

Name of Flower	Present Situation	Character Questionnaire	Final Choice Questionnaire	Your Choice Checklist (after Reading Flower Descriptions)
Agrimony				
Aspen				
Beech				
Centaury				
Cerato				
Cherry Plum				
Chestnut Bud				
Chicory				
Clematis				
Crab Apple				
Elm				
Gentian				
Gorse				
Heather				
Holly				
Honeysuckle				
Hornbeam				
Impatiens				
Larch				
Mimulus				
Mustard				
Oak				
Olive				
Pine				
Red Chestnut				
Rock Rose				
Rock Water				
Scleranthus				
Star of Bethlehem				
Sweet Chestnut				
Vervain				
Vine				
Walnut				
Water Violet				
White Chestnut				
Wild Oat				
Wild Rose				
Willow				

11

Building Blocks to Support the Choice of Individual Flower Combinations

It's difficult to find the exact words to clearly express Inner States. Experience shows that people often hear the same words differently. For example, *duty* has a positive meaning for some people and a negative one for others. Because of this, you may find in an interview that the discussion veers off into arguing intellectually over the meaning of a particular word or phrase while your feeling for the actual state or experience is lost.

To alleviate difficulties like this, the following reference list has been created to provide a common "language" for the Main Problem Areas that tend to come up in a Bach Flower interview. Next to each problem in the list is a page number indicating where in the next section the problem appears with alternative scenarios and the corresponding recommendations for Bach Flower combinations. These recommendations form the Building Blocks that are the result of

my twenty-five years of experience. These Building Blocks may fit your situation precisely or they may speak only to part of it. If you're unable to find your personal scenario among those listed, you may still find it helpful to read through those that have been included; they may help you clarify and understand your individual situation.

Recommendations for Working with the Building Blocks

1. Start by reading through the list of Main Problem Areas and choosing those that most closely match your or your interview partner's situation.

2. Next, locate your chosen Main Problem Areas in the section "Combination Building Blocks" immediately following the list, and read all the scenarios under each of your

Main Problem Areas, selecting those that most closely resemble your specific situation.

3. Now you can put together your or your interview partner's personal Flower combination.

4. If an additional appropriate Flower comes to mind, add it to the combination.

5. This combination should be taken for five days. If you (or your partner) notice any positive reaction, then continue taking the Flowers. If not, the combination of Flowers will have to be reanalyzed.

Here's an example of how the cross-referenced lists work to help you assemble an appropriate Flower combination:

It has become clear to me that I have to change my work style. Things have gotten out of hand and despite this knowledge, I'm failing to implement changes. I don't seem to have any motivation (I'm Unmotivated, Lethargic, Indifferent) and feel as though I don't have the energy to persevere (my Perseverance and Resilience are Weak). In addition, I've noticed that I tend to immediately forget what I had planned (I'm Disorganized; I'm having Concentration Difficulties). I'm also afraid (I'm Fearful) of changing because I cannot see how things will turn out in the end.

After selecting the applicable Main Problem Areas and reading the specific scenarios and suggested Flower combinations for these, I arrive at the following scenarios and combinations for my situation:

Unmotivated, Lethargic, Indifferent, together with extreme fatigue—Wild Rose, Hornbeam, Mustard

Perseverance and Resilience are Weak because you're too exhausted—Olive, Hornbeam

Concentration Difficulties, Disorganized because there are too many things to keep track of—Hornbeam, White Chestnut

Fearful because of the unknown—Aspen, Mimulus

Out of this, I decide that the combination for my situation will contain: Mimulus, Aspen, Wild Rose, Olive, Hornbeam, and White Chestnut.

As a personal Flower I decide to add Vervain because my strong willpower tends to block my energy.

With the help of this combination, in a few days I should be able to find a way to get going with the needed changes in my work style.

Please Note

For making sure that your combination contains the right Flowers, it is recommended that you also read the descriptions for the chosen Flowers in chapter 5. However, please be aware that it is not possible to compare the "Reactions in Blocked State" section directly with the Building Blocks in this chapter. These Building Blocks are a further step in the process and represent constellations of different negative reactions (see beginning of chapter 5) that may or may not come together exactly in your situation.

Main Problem Areas: What Matches My Situation?

Refer to the alphabetized Main Problem Areas in the list below when looking up the appropriate Combination Building Blocks in the alphabetized section directly following the list.

- Acute life crisis
- Adjustment difficulties
- Aggressive, angry
- Authority issues, lacking assertiveness
- Dependent
- Depressed, despondent
- Discipline and self-control are too strong
- Discouraged, quick to give up
- Disorganized, concentration difficulties
- Dissatisfied
- Distracted, scattered, inconsistent
- Doubting
- Exaggerated reactions
- Exhausted, overwhelmed by demands
- Fearful
- Grief
- Homesick
- Indecisive, inconsistent
- Insecure, uncertain

- Learning issues
- Letting go is difficult
- Life transitions
- Lovesick
- Mood swings
- Nightmares
- Offended, touchy, feeling hurt
- Perseverance and resilience are weak
- Resigned, hopeless
- Responsibility issues
- Rigid, inflexible
- Self-blaming, feeling guilty
- Self-centered, egotistical
- Self-worth crisis, feelings of inferiority
- Sensitive in the extreme, possessing a delicate constitution
- Separation difficulty (parting from others)
- Sleeping difficulties
- Socializing and communicating difficulty
- Stressed, nervous
- Stubborn, intolerant
- Test-taking difficulty
- Tense, tight, "blocked"
- Unmotivated, lethargic, indifferent
- Weak-willed, unassertive

Combination Building Blocks

Acute Life Crisis

In the climax	Sweet Chestnut, Rescue
You're still numb	Star of Bethlehem, Sweet Chestnut
You can't decide whether to go along with the circumstances	Scleranthus, Sweet Chestnut
With self-doubt	Sweet Chestnut, Cerato, Larch
With guilt feelings	Sweet Chestnut, Pine
In the moment, nothing makes sense and you're ready to give up	Sweet Chestnut, Gorse, Mustard
You're totally overworked	Oak, Olive, Sweet Chestnut
You don't feel able to adjust to a possible new situation	Honeysuckle, Walnut

Adjustment Difficulties

Motion sickness	Rescue, Scleranthus, Honeysuckle
Weather changes	Scleranthus, Walnut, Hornbeam, Aspen
With new people	Water Violet, Chestnut Bud, Wild Oat, Cerato

Aggressive, Angry

To push through or succeed with your personal will or agenda	Holly, Vine
Because of impatience	Holly, Impatiens
Because of bitterness	Holly, Willow

| Triggered unexpectedly by "insignificant" things | Holly, Cherry Plum |

Authority Issues, Lacking Assertiveness

With anyone in a position of authority	Vine
Because you're determined to keep the upper hand	Vine, Holly
You're set on convincing others to accept your opinion	Vervain
You're determined to force others to accept "what's good for them"	Vervain, Vine
You forget your own wishes around stronger personalities	Centaury
You give in too easily to others' demands because you believe they are more capable	Larch, Cerato
You try to realize your ambitious goals indirectly or through others	Chicory, Vine
You have to learn how to be the boss	Centaury, Vine
When succeeding, you feel guilty	Vine, Pine
You're determined not to hurt others	Agrimony, Centaury, Pine

Dependent

You always ask others what you should do	Cerato
Because you are too weak-willed	Centaury
Because you believe others are more capable	Larch
Because you've gotten yourself caught in all sorts of relationships	Chicory, Willow

Dependent on the moods and capriciousness of others	Star of Bethlehem, Walnut, Willow
Because you believe you are powerless	Willow
Because you mistakenly believe you must sacrifice yourself	Pine, Willow
Dependent on the "atmosphere" of your environment	Agrimony, Aspen
Because you're too strongly connected to another person	Red Chestnut, Walnut
Dependent on a former partner	Honeysuckle, Red Chestnut, Walnut
Because you feel under pressure by the other person	Willow, Vine

Depressed, Despondent

Periodic melancholy, feels like you're sitting in a deep hole	Mustard
Because of failures and disappointments	Gentian
Together with exhaustion	Gentian, Olive
Together with sleeping problems	White Chestnut, Gentian, Mustard
Because you see no alternatives, for instance, in chronic illness	Gentian, Gorse, Mustard
Because you've given up inside	Mustard, Wild Rose
Together with blaming yourself	Mustard, Pine
Because of worrying about another person	Red Chestnut, Gentian
Because of serious past experiences that are still weighing you down	Honeysuckle, Willow, Mustard

Discipline and Self-control Are Too Strong

You're too hard and too strict on yourself   Rock Water

You allow yourself too little out of life   Rock Water, Pine, Wild Rose

You won't give up for any price   Rock Water, Vine, Oak

You try to keep your emotions tightly controlled   Rock Water, Cherry Plum, Vine

You're too critical of yourself   Rock Water, Beech, Vervain

You find yourself swinging between self-discipline and chaos   Rock Water, Clematis

You try hard to discipline yourself but are unable to stick to it   Rock Water, Agrimony, Pine

You wind up exhausting yourself repeatedly   Rock Water, Olive

Discouraged, Quick to Give Up

As soon as things get difficult   Gentian

Because you believe it wasn't meant to be   Aspen, Willow

Because you've lost hope   Gorse

Because you're psychological down   Mustard, Gentian

Because you feel paralyzed   Star of Bethlehem, Willow

Because life is no fun anymore   Willow, Gorse, Wild Rose

Disorganized, Concentration Difficulties (*see also:* "Indecisive, Inconsistent")

Because you're too exhausted   Olive, Hornbeam

Because there are too many things to keep track of   Hornbeam, White Chestnut

Because you're easily distracted	Scleranthus, Clematis
Because you lose interest too easily	Wild Oat, Scleranthus
Because you don't know what you want	Cerato, Wild Oat
Because the mental demand is too taxing	Chestnut Bud, Cerato, Hornbeam, Olive

Dissatisfied

With present life situation	Wild Oat
With a specific life circumstance	Beech
Because you don't live up to your own performance standards	Rock Water, Larch
Because you can't realize your ideas	Vervain, Gentian
For no apparent cause	Mustard
Because others don't follow your well-intended advice	Chicory, Beech
Because you stumble on the same old problem	Chestnut Bud, Gentian
Because your expectations were not met	Chicory, Willow

Distracted, Scattered

Because you are always seeking a better way	Wild Oat
Because of too many little things around you	Crab Apple
Because you get involved in too many things at the same time	Wild Oat, Scleranthus
Because you do things that you really don't want to do	Centaury, Cerato
Because you would rather be doing something else	Clematis, Centaury

Because you act on every impulse	Scleranthus
Because you don't trust you own opinion	Cerato
Because you have too many little fears and anxieties	Aspen, Mimulus
Because you're not really committed	Wild Oat, Cerato, Gentian
Because you want to make everyone happy	Agrimony, Centaury, Scleranthus
Because you always doubt your own decisions	Cerato, Scleranthus
Because you don't have a clear vision for yourself	Wild Oat
Because you don't think you're doing what you really want to do	Gentian, Gorse

Doubting

About a decision you've made	Scleranthus, Wild Oat
About the future	Cerato, Gentian, Gorse
About a spouse or partner	Holly, Gentian, Wild Oat
About your own abilities	Larch, Pine
About people in general	Holly, Gentian, Aspen, Willow
About your strength	Hornbeam, Elm, Larch
Because you don't trust that you will do the right thing	Gentian, Wild Oat, Gorse

Exaggerated Reactions

In your mental and emotional involvement	Sweet Chestnut
Can't stop your actions once started	Vervain

In falling in love	Sweet Chestnut, Vervain, Holly
In your sense of duty	Oak, Vervain, Pine
In your ambitions	Sweet Chestnut, Vine
In showing sympathy	Red Chestnut
In striving for perfection	Vervain, Rock Water

Exhausted, Overwhelmed by Demands

Because of constant pressure to perform well	Oak, Olive
Because of a disliked daily routine	Olive, Hornbeam
Because of excessive demand on mental capacities	Chestnut Bud, Cerato, Hornbeam, Olive
Because you're afraid you lack the ability	Larch, Mimulus
Because of responsibilities in too many areas	Olive, Elm
Because you put too much effort into your work	Olive, Vervain
Because you demand too much of yourself	Olive, Rock Water, Vervain
Together with despondency	Olive, Gorse, Mustard, Gentian
Together with fearfulness	Olive, Mimulus
Because you can't say no	Olive, Centaury
Together with panic	Olive, Rock Rose

Fearful

Fear of a specific situation such as illness or a visit to the dentist	Mimulus
Inner panic felt in every cell of the body	Rock Rose
Of going crazy or becoming violent	Cherry Plum

For a friend or family member	Red Chestnut
Irrational fears—for instance, of the dark	Aspen
Fear of spiders and mice	Aspen, Mimulus
Because of the unknown	Aspen, Mimulus
Because of prophecies	Aspen
Fear of fear	Aspen, Cherry Plum
Fear of contamination	Aspen, Crab Apple
Because of "bad vibes"	Aspen, Crab Apple
To be disappointed	Star of Bethlehem, Mimulus, Gentian
To be hurt emotionally	Mimulus, Agrimony, Holly
To show your true feelings	Mimulus, Agrimony
About being visible to others	Mimulus, Agrimony, Pine
About doing something "wrong"	Mimulus, Cerato, Pine
Fear of failure	Mimulus, Larch, Willow
Fearful thoughts that keep running around in your head	Mimulus, White Chestnut
About getting into a disagreement or quarrel	Mimulus, Star of Bethlehem, Agrimony, Centaury
Of your own unwanted feelings	Agrimony, Cherry Plum
To be alone	Mimulus, Heather
To hurt others	Mimulus, Holly, Pine
To make the wrong decisions	Mimulus, Cerato
Of letting go of or changing a relationship	Mimulus, Honeysuckle, Chicory, Walnut

Fear of exhaustion and strain	Mimulus, Olive, Hornbeam
Of being too close or of close contact	Mimulus, Water Violet
Of not getting enough	Mimulus, Chicory, Holly, Willow
Because you can't keep your thoughts under control (see a specialist!)	Cherry Plum, Sweet Chestnut, White Chestnut
Of flying	Rock Rose, Cherry Plum, Willow, Agrimony

Grief

Deep sadness	Mustard
It makes you lose faith	Mustard, Gentian
It causes bitterness	Mustard, Willow
It causes self-doubt	Mustard, Cerato, Larch
To let go of the past	Mustard, Honeysuckle
If you've lost all hope	Mustard, Gorse
If you've given up	Mustard, Wild Rose
If you feel deeply wounded	Mustard, Star of Bethlehem

Homesick

Occasionally	Honeysuckle
Together with melancholy	Honeysuckle, Mustard
Because you long for someone	Honeysuckle, Red Chestnut

Indecisive, Inconsistent

Because an inner vision for your life is missing	Wild Oat
Because you're vacillating about what to do	Scleranthus
Because you're torn between two options	Scleranthus

Because you're skeptical and repeatedly doubt your decisions	Cerato, Chestnut Bud, Gentian
Because you fear being unable to deal with the consequences	Mimulus, Elm, Scleranthus
Because you're afraid of making the wrong decisions	Mimulus, Cerato, Gentian
Because you haven't come to terms with a situation in the past	Honeysuckle, Walnut
Because you're dependent on somebody else	Red Chestnut, Scleranthus
Because you're still influenced by a shock	Star of Bethlehem

Insecure, Uncertain

You don't want to reveal your insecurity	Agrimony, Vervain
You're easily made uncertain about your decisions and opinions	Chestnut Bud, Cerato, Walnut
It makes you uneasy to be observed by others	Centaury, Larch
Because you're determined to make everybody happy	Agrimony, Cerato, Centaury
Because you don't know what you want	Cerato, Wild Oat
Because you don't trust that you can handle things	Mimulus, Cerato, Larch
Because you have too many sources of advice	Cerato, Walnut
Because you're not sure you that are able to take responsibility	Mimulus, Cerato, Elm
Because you're not sure you are able to make a decision	Cerato, Scleranthus, Wild Oat

Because you're not patient enough	Cerato, Chestnut Bud, Impatiens
Because you're reminded of mistakes you've made in the past	Cerato, Honeysuckle, Pine

Learning Issues

Due to a lack of concentration	Chestnut Bud, Clematis, White Chestnut
Because of earlier setbacks	Chestnut Bud, Honeysuckle, Gentian, Larch
Because of fear of punishment	Aspen, Cherry Plum, Pine
Because you're trying too hard	Chestnut Bud, Vervain
Because you lack motivation	Wild Oat, Wild Rose
With a deeply ingrained mistake pattern	Chestnut Bud, Gentian, Honeysuckle

Letting Go Is Difficult

Because you have to come out the winner	Vine
Because you're driven by an idea	Vervain
Because this is a matter of principle	Rock Water, Vervain
Because you feel obliged to keep a promise	Oak
Because you can't stop working	Vervain, Oak
Because things are never clean enough or orderly enough	Crab Apple, Rock, Water
Because you feel obliged to finish a project once it has been started	Oak, Rock Water
You're determined to do even minor things 150 percent	Vervain, Crab Apple
Because you've made your decision to finish	Vine, Oak

Life Transitions (*see also:* "Insecure, Uncertain"; "Indecisive, Inconsistent"; and "Distracted, Scattered")

Lovesick

In an acute state	Holly, Star of Bethlehem, Willow, Sweet Chestnut
Together with inferiority and guilt feelings	Holly, Pine, Larch
Together with difficulties in deciding	Holly, Wild Oat, Scleranthus
Together with disappointment	Holly, Willow, Gentian, Star of Bethlehem
Together with uncertainty	Holly, Cerato, Walnut
It's secret and you try to hide it	Holly, Agrimony, Cherry Plum
Past memories of someone don't let you sleep	Holly, White Chestnut, Honeysuckle, Red Chestnut
You try to get someone back	Holly, Vervain, Chicory
You can't let go	Holly, Cherry Plum, Honeysuckle

Mood Swings

Moods change depending on "whichever way the wind blows"	Scleranthus
You get angry very quickly	Holly, Impatiens
You're easily thrown off balance by others' remarks	Star of Bethlehem, Walnut, Scleranthus
You're in a dark mood for no apparent reason	Mustard

Nightmares

Together with fearing more nightmares	Aspen, Mimulus
You wake up panic-stricken	Aspen, Rock Rose

| If nightmare cannot be digested | Aspen, Star of Bethlehem |
| Together with guilt feelings | Aspen, Pine |

Offended, Touchy, Feeling Hurt

Because you've been treated unjustly	Holly, Vervain
Because you feel you've been cheated	Holly, Willow
Because you expect others to be more grateful	Holly, Chicory
Because you feel unduly criticized	Beech, Willow
Because of an unexpected dispute	Star of Bethlehem, Agrimony, Willow
You contemplate revenge	Holly, Chicory
You wish to pull back	Holly, Water Violet
Your can't stop thinking about it	Holly, White Chestnut
You're irritated and distrustful because your good intentions were misunderstood	Holly, Willow

Perseverance and Resilience Are Weak

Because you've exhausted yourself	Olive, Hornbeam
Because you've ceased to believe in the future	Cerato, Gorse, Gentian
Because you carry a secret fear or sorrow	Agrimony, Mimulus
Because you're at your wit's end	Sweet Chestnut, Cerato, Rock Rose
Because you're very sensitive	Mimulus, Heather, Star of Bethlehem
Because you're easily distracted	Scleranthus, Clematis
Because something fails to keep your interest	Wild Oat, Scleranthus
Because you'll give up after the smallest of setbacks	Gentian

Because you lack self-confidence in doing a task or are afraid to fail	Larch, Mimulus
Because you've already resigned inside	Gorse, Gentian
Because your mind is somewhere elsewhere	Clematis, White Chestnut

Resigned, Hopeless

Has been going on for a long time	Gorse, Wild Rose
Together with apathy, as if numbed	Star of Bethlehem, Wild Rose
Because of an old disappointment	Honeysuckle, Gentian, Gorse
Together with exhaustion	Wild Rose, Olive
You're gloomy	Gorse, Mustard
Because of undigested experiences	Star of Bethlehem, Honeysuckle, Gorse
Due to repeated setbacks	Chestnut Bud, Willow, Gorse

Responsibility Issues

You're too needy to take responsibility for yourself	Heather
You blame anyone but yourself	Willow
You identify too strongly with tasks and take too much responsibility for them	Elm
You feel guilty and take on responsibilities that aren't yours	Pine
You're can't distinguish between your own responsibilities and those of others	Pine
You take on responsibility so that others will appreciate you	Chicory, Centaury
You'd like to withdraw from being responsible	Water Violet

You're afraid of being responsible	Mimulus, Elm

Rigid, Inflexible

Because you exaggerate principles	Rock Water, Oak
By demanding a dominant position	Rock Water, Vine
Because you fear being taken advantage of	Vine, Chicory
Because you are being dogmatic	Rock Water, Vervain
Because of previous, negative experiences	Honeysuckle, Beech, Gentian

Self-Blaming, Feeling Guilty

Because of another person	Red Chestnut, Pine
You regret having been too harsh	Pine, Vine, Agrimony
Together with criticizing yourself	Pine, Beech
Due to inability to make decisions	Pine, Cerato, Scleranthus
Together with fear and panic	Pine, Mimulus, Rock Rose
Together with tendency to withdraw into yourself	Pine, Water Violet
Together with chewing your nails	Vine, Pine, Agrimony

Self-Centered, Egotistical

You're concerned only about yourself	Heather
You're determined to always succeed	Vine
You talk merely about yourself	Heather
You don't accept anybody else's opinion	Vervain, Vine
You look down on "average people"	Beech, Rock Water
You believe you have the right to expect or	Chicory, Willow

demand things

You believe others are incapable	Beech, Vine
You treat others like pawns	Chicory, Vine
You're overly concerned about taking care of yourself	Heather, Crab Apple
You spend a lot of time worrying about yourself	Heather, Mimulus, White Chestnut
You've been told that you should be more self-centered	Centaury, Red Chestnut

Self-Worth Crisis, Feelings of Inferiority

Together with guilt feelings	Larch, Pine
Together with uncertainty	Larch, Walnut, Cerato
Because you're too good-natured	Larch, Centaury
Because you're slow to learn new things	Larch, Chestnut Bud, Hornbeam
Secret inferiority complex	Agrimony, Larch, Cherry Plum
Fearful moments of insecurity	Larch, Elm, Mimulus
Because of your physical appearance	Larch, Beech, Crab Apple
You fear you're less able than others	Larch, Mimulus
You attempt to cover up feelings of inferiority with defiance	Larch, Vine, Holly
Temporary crisis in self-esteem after overtaxing yourself	Elm
Because of setbacks	Larch, Gentian

Sensitive in the Extreme, Possessing a Delicate Constitution

To feeling insulted	Holly
Because of unfulfilled emotional expectations	Chicory
To disorder and lack of cleanliness	Crab Apple
To criticism	Larch, Beech
To too much light, noise, smells, etc.	Mimulus
To disruptions	Impatiens, Vervain
To fights and quarrels	Agrimony, Mimulus
To being blamed or accused	Pine, Star of Bethlehem
To changing weather	Scleranthus
To "vibrations" you get	Aspen
You feel as vulnerable as a raw egg	Star of Bethlehem, Heather
When others question your plans	Walnut
To being contradicted	Vine, Larch
You're unable to separate personal feelings from those of others	Red Chestnut, Walnut
To resistance from others	Centaury, Mimulus

Separation Difficulty (Parting from Others)

You haven't yet overcome the news	Star of Bethlehem
You feel guilty	Pine
You're afraid about it	Mimulus, Rock Rose
You're afraid you can't start all over again	Mimulus, Aspen, Larch
You're concerned about hurting others	Agrimony, Pine

You believe the other person belongs to you	Chicory
You feel like a victim, are still critical, and can't seem to finish processing it	Willow, Beech, Honeysuckle
You want everything to stay the way it is	Honeysuckle, Chicory
You're still tied energetically	Red Chestnut
You're concerned about losing face	Agrimony, Cerato, Larch
You have doubts about your decision to separate	Cerato, Scleranthus, Wild Oat
You have no idea how things will proceed after the split	Wild Oat, Cerato

Sleeping Difficulties (*see also:* "Nightmares")

Undigested experiences circle in your mind	Star of Bethlehem, White Chestnut, Honeysuckle
Because of suppressed worries	White Chestnut, Agrimony, Cherry Plum
Because of guilt feelings	White Chestnut, Pine, Honeysuckle
Because of fears of nightmares	Aspen, Rock Rose, White Chestnut
Together with depression	White Chestnut, Mustard
Because of too much work and strain	White Chestnut, Elm, Oak, Olive
Because of worries for others	White Chestnut, Red Chestnut
Because of being all wound up inside	White Chestnut, Vervain
Together with grinding your teeth	White Chestnut, Cherry Plum, White Chestnut

Socializing and Communicating Difficulty

Because of false modesty or feelings of inferiority	Mimulus, Larch, Water Violet

Because of heightened sensitivity	Star of Bethlehem, Water Violet
Because of excessive expectations from others	Beech, Chicory, Willow
Because of being impatient	Impatiens, Chestnut Bud
Together with self-reproach	Water Violet, Pine
Because you're too egocentric	Water Violet, Heather
Together with feelings of resignation	Water Violet, Gorse, Gentian
Because of capriciousness or moodiness	Water Violet, Scleranthus, Wild Oat
Because you keep an inner distance from others	Water Violet
Because of shyness	Mimulus
Because you fear doing something wrong	Larch, Cerato
Because you're not quick-witted enough	Mimulus, Star of Bethlehem, Larch
Because you're actually concerned only with yourself	Heather
Because you're impatient and want everything right away	Impatiens
Because you don't feel up to the situation	Aspen, Larch
Because your mind is occupied with another subject	White Chestnut, Clematis
Because you're disappointed and bitter	Gentian, Willow
Because others believe that you're conceited	Water Violet
Because you can't ignore little things about other people such as pronunciation, dandruff	Beech, Crab Apple
Because you have to have the last word	Vine, Larch, Heather

Because you don't expect anything of value from others	Water Violet, Gorse
Because you're afraid being somehow obligated	Mimulus, Elm, Pine
Because you're unable to be spontaneous	Cherry Plum, Agrimony, Chicory
Because you don't let anybody get close	Water Violet, Mimulus
You like to play things close to your chest	Chicory, Agrimony
Because you dislike burdening yourself with the problems of others	Heather, Chicory, Water Violet
Because you dislike disputes	Mimulus, Agrimony, Centaury
Because you've no opinion of your own	Cerato, Wild Oat, Centaury
Because you feel inhibited	Mimulus, Larch, Rock Water
Because of an unexpected dispute	Star of Bethlehem, Willow, Agrimony
You tend to retreat into the role of a victim and blame others	Chestnut Bud, Willow
Because you always find something to criticize	Chestnut Bud, Beech
Because you always start by saying no	Chestnut Bud, Gentian

Stressed, Nervous

Because of minor annoyances	Rock Rose, Crab Apple
Because of fearful expectations	Rock Rose, Mimulus
Because of hidden fears	Rock Rose, Agrimony, Aspen
Because of suppressed urges and feelings	Cherry Plum, Rock Water
Because of too much responsibility	Elm, Rock Rose
Because of inner restlessness	Impatiens

Because of exhaustion	Rock Rose, Olive
Because of inner insecurity	Rock Rose, Scleranthus, Cerato, Walnut
Because you demand too much of yourself	Rock Rose, Rock Water, Vervain, Elm
Because of your stubbornness while being pressured to do something else	Rock Rose, Oak

Stubborn, Intolerant

You expect a very high level of orderliness and cleanliness in others	Crab Apple, Beech
You expect others to react as fast as you	Impatiens
You expect others to have your standards	Beech
You expect others to have your fanatical enthusiasm for an idea	Vervain
You expect others to do what you want; you'd even force them to	Vine
Your principles don't allow you to give in	Vine, Rock Water
You don't allow any exceptions to the rule	Rock Water, Oak

Test-Taking Difficulty

Typical testing situations	Rock Rose, White Chestnut, Elm, Clematis, Gentian
In cases where you failed the last time	Honeysuckle, Chestnut Bud, Larch, Gentian
Feeling like a sacrificial lamb on the way to the slaughterhouse	Rock Rose, Willow, Centaury, Clematis
If you tend to get blocked or can't think straight	Chestnut Bud, Clematis, Aspen

Tense, Tight, "Blocked"

Because you fear others' expectations	Agrimony, Mimulus
Because of an intense inner push to "do it now"	Impatiens
Because of exaggerated enthusiasm	Vervain
Because of high personal performance expectations	Rock Water, Vervain
Because you're in shock	Star of Bethlehem, Cherry Plum
Because you're extremely goal-oriented and ambitious	Vine
Because you're totally fixated on a certain goal	Rock Water, Vine, Vervain
Because of your intense determination to persevere	Oak
Because you overcompensate for your openness and flexibility	Aspen, Scleranthus, Vervain
Because you're too hard on yourself	Rock Water
Because you desire something too much	Vine, Vervain
Because you're still stuck in an old situation yet	Star of Bethlehem, Cherry Plum

Unmotivated, Lethargic, Indifferent

You are indifferent and apathetic	Wild Rose
Following a stroke of fate	Willow, Wild Rose
Together with extreme fatigue	Hornbeam, Wild Rose, Mustard
Together with resistance to routine work	Wild Rose, Hornbeam
Because of resignation and feeling victimized	Gorse, Willow

Because of resignation and pessimism	Gorse, Gentian
Because of an unprocessed disappointment	Star of Bethlehem, Gentian, Willow
Because of the loss of a loved one	Honeysuckle, Red Chestnut, Wild Rose
Because of an extended period of overwork	Oak, Olive, Wild Rose
Because you no longer believe in the goodness of others	Gentian, Wild Rose
You'd like to retreat from everything	Water Violet, Clematis

Weak-willed, Unassertive

You can't say no	Centaury
Because you don't want to hurt anyone	Centaury, Agrimony
Because you have no personal direction	Centaury, Wild Oat
Because others can easily make you unsure of yourself	Centaury, Walnut, Cerato
Because you're shocked and disappointed	Centaury, Star of Bethlehem, Gentian
Because you don't want to repeat past mistakes	Centaury, Chestnut Bud, Honeysuckle, Pine
Because you don't know what you really want	Centaury, Cerato, Wild Oat
Because you feel guilty from asserting your will	Pine, Vine
Because you fear a conflict or fight	Centaury, Mimulus, Agrimony
Because of false tolerance	Centaury, Beech

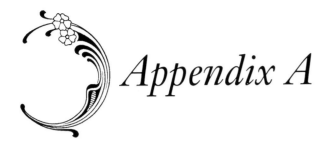

Appendix A

Important Key Words and Answers to Frequently Asked Questions

If you are unable to locate below a reference to a specific area of application for Bach Flowers, please turn to the Questionnaires and Checklist in chapter 11 and the Building Blocks in chapter 10 for more detailed information.

Acne. *See* **page 237**

Acupuncture. *See* **page 231**

Addiction. *See* **page 245**

Addiction to Bach Flowers. *See* **Habit-forming**

Additional Methods of Diagnosis

What are the advantages and disadvantages of additional methods of diagnosis?

Beginners tend to believe that nonverbal methods such as kinesiology, dowsing, and electronic measurements will make it easier and give them more security in making choices. They often seek to completely avoid an interview and the conscious study of the Flower principles.

In individual cases the benefit of such methods may be that an important Flower pattern that had been previously overlooked suddenly becomes apparent. The interview will then be the deciding factor as to whether or not to incorporate it.

Still, these nonverbal diagnosing methods are generally overvalued. They are not more objective, as some believe, because they are dependent on the daily form, talent, and ability of the person who is using them. To accept their results without critical review would be a mistake. Chapters 7, 9, 10, and 11 contain tried-and-true practical help to determine the most appropriate Bach Flower combinations.

Another group of diagnostic methods employs fixed structures for interpretation such as skin zones and energetic tracks. Still others use predetermined correlations to systems such as color spectrums, astrology, and the I Ching to help with the choice of Bach Flowers.

These methods will generally result in contradictions or confusion. Any such system can come between you and your partner and can distort your direct, intuitive perception. The therapist who uses these methods hinders the development of his or her diagnostic skills.

It's important to understand that while different systems do have their place, no system can ever simply be laid over another. When doing this, both systems are distorted and the full potential of each is lost.

Administering Flowers without a Person's Awareness. *See* **Awareness of Administration**

Aggressiveness. *See* **pages 242, 302**

AIDS. *See* **page 237**

Alcohol and Taking Bach Flowers. *See* **Coffee, Alcohol, and Nicotine**

Alcohol Content

Does the alcohol content in the stock bottles have a negative effect on babies?

No. When mixed with water, the amount is so minute that it has no effect. The mixture contains one drop of concentrated Essence to ten milliliters of water, which is less alcohol than you'll find in regular homeopathic drops. It can be given without concern.

Alcohol Used in the Bach Flower Mixtures. *See* **page 227**

Alcoholic. *See* **page 246**

All Thirty-eight Flowers

Is it possible to take all thirty-eight Flowers in just one combination?

Bach would have applied this method had he found it useful. It was his goal to make Flower Therapy available to as many people as possible in the shortest possible time. Our energy system is able to deal with only a limited number of impulses at any given time. To take all thirty-eight Flowers at once would be like simultaneously playing thirty-eight keys on a piano, which would only result in a jumble of noise. Experience shows that up to twelve Flowers will yield specific results.

Allergies

Can a person with allergies take Bach Flowers?

Taking Bach Flowers does not cause any problems for people with allergies. The Essences do not contain any material substance deriving from the Flowers; thus they contain no allergens. They carry only the energetic information of each Flower. The treatment of allergies with the support of Bach Flowers has been clearly successful.

Alzheimer's Disease. *See* **page 237**

Aromatherapy

How compatible are the subtle frequencies of Bach Flowers and the oils used in aromatherapy?

Ethereal oils have a harmonizing effect on physical and spiritual-mental levels. Compared to the

Bach Flowers, they affect a wider spectrum but are less specific. A vapor lamp with ethereal oils will provide a supportive atmosphere in a Bach Flower session. Evaporating Bach Flower Essences in such a lamp is of no benefit, however.

Asthma. *See* **page237**

Awareness of Administration

Is it advisable to give a dose of Flowers without a person's awareness of the administration?
No. If you put a few drops of Essence into your partner's drinking water because you might like to change his or her character, it contradicts the Heal Thyself principle of Bach Flower Therapy.

Exceptions can be made for small children, who are not yet responsible for themselves, and adults who are in emergency situations. Rescue Remedy (or other Flowers if called for) should be administered here as a form of first aid.

Bach Didn't Include Certain Flowers

Do we know why Bach didn't include certain flowers in his system that may have fit his criteria, such as linden flowers?
No. There are many theories, but nothing is certain.

Bach Flowers and Positive Potential. *See* **Positive Potential.**

Bach Flowers at the Bedside. *See* **Bedside or Under Your Pillow**

Bach Flowers in Globuli (Pellet) Form. *See* **Globuli (Pellet) Form**

Bach Flower Production. *See* **Produced Today**

Basic Flowers. *See* **Type-Specific Remedies**

Baths with Bach Flowers. *See* **page 228**

Bedside or Under Your Pillow

Is it useful to put Bach Flowers at your bedside or under your pillow?
This can be done only in addition to taking the drops, very occasionally and for a short time when you're treating deeply rooted, long-term negative behavior patterns and you feel that you have little or no opportunity during the day to work on them consciously. This practice is not recommended for children or highly sensitive people.

Bed-wetting. *See* **page 242**

Blood Pressure Problems. *See* **page 237**

Boiling Method. *See* **pages 30–31**

Cancer. *See* **page 237**

Cancer Surgery. *See* **page 245**

Carry Bach Flower Remedies Close to the Body

Is it useful to carry Bach Flower remedies close to the body all day?
If useful at all, it is only useful during unusual—and brief—circumstances, perhaps during a court case (Rescue Remedy) or during a family crisis (Holly and Willow). Keeping the bottles near you all the time will ultimately have a weakening

effect on the potential energy of the Bach Flower Essences.

Changes in the Earth's Energy Field

Is the effectiveness of Bach Flowers influenced by changes in the earth's energy field?

Energy frequencies are constantly changing on earth and so are the analogous frequencies in plant and animal energy fields. These changes occur within a system that maintains its own overall balance. These changes pose no threat to the effectiveness of the Flowers.

Childlessness. *See* page 244

Children and Healing Crises. *See* Healing Crises Common for Children

Cigarettes and Bach Flowers. *See* Coffee, Alcohol and Nicotine

Coffee, Alcohol, and Nicotine

Do coffee, alcohol, and nicotine have adverse effects on Bach Flowers?

Generally these drugs do not have a negative influence on the effect of Bach Flowers. On the contrary, Bach Flowers help to regulate the use of these substances.

Combinations, Finishing Those No Longer Needed. *See* Personal Combination That Is No Longer Needed

Combinations, Knowledge of the Flowers in Yours. *See* Consciously Study the Flowers in My Combination

Combinations, Number of Flowers in Each. *See* How Many Flowers

Combine Drugs or Other Medicines with Bach Flowers

Is it possible to combine drugs or other medicines with Bach Flowers?

Due to the nonmaterial level of effect of Bach Flowers and according to fifty years of experience, other drugs and medicines show no significant influence on therapy with Bach Flowers, nor do the Essences have a negative effect on them. This is true for all kinds of drugs and medicines including naturopathic, allopathic, and neurological treatments as well as psychopharmaceuticals. On the contrary, supportive treatment with Bach Flowers is useful in combination with natural or allopathic treatments. However, it's recommended that if you take high potencies in homeopathic treatments, you should wait at least two weeks before using Bach Flowers in order to better observe the progress of either treatment.

Combined with Other Forms of Therapy. *See* pages 230–31

Combining all Bach Flowers. *See* All Thirty-eight Flowers

Compatability

What is the compatibility of each Bach Flower with the others?

All thirty-eight Flowers may be combined with each other. In comparison with homeopathic remedies, for instance, Bach Flowers form a harmonious group or family. Bach called them "the happy fellows of the plant world." Even Flowers that represent opposite states of mind can and sometimes must be used together when both states are present at the same time. The coexistence of two opposite behavior patterns is a common problem because one pattern frequently compensates for the other. For example, a person may be the one who gives in at home (Centaury) and the one who is demanding and bossy at work (Vine). With the help of Bach Flowers both traits may be harmonized so that at home this person is able to say what he or she needs (Centaury) and thus doesn't feel the pressing need to impose opinions at work (Vine).

Compresses and Pads. *See* **page 228**

Consciously Study the Flowers in My Combination

Must I consciously study the flowers in my combination in order for them to work?

No, this isn't really necessary. In cases where the combination has been given by a therapist, you needn't understand the specifics of your state in order for the Bach Flowers to show a harmonizing effect. Don't push yourself to read about all the Flowers at the beginning of your Bach Flower Therapy. It might even be very confusing to study detailed descriptions when you're in a difficult situation. It may also be difficult to imagine how combinations of Flowers work synergistically to address certain states. In this context many of us make the mistake of compiling the details in all the descriptions and looking for them in ourselves. This can leave you feeling as though there's too much to deal with or, if you don't see the connections, can convince you that the Flowers don't apply to you. Specialists have related that at the beginning of therapy in acute situations, many patients don't care about the content of the combination they are taking. However, as soon as they notice progress, they become more interested. Thus step by step, more awareness and responsibility develops.

Continuous Intake of Bach Flowers

Is it a good idea to suggest a continuous intake of Bach Flowers for children so their life will be better later?

No—it's misleading to believe that taking Bach Flowers continuously will harmonize the character of a child and grant an adult life without conflict. Children will indicate clearly when the time has come for them to benefit from Bach Flowers. A six-year-old, for example, might like taking a combination that helps him with problem in school, but a few years later when he experiences a comparable problem, he may refuse to take the same combination. Perhaps he might feel instinctively that the time had come to deal with the problem in a different way.

Correct or Incorrect Combination

Is there such a thing as a correct or incorrect combination?

An incorrect combination can be suggested

whenever a situation is not perceived correctly, and while not dangerous, the more precise the assessment of a situation and the choice of Flowers are, the more effective the combination will be. When, for example, six specific Flowers are needed in a combination but only three of them are used and three "less correct" ones are also used, the results may still be positive but the progress will be slower.

In practice, each combination can be more or less precise in addressing a specific situation. A problem can be approached from many different angles; one therapist may prescribe a slightly different combination than another does for the same person and the same reasons—and both may lead to positive results. However, it is not advisable to take more than one combination at a time. In Bach Flower Therapy it has proved to be more effective to work with one partner or therapist and one issue at a time.

Cortisone. *See* **page 231**

Dependency. *See* **Habit-Forming**

Difficult Teething. *See* **page 242**

Difficulties at School. *See* **page 242**

Dosages for Children and Adults. *See* **pages 228–229**

Dreams. *See* **page 235**

Drugs and Bach Flowers. *See* **Combine Drugs or Other Medicines with Bach Flowers**

Duration of Bach Flower Therapy
What should the total duration of Bach Flower Therapy be for a given situation or behavior pattern? The harmonization of acute situations such as tensions among colleagues will usually require one to three mixtures or three to six weeks. A positive effect on chronic negative behavior patterns usually takes at least ten to twelve combinations or twelve to fifteen months. These are average numbers, which may be individually lower or higher. The longer a negative behavior pattern has existed, the longer it usually takes to resolve it. The treatment is finished at the point when the individual has a clear sense of not needing the Flower Essences any longer.

Dyslexia. *See* **page 242**

Earth's Energy Field. *See* **Changes in the Earth's Energy Field**

Eating and Digestion Problems. *See* **page 242**

Eating Flowers of Bach Plants. *See* **Tea**

Eczema, Psoriasis. *See* **pages 237, 242**

Effects of a Combination. *See* **First Effects**

Epileptic Seizures. *See* **page 207**

Family Combination. *See* **page 243**

Fasting. *See* **pages 230, 234**

First Effects
How long does it take to see the first effects from taking a combination?

In an acute situation such as trouble with colleagues, you should feel a clear harmonizing effect or a healing crisis within two or three days. If neither develops, it becomes necessary to reevaluatee the combination of Flowers. When treating chronic negative behavior patterns such as a lack of self-esteem rooted in childhood, it may take two to three weeks to observe an effect.

Gastritis. *See* **page 237**

Gastrointestinal Problems. *See* **page 237**

General Mixture for Starting Treatment

Is there a general mixture for everyone starting treatment?

No. None of the recommendations of this kind has generally been successful. At any given time every person who comes to Bach Flower Therapy has his or her own unique situation, and only this specific situation should be addressed. One case may present as a deep spiritual exhaustion, another as indecision about a course of action, a third as despair. Although many people who turn to Bach Flower Therapy have experienced shock in their lives, there is still no absolute requirement for Rescue Remedy or Star of Bethlehem to be part of the first mixture taken; these experiences of shock may already have been digested and thus do not affect each person's present situation.

In some cases the emotional equilibrium is so seriously disturbed that there is no clear experience of any particular state (for instance, a person reporting, "I can't say anything, I need all the Flowers"). It would then be beneficial to take Rescue Remedy for a few days before going any further.

Globuli (Pellet) Form

Are Bach Flowers in globuli (pellet) form useful?

This form of medication is recommended only for exceptional cases, such as alcoholism, and is for immediate use only. Experience has shown that the energy charge of the mixture that is sprayed onto the globuli (milk-sugar pellets) dissipates quickly.

Habit-Forming

Is it possible for Bach Flowers to become habit-forming?

Bach Flower Essences are not habit-forming, since they consist of no physical substance and are merely taken to reestablish harmony. When a person's balance has been restored, an Essence has no further effect. At this point a person may lose interest, forget to take the drops, or misplace the bottle—all signs that the treatment has succeeded.

Even psychological dependence is impossible because a well-chosen combination has the effect of strengthening Inner Guidance. Step by step these measures lead to increased inner freedom, independence, and self-reliance. Thus the Flowers' effect creates the opposite of dependency.

Hay Fever. *See* **page 237**

Headaches and Migraines. *See* **pages 237, 242**

Healing Crises Common for Children

Are healing crises common for children during Bach Flower Therapy?

Children, more than adults, have primarily acute states and therefore healing crises are very rare. However, a healing crisis may occur when treating a recurring problem such as eczema or bronchitis. The natural concern at this point is that a child may be experiencing the parent's distorted state. In this case it becomes necessary to also treat at least one of the parents.

Healing Crisis as a First Reaction. *See* pages 231–235

Should I always expect a healing crisis as a first reaction?

Whether or not you experience a healing crisis as a first reaction depends on individual circumstances such as, the tenacity of the negative pattern, your own resistance to change (which you may not be aware of), or whether or not a chronic problem is part of a current acute situation.

Heart Problems. *See* pages 237–238

Higher Self, Inner Guidance. *See* page 19

Homeopathic Potentization

Are Bach Flowers even more effective in homeopathic potentization?

This does not increase their effectiveness. On the contrary, the energetic patterns in the Essences are broken up by homeopathic potentization.

How Long Should I Take a Combination? *See* pages 229–230

How Many Flowers

How many Flowers should be combined into a single mixture?

The number varies according to each situation. Generally speaking, a mixture should not contain more than six Flowers. However, when putting together a mixture for initial treatment, there are frequently too many states present to hold to this limit and the number is often closer to ten. If you cannot decide between two Flowers even after a thorough study, both Flowers should be included in the mixture. Often it turns out that the Flower you felt was less important is the one that's needed more. A large initial combination will result in a general clearing out or a basic clarification of the person's inner terrain. In the following interviews the crucial reaction patterns will then be significantly more evident. Despite the fact that "wrong choices" have no effect, it's still desirable to reduce the number of Flowers in subsequent mixtures so that you are able to focus on a few, specific reaction patterns and deal with them more effectively.

Hyperkinetic Syndrome. *See* page 242

Libido Dysfunction. *See* page 244

Life Plan. *See* pages 18–19

Manipulate Children

Is it possible to manipulate children through the use of Bach Flowers?

In principle Bach Flowers cannot be an instrument of manipulation for either adults or children. Bach Flowers have an effect only when they are needed. Because their effect is to strengthen connection to Inner Guidance, those taking Essences are ultimately less subject to manipulation.

Even if Bach Flowers were to be used to transform a very lively child into one who is better adapted to a situation or environment, the treatment would not be successful because the child's true nature is lively. It isn't possible to create an entirely new character trait in a child.

Menopause. *See* **pages 244–245**

Mental Retardation. *See* **page 246**

Miscarriage. *See* **page 244**

Mixing Bottle. *See* **page 227**

Multiple Sclerosis. *See* **page237**

Near Death, *See* **pages 239–240**

New Flower Essences. *See* **page 209**

No Reaction

Do some people show no reaction to Bach Flowers?
Theoretically the answer is no, but in practice the answer is yes. Everything happens at the proper moment. People will be intuitively drawn to and also benefit from different kinds of therapy at various stages of their development. In Bach Flower Therapy too, there are ideal times when the seeds will fall on fertile ground. It is possible to cause someone to miss a healing opportunity by trying to talk him or her into Bach Flower Therapy at the wrong time. Choosing the right moment should remain an individual's personal decision.

Nursing Babies. *See* **page 240**

Original Locations

In what ways do the locations of Bach's original plants differ from other locations where the same plants grow?
The spiritual energetic field that has been in these places since Bach's time remains unchanged even today. Additionally, the curators have been producing mother tinctures continuously from these same locations that Bach selected and in the same fashion as did Bach himself.

Overdose

Is it possible to overdose with Bach Flowers?
According to the principle of how Bach Flowers work, an overdose is theoretically impossible. *See also* Dosages and First Reactions in chapter 8

Overweight. *See* **page 213**

Perishability. *See* **page 228**

Personal Combination That Is No Longer Needed

Is it necessary to finish a personal combination that is no longer needed?
No. The energy impulse of the Flowers is no longer needed as soon as the best possible harmonization has been achieved. There can be no

further reaction in the bio-energetic field after this point has been reached. Children, for example, may suddenly say that they don't like the drops anymore once they have achieved this harmonization, or they may refuse to take them, or say that they taste bad.

Any unfinished drops can be used to water plants or can be added to your bath.

Physical Illness. *See* **pages 237–240**

Physical Proximity to Bach Flower Essences. *See* **Bedside or Under Your Pillow; and Carry Bach Flower Remedies Close to the Body**

Placebo Effect

How strong is the placebo effect with Bach Flowers?
Clearly, anything can have a placebo effect. However, positive effects, particularly in babies and small children, animals, and plants, speak for themselves—children, animals, and plants have no conscious expectations when taking the Flowers. Of course, an open and positive embrace of Bach Flower Therapy is always beneficial during its course, but this is not necessary. On the other hand, even a very optimistic attitude will not lead to improvements as long as an inappropriate combination of Flowers is chosen.

Plants

Is it advisable to treat plants with Bach Flower Essences?
All plants show excellent responses, inside and out, to the harmonizing energy of Bach Flowers. Three or four drops of Rescue Remedy from the stock bottle can be added to plant water, particularly when the plant is being moved, transplanted, or is recuperating from a fall. Indoor plants also profit from combinations that the owner is no longer taking. To combat pests, it sometime helps to give Crab Apple.

Pollution

Does the quality of Bach Flowers suffer because of pollution?
Not according to experience up to this point. In Bach Flower Therapy, it is not the material body of the plant but rather its energetic information that is used. Environmental influences such as acid rain and pollution do not seem to have an effect on this energetic information or true character of the plant.

Positive Potential

Is it possible to choose Bach Flowers according to their positive potential?
This has not been seen to be effective. The positive potentials of the Flowers are ideal aspects of the divine nature of humanity. This is a collective unity and contains all the potentials in an undifferentiated state. The negative behavior patterns are distortions that have become separated from the whole and can therefore be observed, described, and diagnosed precisely in their separate expressions. *See also* The Healing Strategy of Edward Bach, in chapter 3.

Postnatal. *See* **page 244**

Pregnancy. *See* **page 244**

Premenstrual Syndrome (PMS). *See* **page 244**

Preventive Measure

Is it possible to take specific Flowers as a preventive measure?

No. Bach Flowers are used to restore balance and harmony when they have been lost. When all is balanced there is nothing to restore; Bach Flowers have nothing to affect.

Rescue Remedy is the one exception to this rule. *See* Rescue Remedy as a preventive measure.

Primary Diseases of Mankind. *See* **pages 19–20**

Produced Today

How are the Bach Flowers produced today?

The present curators of the Dr. Edward Bach Centre, John Ramsell and Judy Howard (John was appointed by Bach's successors, Nora Weeks and Victor Bullen), were personally producing the mother tinctures until John retired. Now Judy Howard and her husband, Keith, prepare them according to original specifications. The mature Flowers are primarily collected at the original locations chosen by Bach himself, though today Vine and Olive are harvested in Spain.

For reasons based on pharmacological law, the Bach Centre appointed Nelson & Co., Ltd., to take up production of the stock bottles and distribute these worldwide as Bach Flower Remedies. Nelson is a company with a long history of producing homeopathic medicine and was one of two apothecaries that Bach allowed to sell his first mother tinctures.

Prone to Infections. *See* **page 242**

Psychiatric Patients. *See* **pages 246–247**

Psychopharmacological Drugs. *See* **page 247**

Psychotherapy. *See* **page 230**

Puberty Problems. *See* **page 243**

Reaction Records

How do I set up reaction records?

When you're taking a combination of Bach Flowers that has been well chosen, you will—particularly in the beginning—experience a number of interesting reactions, which you may take for granted or quickly forget. These might include new thoughts, changed behavior, interesting dreams, a need for more or less sleep, and changed eating habits. A conscious effort to observe and record these reactions will train your perception (Heal Thyself!) and solidify the results of Bach Flower Therapy. This technique is also good preparation for the next Bach Flower interview and the selection of your next combination.

Make your record each day at the same time and note, in one or two sentences, what you've observed about your behavior. When writing down your dreams, try to include the overall story line and as many specific details and symbolic references as possible. Make a special note if you recognize a connection between your dream and any Flowers in your combination.

You should also note days when you observe no new reactions.

When you finish taking the combination, summarize the steps you've taken, answering questions such as: "How has my behavior changed?"; "What insights have I gleaned?"; and so forth. Here are some typical record entries from the start of taking a new combination:

Combination: Honeysuckle, Red Chestnut, and White Chestnut

Beginning date: 9/17

Wednesday, 9/18: Slept more deeply than usual; didn't feel like getting up.

Thursday, 9/19: When doing my daily writing, I noticed that I didn't have thoughts spinning around in my head about all the things that I still had to do (White Chestnut).

Reactions, Lack of. *See* **No Reaction**

Rehabilitation. *See* **page 239**

Rescue Remedy and the Elderly. *See* **page 245**

Rescue Remedy and Painkillers

Is it possible to combine Rescue Remedy with painkillers?

Yes, because Rescue Remedy and all other Bach Flowers work on a level different from pharma-

ceutical drugs. The drops begin a stabilizing effect in the psycho-energetic systems that often helps to reduce pain.

Rescue Remedy Applications

What are the most common Rescue Remedy applications?

Typical psychological situations

- Before and after surgery

- After family disputes

- Before personal confrontations

- Before a funeral

- Before a court case

- Before a difficult parting

- Before a public performance, premiere, and so on

- Before a feared dentist visit

- Before a feared airplane flight

- With a crying baby in public

- After disappointing news

- When children are upset by brutality on TV

Typical physical situations

- After a car accident

- After a domestic, home-improvement, or sports accident

- After insect or dog bites

- After a sunburn

- After bruises or burns

- After choking, serious allergic reaction, stroke, and the like

Typical situations for animals

- When they need to be transported in a car or plane

- When a bird has flown into a windowpane

- When a pet suddenly becomes ill and you don't yet know the reason

Rescue Remedy as a Preventive Measure

Is it possible to take Rescue Remedy as a preventive measure?

Generally yes because it often happens that merely the expectation of some stressful event can cause an imbalance on the psychological level. The timing of this varies from person to person. To understand your own tendencies, observe when your internal response to expected stress sets in. Does it come days ahead of time, or only an hour before? Taking Rescue Remedy immediately when you feel your response will help you to be more relaxed so that you can better deal with the situation.

However, beware of viewing Rescue Remedy as a miracle cure or a way to avoid all difficulties in life. This kind of expectation is certain not to be fulfilled. Bach Flowers are not meant to pre-vent experiences, but to support their healthy integration.

Rescue Remedy as Part of a Combination

Is it possible to use Rescue Remedy as part of a combination?

Normally Rescue Remedy is not meant for long-term intake, but it may on occasion be useful to add to a combination. It might be indicated particularly at the beginning of therapy, when someone may be quite out of balance and unable to describe his or her problem clearly. In such cases it will help the person become more aware of the problem and communicate it more clearly.

Rescue Remedy Cream

How is Rescue Remedy Cream applied?

Like any other cream, Rescue Remedy is applied thinly on the parts of the body that are afflicted. Immediate application of the cream usually brings about a rapid improvement. If there are no noticeable improvements after one or two days, it is clear that Rescue Remedy Cream is the wrong choice. It has been helpful in massage (apply it before the lubricant), and is also beneficial in the prevention of irritation to the skin.

Scanners at Airports

Do baggage scanners at airports affect Bach Flowers?

According to present knowledge, security controls at airports do not have a negative affect on Bach Flowers.

Scars. *See* **pages 27, 206**

Single-Flower Essences. *See* **Taking Single-Flower Essences**

Smoking Habit. *See* **pages 213, 246**

Spontaneous Choice

What can I expect from a spontaneous choice?

Often overvalued, misunderstood, or even misused, spontaneous choice is best employed as an additional diagnostic tool during Bach Flower interviews. In this technique a quick choice of bottles is made from an unpacked collection of all thirty-eight Essences. The spontaneous choice shows a snapshot of the current subconscious state. It has been particularly effective with children (up to eight or nine years old) who have shown a remarkable accuracy in picking what they need. One explanation of this phenomenon is that their natural sensitivity is still working clearly. Children will spontaneously pick those Flowers that will create a balance where there is current disharmony. With adults a spontaneous choice does not always have the same reliable results, so it's not advisable to rely on this method alone. It may suggest a new Flower to think about, but the appropriateness of this Essence would need to be clarified through further discussion. *See also* pages 114, 135, 187, 199.

Spray Form

Is it possible to use Bach Flowers in spray form?

Spraying Bach Flowers into the energy field rather than taking them as drops is much less effective than you might think. If used at all, the spray should be pointed directly into your mouth or nose.

Standard Combinations

Are there standard combinations for specific problems or situations?

Much has been written on this subject, yet apart from Rescue Remedy, which addresses an overall typical reaction pattern by itself, no other standard combinations exist at this time that show the same positive results in all people. A standard Bach Flower combination can be compared with a homeopathic mix such as "flu-tincture," that works only on some people but not on others. Even in an individual, although a recurring problem may appear to be the same each time it comes up, it is never exactly the same.

To begin learning how to put together combinations for specific situations, start by studying the Building Blocks in chapter 10.

Stopping Bach Flower treatment. *See* **When to Stop Taking a Specific Combination**

Stuttering. *See* **page 242**

Sun Method. *See* **page 30**

Supplies from Original Locations

How long will the supplies from the original locations of Bach Flowers last in anticipation of increasing worldwide use of the Essences?

At this point it is not expected that Bach Flowers will become scarce. The volume of material (Flowers) needed to produce the mother tinctures is so small that such a situation is difficult to imagine. With the Sun Method, each essence produced every year requires only a few water bowls filled with Flowers. Stock bottles of remedies are made from a dilution of two drops of mother tincture to thirty milliliters of brandy—thus each stock bottle of ten milliliters contains less than one drop of mother tincture. Due to the weather, it is not possible to produce mother tinctures for all thirty-eight Flowers every year, but in good years production is increased. At this time the reserve supply is enough to last for at least five years.

Taking Single-Flower Essences

Is taking only single-Flower Essences more effective than taking combinations?

This question is frequently asked by classical homeopaths, and the answer is basically no. According to Bach Flower Therapy, every crisis situation is characterized by a constellation of different negative behavior patterns. The more complete the analysis of the constellation of patterns, the more precise will be the harmonizing effect of the Flower combination.

One exception can be found in later stages of Bach Flower Therapy, when a patient concentrates for a longer period of time on dealing with a specific problem such as guilt. This becomes a practical option only after you have worked extensively on your personal behavior patterns.

Tea

Is it effective to make tea from the Flowers of Bach plants or to eat them raw?

Neither is effective. The specific information in the Essence is released from them only through the Sun Method or the Boiling Method.

Therapy Blocks. *See* pages 235–236

Times of Day for Dosage. *See* page 229

Toddlers. *See* pages 240–241

Type-Specific Remedies or Basic Flowers

What are type remedies or basic Flowers?

In his first series of Flowers, the Twelve Healers, Bach initially assigned twelve personality types to match each of the "healers." He called these Flowers type remedies. This caused misunderstandings because not everyone could identify with being classified as a character type. Today this term is used less and less.

In the meantime, my practical experience of thirty years and thousands of patients has shown the following: All patients exhibit between six and fifteen deeply rooted, negative behavior patterns that repeatedly become problematical for them. I call the Flowers that address these patterns each person's basic Flowers. Each of the thirty-eight Flowers can be a basic Flower for someone. If you wonder what your basic Flowers are, you will recognize them when you use Bach Flower Therapy for at least a year because they will show up in your combinations again and again.

However, the effectiveness of a combination doesn't hinge on whether or not a Flower is a basic one, and not every combination must include one or more of your basic Flowers. A basic Flower is simply one that's needed more frequently than others. It reflects a principle that you have to work with more deeply, one that is clearly important in your Life Plan.

Typical Behavior Patterns. *See page 209*

Vices. *See page 19*

Virtues. *See page 19*

Water for the Mixtures. *See page 227*

Water Glass Method. *See page 226*

Weaning, Stopping Breast-feeding, When Nursing Ends. *See page244*

When to Stop Taking a Specific Combination

How will I know when I can stop taking a specific combination?

You will note a sense of overall well-being, a sense that you are harmonized and stable. Usually you don't feel the need to take the combination anymore, or you simply "forget" to take the drops. If the combination has been chosen well, this usually happens after eighteen to twenty-six days, though there is no fixed rule for the length of time it takes to reach this point. As long as you feel like taking the mixture, you should do so.

Workaholic. *See page 213*

Wrong Choice of Bach Flowers
What happens if I take the wrong choice of Bach Flowers?
Nothing. Where there is no disharmony, an Essence taken finds no resonance and can have no effect. The wrong Flowers neither negatively nor positively affect the bioenergetic field. Homeopathic substances, in contrast, will cause a reaction if not chosen correctly. *See also* Correct or Incorrect Combination.

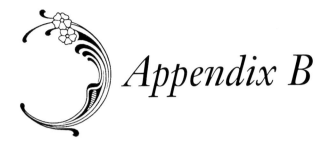

Appendix B

Resources

Mechthild Scheffer's Institutes for Bach Flower Therapy Research and Education
Postfach 20 25 51,
D-20218 Hamburg
Germany
Phone: +49 (40) 43 25 77 10
Fax: +49 (40) 43 52 53
e-mail: info@bach-bluetentherapie.de

Börsegasse 10,
A-1010 Vienna
Austria
Phone: +43 (1) 533 86 40 0
Fax: +43 (1) 533 86 40 15
e-mail: bach-bluetentherapie@aon.at

Mainaustrasse 15
CH-8034 Zürich
Switzerland
Phone: +41 (1) 382 33 14
Fax: +41 (1) 382 33 19
e-mail: bach-bluetentherapie@swissonline.ch

Mechthild Scheffer travels internationally. Her institutes provide training, coaching, special seminars in English, and mail-order books in a number of languages

Dr. Edward Bach Centre/Dr. Edward Bach Foundation
Sotwell, Wallingford
Oxon
OX10 OPZ, United Kingdom
www.bachcentre.com

For further information in the United States:
Nelson Bach USA
100 Research Drive
Wilmington, MA 01887
Phone: (978) 988-3833 or (800) 319-9151
Fax: (508) 988-0233
www.nelsonbach.com

Nelson Bach USA is the official U.S. distributor of Bach Flower Remedies prepared from mother tinctures at the Dr. Edward Bach Centre. It also provides information on official courses in the United States.

Bibliography and Recommended Reading

Bach, Edward. *The Twelve Healers and Other Remedies* (Saffron Walden, Essex, England: C. W. Daniel Company, 1933).

Bach, Edward. *Heal Thyself.* (Saffron Walden, Essex, England: C. W. Daniel Company, 1931).

Weeks, Nora. *Medical Discoveries of Edward Bach Physician* (Saffron Walden, Essex, England: C. W. Daniel Company, 1940). A biography of Dr. Edward Bach.

Howard, Judy and John Ramsell. *The Original Writings of Edward Bach* (Saffron Walden, Essex, England: C. W. Daniel Company, 1990). Text compiled from the archives of the Bach Centre by its curators and trustees.

Weeks, Nora and Victor Bullen. *The Bach Flower Remedies: Illustrations and Preparations* (Saffron Walden, Essex, England: C. W. Daniel Company, 1964).

Scheffer, Mechthild. *Keys to the Soul* (Saffron Walden, Essex, England: C. W. Daniel Company, 1998). A workbook for self-diagnosis using Bach Flowers; available in English, German, French, and Italian.

———. *Original Bach-Blütentherapie: Lehrbuch für die Arzt- und Naturheilpraxis* (Munich: Krone and Fischer, 1999). A teaching book for professionals with over one hundred case studies; available in German, Spanish, Italian, and Portuguese.

Scheffer, Mechthild and Wolf-Dieter Storl. *Die Seelenpflanzen des Edward Bach. Neue Einsichten in die Bach-Blütentherapie* (München: Heinrich Hugendubel Verlag, 1995). Explores ancient and folk medicine uses of Bach's plants; available in German, Spanish, and Italian.

About the Author

Mechthild Scheffer is an internationally known pioneer in Bach Flower Therapy and the author of a number of standard texts on the subject, which have been translated into many languages. She introduced the work of Dr. Edward Bach to German-speaking countries over twenty-five years ago and has continued to expand on this work ever since. For two decades she represented England's Dr. Edward Bach Centre in Germany, Austria, and Switzerland, and is now active in the Bach Foundation Network.

In 1982 she created the first training program for Bach Flower Therapy, which has been completed by several thousand practitioners as well as by those who incorporate the knowledge gained there in their own private use.

She is also the founder of the Institutes for Bach Flower Therapy Research and Education in Hamburg, Vienna, and Zurich.

Currently the most important focus of her activity is the further development of Bach Flower Therapy and its integration with other future-oriented preventive health care initiatives.